Molecular Endocrinology
of the
Steroid Hormones

Molecular Endocrinology
of the
Steroid Hormones

Dennis Schulster

*School of Biological Sciences, University of Sussex,
Brighton, England*

Sumner Burstein

*Worcester Foundation Experimental Biology,
Shrewsbury, Massachusetts, U.S.A.*

Brian A. Cooke

*Medical Faculty, Erasmus University,
Rotterdam, The Netherlands*

JOHN WILEY & SONS

London · New York · Sydney · Toronto

Library of Congress Cataloging in Publication Data:

Schulster, Dennis.
    Molecular endocrinology of the steroid hormones.

    1. Steroid hormones. I. Burstein, Sumner H.,
joint author. II. Cooke, Brian A., joint author.
III. Title. [DNLM: 1. Sex hormones. 2. Steroids.
WK150 S386M]
QP572.S7S38   599'.01'927   75—31525

ISBN 0 471 76582 1 (Cloth)
ISBN 0 471 76583 X (Pbk)

Typeset in IBM Journal by Preface Ltd., Salisbury, Wilts.
and printed in Great Britain by The Pitman Press, Bath

To our wives
and parents

Foreword

It is remarkable how many classical questions in steroid endocrinology, such as the cellular origin of adrenal and testicular androgens, still remain unanswered. In this respect perhaps this book is a little optimistic as to the completed nature of the most popular questions in the field put in the first half of this century. Nevertheless, in the last twenty years, the centre of interest for most steroid biochemists has moved away from the nature of the secretions and metabolites of steroid hormones and even from consideration of broad theoretical hypotheses as to their mode of action. Attention has now settled on the detailed examination of these mechanisms of action, which are certain to be significant processes. The role of the two most influential hypotheses guiding such studies, cyclic AMP as a second messenger and the binding of a hormone to components of a target cell as essential processes in the action of hormones, has been invaluable in this respect. Most investigators are quite appropriately interested in finding out when such an ambitious hypothesis is not applicable and yet the second messenger theory is still dominant as a general guide to work on the mode of action of peptide hormones. Also, the unravelling of the details of the binding of steroid hormones has revealed processes quite remarkably universal for different target cells. In fact, the danger now is that these hypotheses and findings have been so generally effective that they might become dogma and inhibit progress in the field. However, the authors of this book are well-qualified as teachers and researchers not only to explain these theories clearly but also to examine them critically and objectively. They have also been in intimate contact with recent developments in methodology particularly the preparation, superfusion and purification of isolated cells. Such preparations are rapidly becoming a major 'physiological' tool of the modern steroid biochemist with purity of the cell now being regarded as important as that of the isolated enzyme.

PROFESSOR JAMES F. TAIT, F.R.S.,

Middlesex Hospital Medical School,
London.

Preface

In a rapidly developing scientific field, it is often difficult for the student to acquaint himself with the fundamentals of a subject without becoming lost amidst the complexities of new ideas and seemingly unrelated data. The number of publications concerned with the biochemistry of steroids has followed the proliferative trend of biochemistry in general and shows no sign of decreasing. We feel that now is as good a time as any to pause and review the present state of our knowledge of steroid biochemistry. The attempt has been to provide as broad a coverage of the subject as possible with the minimum of fine detail. The emphasis of the book however is on our present understanding of the biochemical control mechanisms in this field, operating at the cellular level. This relates both to the regulation of steroid hormone production and to their mechanism of action (Sections III and IV). The earlier sections of the book are intended as a basis for these later chapters. Where possible, the main references are to review articles, monographs and books which provide depth in particular topics; only where it is of obvious importance is the original literature cited.

This book is intended primarily for the student of biochemistry or medicine who seeks an understanding of what steroid hormones are, how they are formed, what they do and how they do it. Although it is not intended as a reference text for researchers in the field, it is hoped that it may be of some value in this respect, and to specialists in other topics who, in the furtherance of their work find a need to become acquainted with this subject.

A knowledge of steroid hormones involves an understanding of the principles of their chemistry, biochemistry and endocrinology. In a book of this size, it is impossible to provide a detailed background in each of these subjects, but as far as possible, the approach is from first principles and assumes no great specialized knowledge on the part of the reader.

In the preparation of this book we were fortunate in having the generous help and expert advice of many friends and colleagues, who read drafts of the manuscript or provided pre-publication copies of their own articles. To them we owe a great deal, not only for their active encouragement but also for their valid criticisms. We wish to express our thanks to all of these and in particular to: Dr. Andrzej Bartke, Dr. Robert Bing, Dr. Angela Brodie, Dr. Harry Brodie, Prof. C. L. Foster, Dr. Mary Harris, Dr. Brigid Hogan, Prof. Vivian James, Dr. Chris Longcope, Dr. Caroline Mackie, Dr. David Maudsley, Dr. John McCracken, Dr. Eppo Mulder,

x

Dr. Fernie Peron, Dr. Evan Simpson, Mrs. Sylvia Tait, Prof. James Tait, Prof. Henk van der Molen, Dr. Mike Wallis and Dr. Gerard Zeilmaker. We would also like to thank Willie Bakhuizen, Marja Decae-van Maanen and Diana King for their patience and expertise in typing various parts of the text, and our deep appreciation to our wives and families for their continued help and their forbearance throughout the long gestation of this book. It is, however, inevitable that errors of fact, omission, interpretation and emphasis still remain, and for these shortcomings we alone are accountable. In this regard comments, criticisms and notice of errors from our readers would be greatly appreciated.

October 1975

D. S.
Sussex, England
S. B.
Shrewsbury, Mass., U.S.A.
B. A. C.
Rotterdam, The Netherlands

Contents

Introduction

Among the many fascinating areas of present day scientific research, one which undoubtedly has captured the imagination and interest of many is that involving the mode of hormone action in living organisms. The complex mechanisms whereby these biological molecules regulate, organize and manipulate the whole organism is only just beginning to be appreciated.

It is now clear that within this field, an understanding of the role of the steroid hormones has a fundamental importance and significance with wide ramifications in many other disciplines. Since the characterization and identification of the steroid hormones in the first half of this century, recent research effort has placed considerable emphasis on discovering both how steroid biosynthesis in endocrine tissues is controlled, and the details of the intracellular mechanisms by which the steroid hormones act within their target tissues.

It follows that these studies interrelate with those on many other hormones and biomolecules. Thus in this book the role of pituitary hormones and hypothalamic releasing hormones are examined as part of the steroidogenic control system and this is of direct interest to other hormone secreting and hypothalamic-pituitary-endocrine tissue control systems. Central to such studies are the interactions between receptors for steroidogenic protein hormones in the outer plasma membranes of steroid-producing endocrine cells, with consequent relevance to other plasma membrane studies in fields ranging from biophysics to immunology. Moreover the characteristics of the involvement of adenosine $3'$, $5'$-cyclic monophosphate (cyclic AMP) in the control of steroidogenesis has implications not only in a variety of other hormonal responses but also in the understanding of the processes for control and integration of cellular growth. Much of our (still somewhat limited) knowledge of cyclic AMP involvement in normal and tumour cell growth, stems from earlier studies on hormonal control systems.

Similarly the mechanism of steroid hormone action covers a vast field, embracing not only the fundamental aspects of molecular biology, including the role of receptors, protein and RNA synthesis and events at the chromosomal level, but also the control of biological differentiation, processes regulating tissue growth and the more recently high-lighted field of sexual differentiation in the brain.

However, long before it was possible to undertake studies relating to the mechanism of hormone action, it was necessary to establish the characteristics of steroid hormone production by the adrenal cortex, gonads and placenta, together

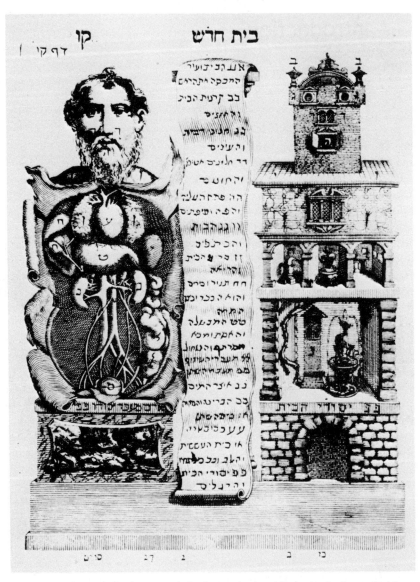

A comparison of the features of the human body with those of a house (Tobias Cohn, 1711; from the Bettman Archive). Our understanding of the processes within the living organism has increased dramatically since these early days of scientific investigation. Reproduced by permission of The Bettman Archive Inc.

with the chemistry and biochemistry of steroid hormone metabolism. Our current knowledge of these aspects of the steroid hormones is probably fairly complete, and the earlier chapters of this book attempt to cover these fundamentals. It should be emphasized that this well-established knowledge, gained by the hard efforts of earlier generations of scientists, is not just history but still plays an essential role in elucidating problems of current interest. In the words of Sir Isaac Newton: 'If I have seen further than most men, it is by standing on the shoulders of giants'.

Our understanding of endocrinological mechanisms has come a long way since 1711 when physician Tobias Cohn compared the organs and processes within the human body with the structure and organization of a house. Advances in the treatment of endocrine disorders has followed hand-in-hand with the rapid advances in our understanding of the normal patterns of secretion and actions of steroid hormones. Methods available for the treatment of endocrine disorders are still far from ideal, nevertheless there is a continuing improvement in the biochemical and analytical procedures available to aid accurate diagnosis and therapy. Notable recent achievements have been made particularly in the fields of adrenal endocrinology, female infertility and contraception, and the application of recently acquired knowledge on the mode of action of hormones is perhaps beginning to make significant inroads into the problems of cancer in endocrine and related tissues. We are also now aware of the extraordinarily wide spectrum of steroid hormone effects (ranging from the general metabolic effects of the glucocorticoids to the effects of androgens and estrogens on secondary sex organs) together with the multiplicity of disorders that can result from disruption of the steroid hormone production system. Just taking one steroid as an example it is now recognized that aldosterone plays a significant role in cardiovascular-hypertensive disorders that affect millions of patients.

SECTION I

Methodological and Molecular Aspects of Steroid Hormones

CHAPTER 1

Structure and nomenclature of steroids

I. INTRODUCTION

More and more biological phenomena are being explained at the molecular level, hence a knowledge of structural features becomes necessary for a full understanding of modern theories. The stereochemistry of steroidal substrates, for example, play a critical role in their interactions with enzymes and other proteins. The vast literature dealing with the structure proofs and syntheses of steroids is of no direct importance to the intended reader of this text. For the most part, these reactions will throw little light on the biological processes involving steroids. However, it is relevant to an understanding of the succeeding chapters, firstly to discuss the structure and nomenclature of the steroids.

II. THE STRUCTURAL FORMULAE OF THE STEROIDS

The steroids are a large class of lipids which are synthesized mainly in the adrenal gland, testis, ovary and liver. They all have a common ring structure which consists of three six-membered rings and one five-membered ring joined to each other by common sides as shown below:

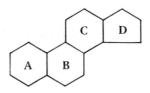

They differ from each other in the position, number and structure of the functional groups (e.g. hydroxyl and ketone groups, degree of unsaturation, length of side chain, and so forth). The formulae of some of the more common steroids are given in Figure 1.1 and the numbering of the carbon atoms in Figure 1.2

III. STEREOSTRUCTURES

A knowledge of the three-dimensional arrangement of atoms in a steroid (or any molecule) is essential for an understanding of the reactions of the substance. This is especially true for biological reactions since enzymes are highly sensitive to steric factors. Even such properties as chromatographic mobility are influenced, to varying degrees, by the steric arrangement of the molecule.

The angles between atoms are determined by the directions of the bonds which, in turn, depend on the orbitals of the bonding electrons of the atoms. The double bond has an sp^2 planar trigonal arrangement in which the angles are each $120°$. The triple bond has an sp orbital which is linear. Saturated carbon, however, has its electrons in an sp^3 orbital which forms a regular tetrahedron with an angle of about $109°$ between each pair of bonds.

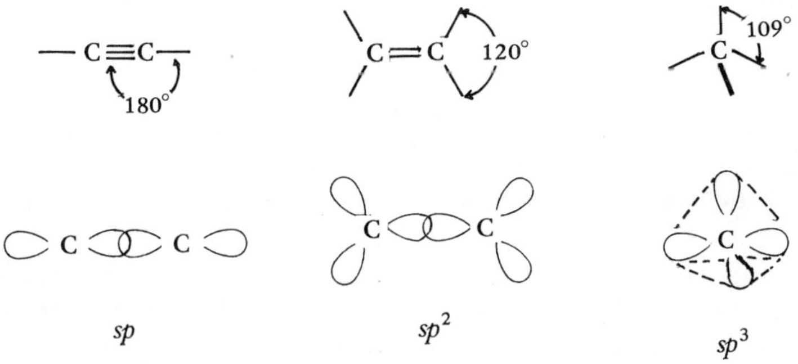

As a result of this geometry, molecules made up mainly of saturated carbon atoms have three-dimensional structures which are quite different from the planar representation given on paper.

For example, in the situation where six carbons are arranged in a ring, the angle between each pair of carbon–carbon bonds is about $109°$ because of the orbital requirements. This gives rise to a staggered arrangement of the atoms where alternate carbons are in parallel planes. This is the most stable arrangement of

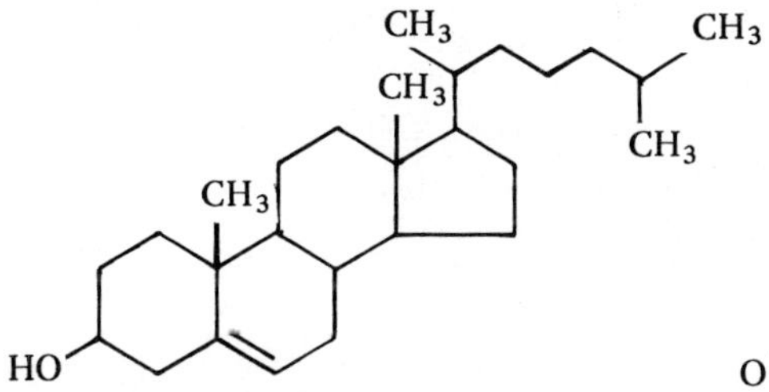

Cholesterol

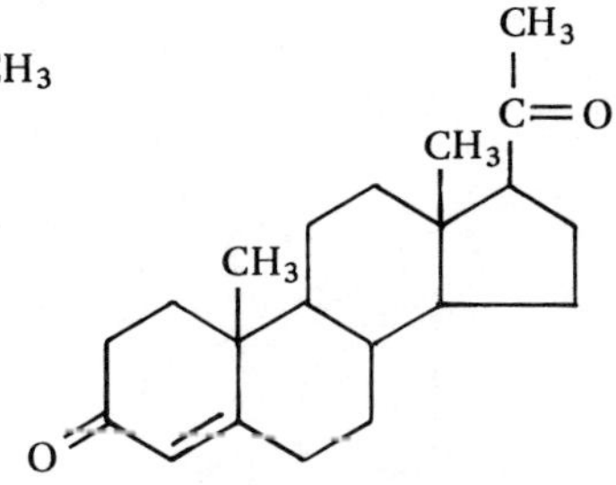

Progesterone

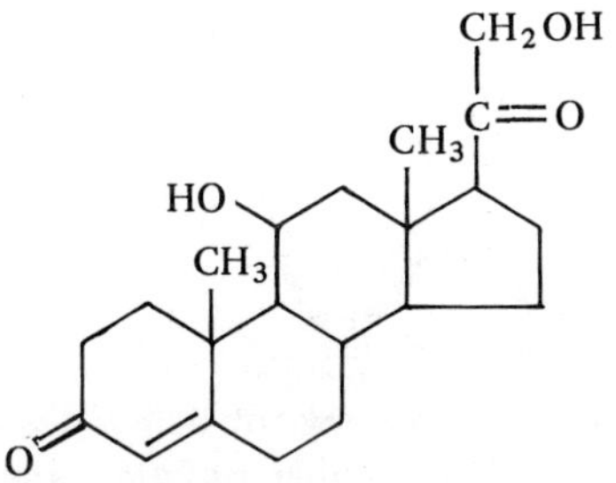

Corticosterone

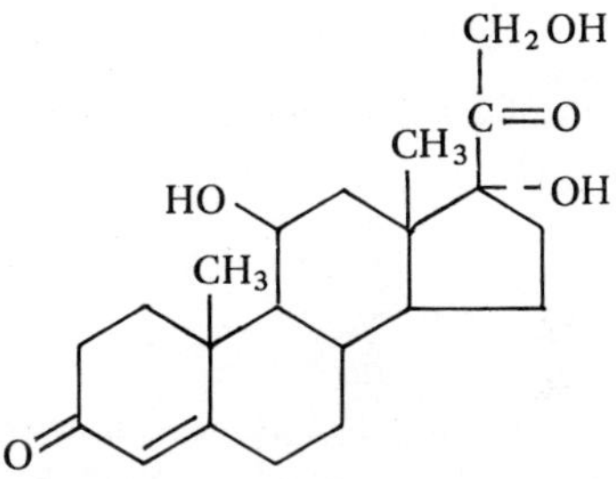

Cortisol

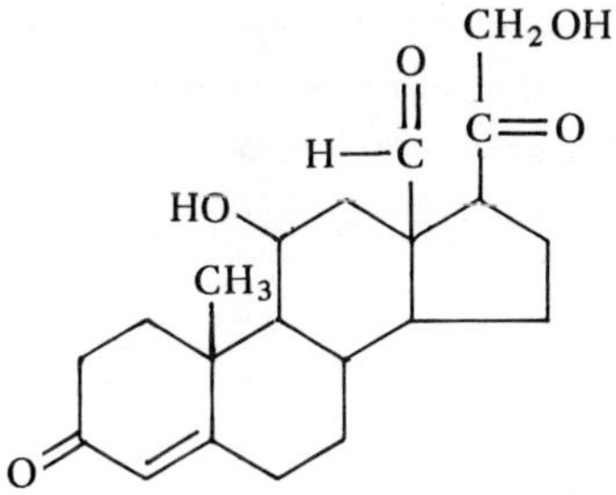

Aldosterone

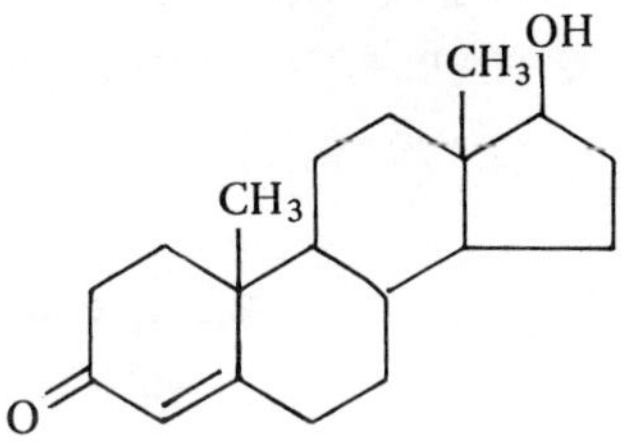

Testosterone

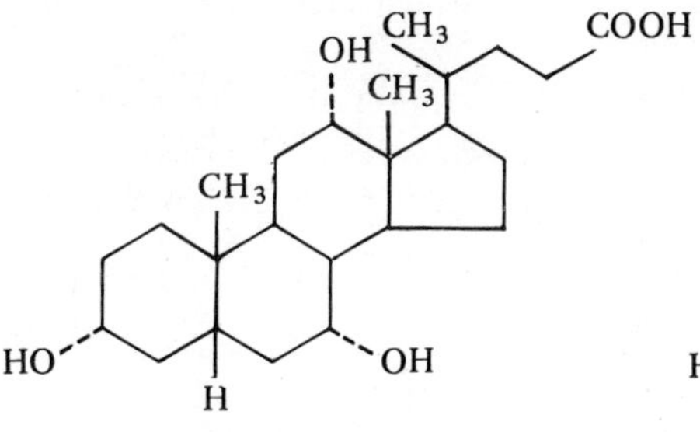

Cholic Acid

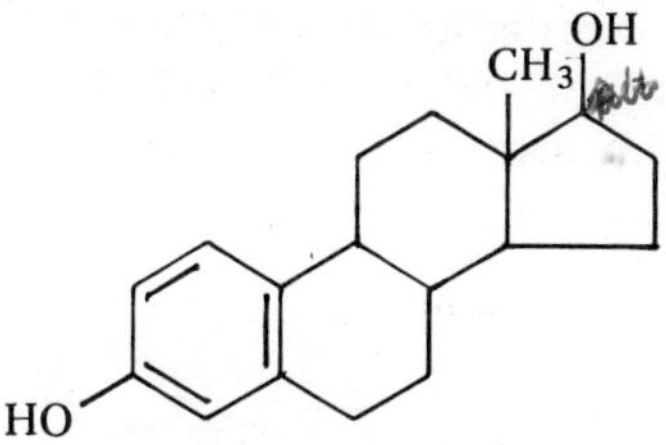

Estradiol-17β

Figure 1.1 Formulae of some of the common steroids.

6

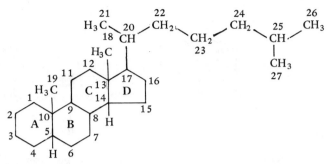

Figure 1.2 The numbering of the carbon atoms in the steroid molecule.

atoms in a six-membered ring and is referred to as the 'chair'

conformation. The atoms can be rearranged without breaking any bonds to give the so-called 'boat' conformation; however, this is a less stable situation and only occurs under special conditions.

The remaining bonds of the atoms in the ring are oriented in two general directions. One bond of each atom is perpendicular to the plane of the ring; the other points away from the centre of the ring and forms an angle of 30° with the plane. The former are called axial and the latter equatorial bonds.

Unsaturation leads to changes in the conformations of the rings which will be discussed later on. The five-membered ring does not possess clear axial and equatorial substituents but intermediate types which are at angles of between 30—90° with the plane of the ring.

Rings A and B can be joined in either a *cis* or *trans* fashion. That is the angular substituents (R) are either on the same or opposite sides of the rings. In the *trans* situation both substituents are axial with respect to both rings. However, in the *cis*

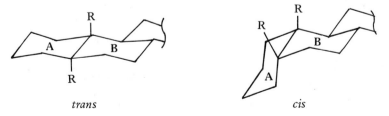

trans   *cis*

case each substituent will be axial to one ring and equatorial to the other. The B and C rings are joined in a *trans* fashion with the exception of a few synthetic compounds. Also the C and D rings are *trans* in almost all cases. The result of these ring fusions in the AB *trans* situation is a molecule in which all the rings lie in about the same plane. The AB *cis* compounds, on the other hand, present a somewhat different steric picture as seen in the diagram below:

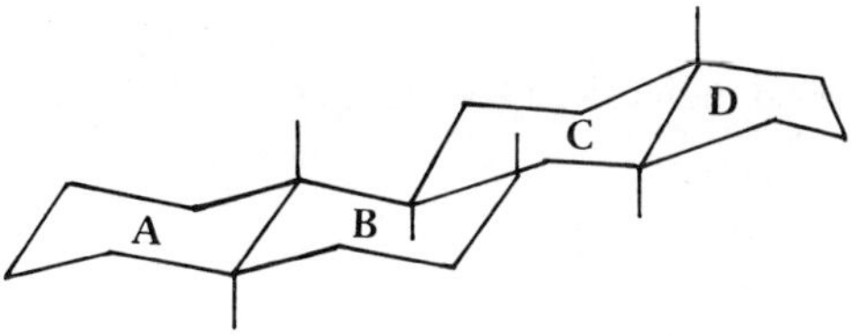

all *trans* 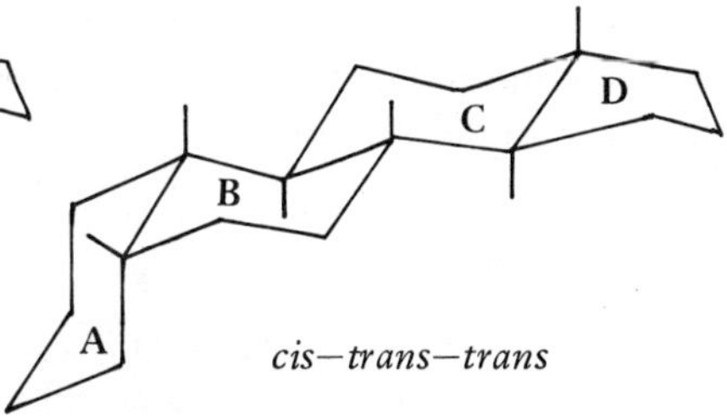   *cis—trans—trans*

The axial substituents will be situated above or below the plane of the molecule (except in Ring A of the *cis* series) while the equatorial ones extend outward from the molecule. There is a good deal of interaction between alternate axial groups, namely, those on the same side of the molecule and located 1,3 to each other. These are the so-called 1,3 diaxial interactions and are due to the spatial requirements of the groups. In general, they will be proportional to the sizes of the groups. 1,3 interactions between hydrogens are mild but between methyls are quite pronounced; between larger groups they will be even more severe. The interactions between equatorial groups, in general, are small, however with very bulky groups there is some interaction.

Equatorial groups are more accessible to reagents or other molecules and in many cases react faster than the corresponding axial groups. On the other hand, if relief of steric interaction is a factor in the rate-limiting step of a reaction, then axial groups will proceed at a faster rate. In the Appendix several comparisons between axial and equatorial substituent reactions are given which illustrate this point.

The introduction of double bonds into the ring system of a steroid will have a pronounced steric effect in the immediate vicinity of the unsaturated system. There can even be so-called 'long-range effects' where bond angles quite distant from the double bond are slightly affected. In general, there will be a flattening effect since the four atoms connected to the double bond as well as the unsaturated carbons themselves must be coplanar. An aromatic ring is completely planar and atoms connected to it will also lie in its plane. As a result of this, molecules in the estrogen series are quite planar.

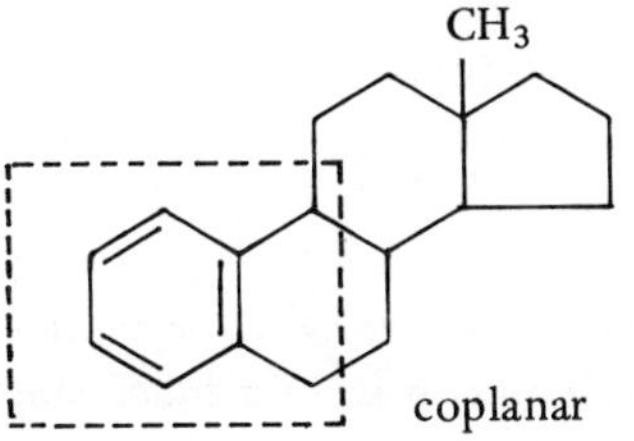

CH_3

coplanar

IV. FUNCTIONAL GROUPS

The carbon skeletons of the steroids (Figure 1.2) can be substituted with practically all of the groups known to the organic chemist. The steroids found in nature, however, contain only a few types which we shall discuss. An important aspect of steroid chemistry is that the molecule usually contains two or more functional groups so that the polyfunctional nature of these compounds must be considered in any reaction carried out in the laboratory. Steroid enzymes can readily select for reaction one group of several on the steroid molecule, a feat which still offers many problems to the chemist.

A. Double Bonds

The *carbon—carbon double bond* is a common functional group for a steroid. Double bonds are known at all of the possible positions in the steroid molecule, however most of them are synthetically produced. The hormonally important compounds which contain double bonds usually have them between carbons 4 and 5, or between 5 and 6. In the sterol field a number of other types are found both in the rings and side chain.

Two or more double bonds at adjacent positions give rise to conjugated systems which usually are more reactive than either of the bonds when isolated. They also have characteristic ultraviolet spectra which are useful for identification and analysis.

A special case of a conjugated system occurs when three double bonds are located in a six carbon ring. The π electrons distribute themselves into two doughnut-shaped clouds above and below the plane of the ring and give rise to a so-called *aromatic system*. The A ring of the estrogens contains such an aromatic

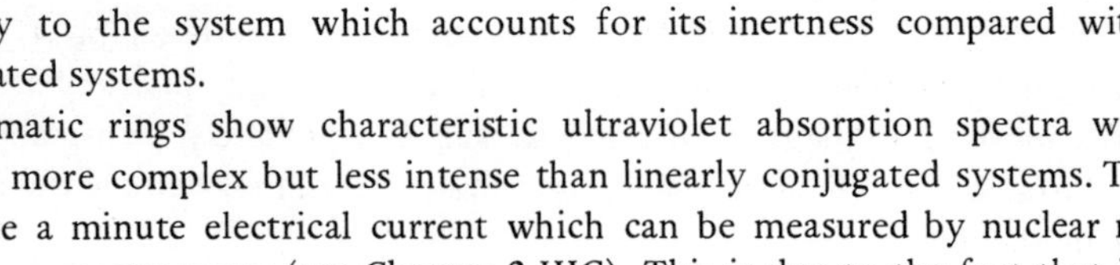

system. This delocalization of the electrons around the ring confers a great deal of stability to the system which accounts for its inertness compared with other conjugated systems.

Aromatic rings show characteristic ultraviolet absorption spectra which are usually more complex but less intense than linearly conjugated systems. They also generate a minute electrical current which can be measured by nuclear magnetic resonance spectroscopy (see Chapter 2.IIIC). This is due to the fact that in such a system there is a stream of electrons following in a closed path.

B. Hydroxyl Groups

Almost every steroid molecule contains one or more *hydroxyl* groups, and their reactions are of great importance in steroid biochemistry. Examples of primary, secondary and tertiary hydroxyls are all to be found among the various steroids, however secondary alcohols are the most prevalent. In general, steroidal alcohols behave like their non-steroidal counterparts except for the stereochemical influences (see Appendix).

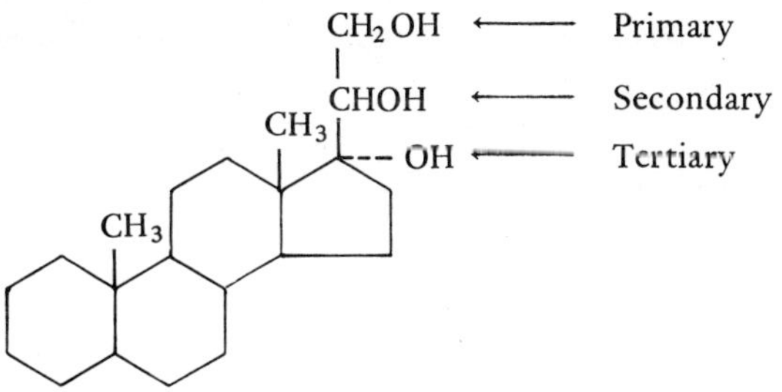

CH_2OH ⟵ Primary

$CHOH$ ⟵ Secondary

OH ⟵ Tertiary

The estrogens contain an *aromatic hydroxyl* which reacts in a similar manner to other phenols. Another special type of hydroxyl

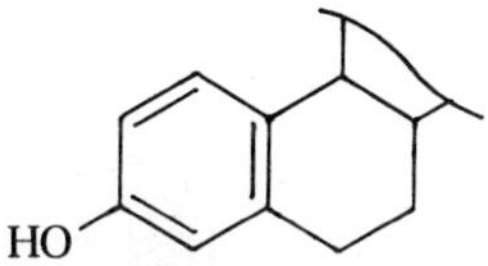

Aromatic

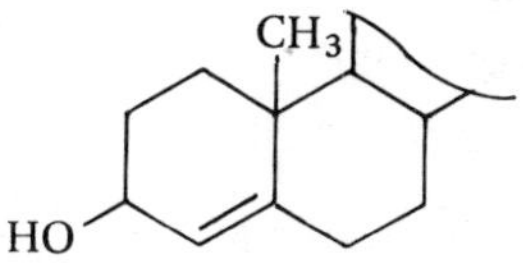

Allylic

found occasionally in steroids is an *allylic alcohol*. Like other examples of this class of alcohols, it is rather reactive and is easily oxidized to a ketone or dehydrated to a diene system (see Appendix). There are examples of glycol systems in the steroid field, both of the 1,2 and 1,3 variety. Many of the reactions of these compounds are similar to their counterparts in the carbohydrate field where such glycol systems are common.

C. Ketone Groups

Ketone groups (carbonyl functions) are as prevalent amongst the steroids as hydroxyl groups and are also involved in many biological reactions. Very often they are found in conjugation with a double bond and are referred to as α,β *unsaturated ketones;* as might be expected these have special properties due to the mutual interaction of the two functional groups. As with the double bonds and hydroxyls, ketone groups are to be found at every possible position, however only some are of interest in the hormone field (see Figure 1.1).

Although the *aldehyde group* is not very common amongst the steroids, one important example is known. Aldosterone (see Figure 1.1), the hormone which controls the body's salt balance, has an aldehyde group at the 18-position. In general, aldehydes undergo the same reactions as ketones but much more rapidly. Since there are no hydrogens next to the aldehyde group of aldosterone, it cannot enolize.

D. Carboxyl Groups

The *carboxylic acid group* is to be found mainly in the bile acids such as cholic acid (Figure 1.1). These behave for the most part like other organic acids except for certain physical properties attributable to the rest of the molecule. Bile acid chemistry is in many ways a field of its own and will not be discussed further in this text.

V. STEROID NOMENCLATURE

The following is an abbreviated version of the IUPAC — IUB *Revised Tentative Rules for Steroid Nomenclature*. Only nomenclature which is relevant to the steroid hormones discussed in this book has been included. Steroids are numbered and rings are lettered as shown in the formula in Figure 1.2.

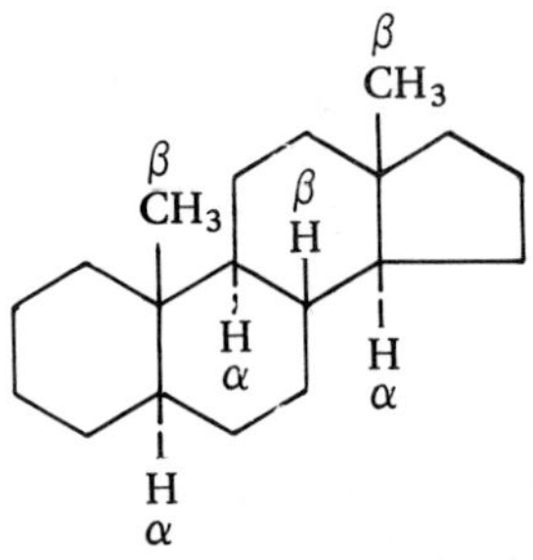

A. α and β Groups

An atom or group attached to a ring is termed α (alpha) if it lies *below the plane* of the paper or β (beta) if it lies *above the plane* of the paper. In formulae, bonds to atoms or groups lying below the plane of the paper are shown as broken (− −) lines and bonds to atoms or groups lying above the plane of the paper are shown as solid lines (——). Bonds to atoms or groups whose configuration is not known or is unspecified are denoted by wavy lines (∼∼) and indicated by the Greek letter ξ.

All hydrogen atoms and methyl groups attached at ring junction positions must always be inserted as H or CH_3 respectively (Me may also be used). The practice of denoting methyl groups by bonds without lettering is liable to cause confusion and it has been recommended that this be abandoned.

Unless implied or stated to the contrary, use of a *steroid name* implies that atoms or groups attached at the ring-junction position 8, 9, 10, 13 and 14 are oriented as shown in the formula above (i.e. 8β, 9α, 10β, 13β, 14α) and a carbon chain attached at position 17 is assumed to be β-oriented. The configuration of hydrogen (or a substituent) at the ring-junction 5 should always be designated by adding α, β or ξ after the numeral 5, this numeral and letter being placed immediately before the stem name, e.g. 5α-pregnane (see below for explanation of pregnane).

When the configuration at position 20 in the side chain of a pregnane derivative is depicted as in the formula below, substituents shown to the right of C-20 are termed α and those to the left are termed β.

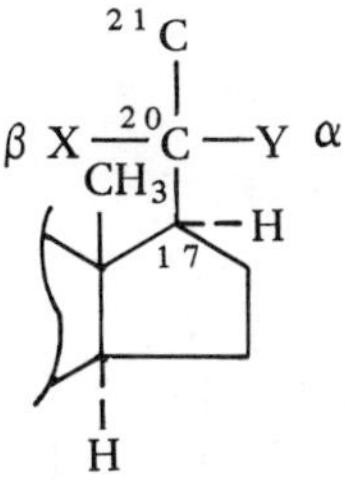

e.g.

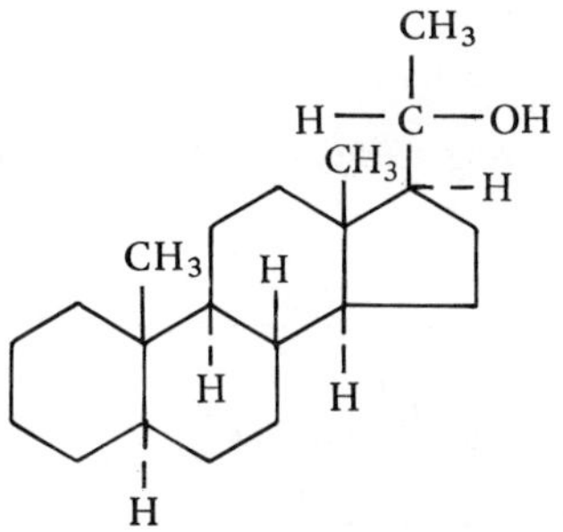

5α-Pregnan-20α-ol

The Ingold system or *Sequence Rule procedure* for nomenclature of substituents in the C-17 side chain relates to the three-dimensional position of each substituent on any particular carbon atom. The symbols R for right (*rectus*) and S for left (*sinister*) are used. For 20-hydroxy, 20-amino, 20-halogeno and 20-alloxy derivatives of pregnane without a substituent on C-17 or C-21, 20α is equivalent to (20S)-, and 20β to (20R)-. These relationships may be reversed when additional substituents are present (see Section VB). For a description of the application of the Sequence Rule procedure for the R and S nomenclature of steroids, see Briggs and Brotherton (1970).

B. Fundamental Carbocycles

The parent tetracyclic hydrocarbon without methyl groups at C-10 and C-13 and without a side chain at C-17 is named *gonane*.

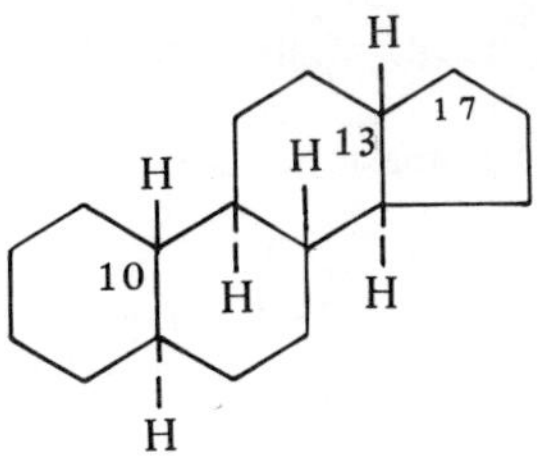

5α-Gonane

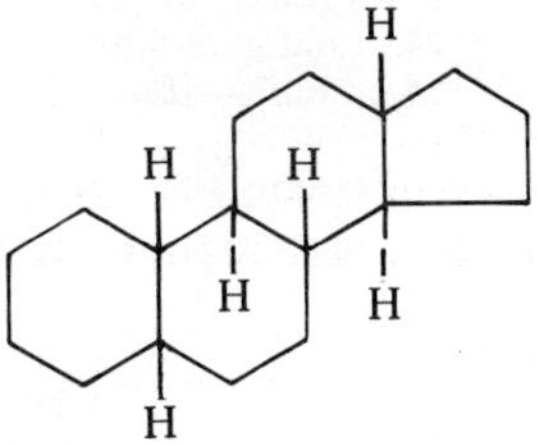

5β-Gonane

The hydrocarbon with a methyl group at C-13 but without a methyl group at C-10 and without a side chain at C-17 is named *estrane*.

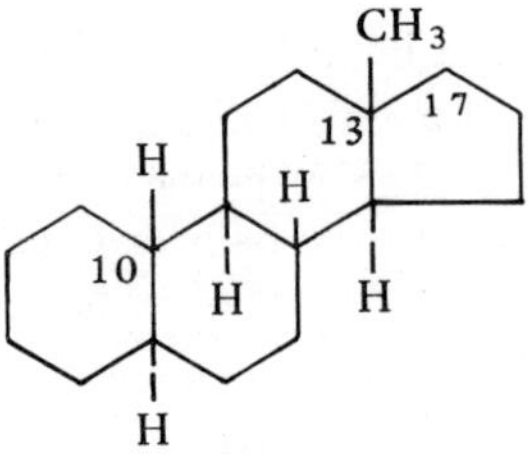

5α-Estrane 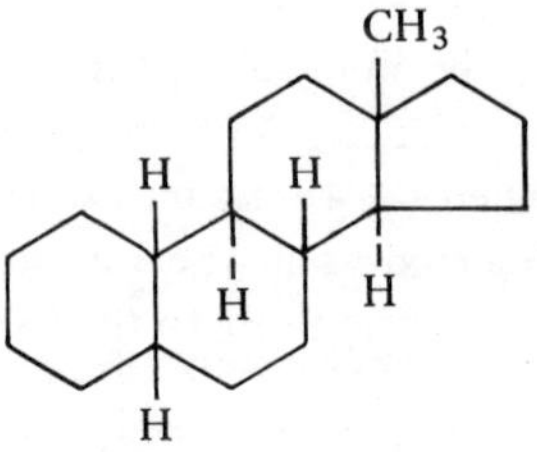   5β-Estrane

The following names are used for the hydrocarbons with methyl groups at both C-10 and C-13.

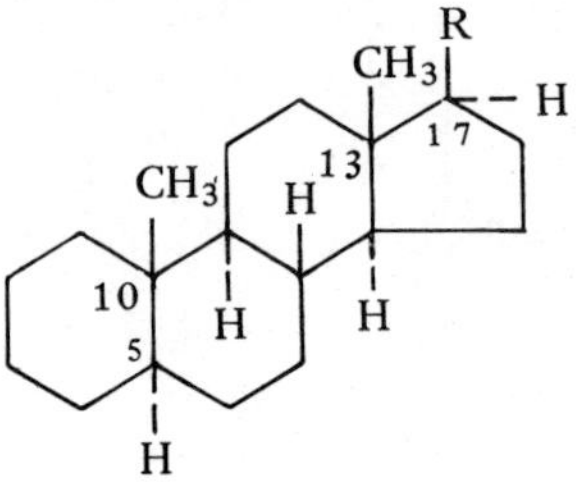

Structure I (5α) 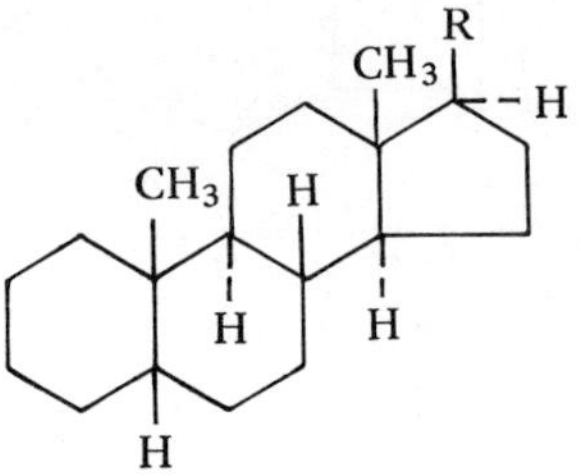   Structure II (5β)

R : the side chain at C-17	5α-Series (Structure I)	5β-Series (Structure II)
H	5α-Androstane	5β-Androstane (*not* testane)
C_2H_5	5α-Pregnane (*not* allopregnane)	5β-Pregnane
*CH(CH$_3$)CH$_2$CH$_2$CH$_3$	5α-Cholane (*not* allocholane)	5β-Cholane
*CH(CH$_3$)CH$_2$CH$_2$CH$_2$CH(CH$_3$)$_2$	5α-Cholestane	5β-Cholestane (*not* coprostane)
*CH(CH$_3$)CH$_2$CH$_3$ $\overset{24**}{CH}$(CH$_3$)CH(CH$_3$)$_2$	5α-Ergostane	5β-Ergostane
*CH(CH$_3$)CH$_2$CH$_2$ $\overset{24***}{CH}$(C$_2$H$_5$)CH(CH$_3$)$_2$	5α-Stigmastane	5β-Stigmastane

  *20R Configuration.
 **24S Configuration.
***24R Configuration.

The names 'cholane', 'cholestane', 'ergostane' and 'stigmastane' imply the configuration at C-20 shown in the partial formula below:

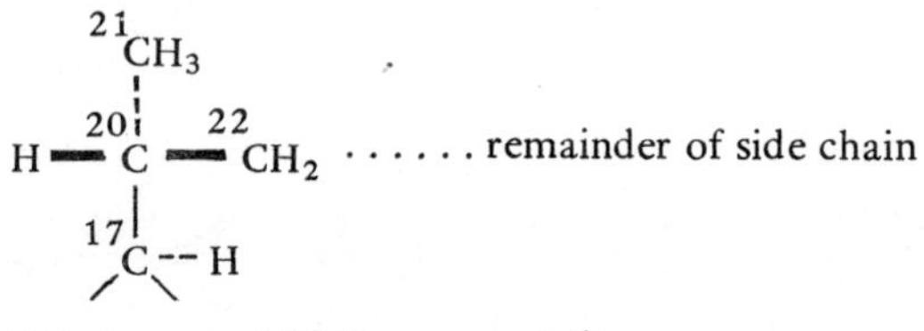

(this is termed 20R; see page 11)

C. Derivatives

1. Unsaturation

Unsaturation is indicated by changing terminal '-ane' to '-ene' (one double bond), '-adiene' (two double bonds), '-yne' (triple bond), or '-an' to '-en' (one double bond), '-adien' (two double bonds), '-yn' (triple bond), e.g. 5α-cholest-6-ene.

2. Substituents

Most substituents can be designated either as suffixes or as prefixes; a few can be named only as prefixes, the commonest of these being halogens, alkyl and nitro groups. When possible, one type of substituent must be designated as suffix. When more than one type is present that could be designated as suffix, one type only may be so expressed and the other types must be designated as prefixes.

Choice for suffix is made according to the following decreasing order of preference: 'onium salt, acid, lactone, ester, aldehyde, ketone, alcohol, amine, ether.

Suffixes are added to the name of the saturated or unsaturated parent system, the terminal 'e' of '-ane', '-ene', '-yne', '-adiene', and so on being deleted before a vowel (presence or absence of numerals having no effect on such deletions). The following examples illustrate the use of these principles:

a. *Esters of steroid alcohols.* For esters of *monohydric* steroid alcohols the steroid radical name is formed by replacing the terminal 'e' of the hydrocarbon name by 'yl' and inserting before this the locant and Greek letter, with hyphens, to designate the position and configuration; e.g. 5α-cholestan-3β-yl acetate. For esters of polyols the name of the polyol is followed by that of the acyloxy group(s) in its anionic form, with locants when necessary; e.g. 5β-cholestane-3α,12α-diol diacetate; 5β-cholestane-3α,12α-diol 3-acetate 12-benzoate; estradiol-17β 17-monoacetate.

b. *Aldehydes.* Suffix: -al (denotes change of $-CH_3$ to $-CHO$, i.e. without change in the number of carbon atoms); -aldehyde (denotes change of $-COOH$ to $-CHO$, i.e. without change in the number of carbon atoms; name derived from that of the acid). Prefix: oxo- (denotes change of $>CH_2$ to $>CO$, thus also of $-CH_3$ to $-CHO$, with no change in the number of carbon atoms); e.g. 5α-androstan-19-al; 5α-cholan-24-aldehyde; 19-oxo-5α,17(αH)-etianic acid. Other methods are used for introduction of additional carbon atoms as $-CHO$ groups.

c. *Ketones.* Suffix: -one; Prefix: oxo-; e.g. 5β-androstan-3-one; 5-pregnene-3,20-dione; 11-oxo-5α-cholan-24-oic acid.

d. *Alcohols.* Suffix: -ol; Prefix: hydroxy-; e.g. 5β-cholestane-3α,11β-diol; 3α-hydroxy-5α-androstan-17-one.

e. *Ethers.* Ethers are named as alkoxy derivatives when another group is present that has priority for citation as suffix; e.g. 3β-ethoxy-5α-cholan-24-oic ·acid;

17β-methoxy-4-androsten-3-one. When no other such group is present the word 'ether' may be used; e.g. 5α-androstane-3β-yl methyl ether; 5α-pregnane 3β,17α,20α-triol trimethyl ether; cortisol 21-methyl ether.

D. Trivial Names

The following are examples of trivial names retained for important steroid derivatives, these being mostly natural compounds of significant biological activity (Table 1.1).

Some of the trivial names found in the literature are misleading or wrong. For example 'epi' is often used with trivial names to denote inversion at one centre: the name 11-epicortisol defines the compound fully since cortisol is already defined as the 11β-alcohol; but the name epi-cortisol does not define the compound and is inadequate. Similarly 20α- or 20β-hydroxy progesterone is often used to denote reduction of the 20 carbonyl group. This is wrong; 20α- or 20β-dihydroprogesterone are acceptable trivial names. The term '17-keto steroids' to denote all androstane derivatives containing a 17-ketone group is still extensively used; the new nomenclature recommends the term '17-oxosteroids'. Androstane-17-carboxylic acids may be called 'etianic acids' although the former (systematic) name is preferred. For steroids with additional double bonds the prefix 'dehydro' is used; e.g. 11-dehydro-estradiol. The prefix 'allo' to denote '5α' isomers and the marking

Table 1.1

Aldosterone	18,11-Hemiacetal of 11β,21-dihydroxy-3,20-dioxo-4-pregnen-18-al
Androsterone	3α-Hydroxy-5α-androstan-17-one
Cholecalciferol*	9,10-Seco-5,7,10(19)-cholestatrien-3β-ol[†]
Cholesterol	5-Cholesten-3β-ol
Cholic acid	3α,7α,12α-Trihydroxy-5β-cholan-24-oic acid
Corticosterone	11β,21-Dihydroxy-4-pregnene-3,20-dione
Cortisol	11β,17α,21-Trihydroxy-4-pregnene-3,20-dione
Cortisol acetate	Cortisol 21-acetate
Cortisone	17α,21-Dihydroxy-4-pregnene-3,11,20-trione
Cortisone acetate	Cortisone 21-acetate
Deoxycorticosterone	21-Hydroxy-4-pregnene-3,20-dione (i.e. the 11-deoxy derivative of corticosterone)
Ergocalciferol*	9,10-Seco-5,7,10(19)22-ergostatetraen-3β-ol[†]
Ergosterol	5,7,22-Ergostatrien-3β-ol
Estradiol-17α	1,3,5(10)-Estratriene-3,17α-diol
Estradiol-17β	1,3,5(10)-Estratriene-3,17β-diol
Estriol	1,3,5(10)-Estratriene-3,16α,17β-triol
Estrone	3-Hydroxy-1,3,5(10)-estratrien-17-one
Lanosterol	8,24-Lanostadien-3β-ol
Lithocholic acid	3α-Hydroxy-5β-cholan-24-oic acid
Progesterone	4-Pregnene-3,20-dione
Testosterone	17β-Hydroxy-4-androsten-3-one

*Included in the List of Trivial Names for Miscellaneous Compounds published by the IUPAC-IUB Commission of Biochemical Nomenclature; see, for example, IUPAC Inform. Bull., (1966) **25**, 19, or *J. Biol. Chem.*, (1966) **241**, 2987, or *Biochim. biophys. Acta*, (1965) **107**, 1.
†Fission of a ring with addition of a H atom at each terminal group thus created is indicated by the prefix 'seco-'.

of double bonds with 'Δ' are not recommended in the new nomenclature. Single letter abbreviations for steroids are also not acceptable.

E. Shortening of Side Chains and Elimination of Methyl Groups

Elimination of a methylene group from a steroid side chain (including a methyl group) is indicated by the prefix 'nor-', which in all cases is preceded by the number of the carbon atom that dissappears;

19-Nor-testosterone
(19-nor-17β-hydroxy-4-androsten-3-one)

VI. REFERENCES

Nomenclature

IUPAC — IUB Rules: *Steroids*, **13**(3), 227–310 (1969); or *Biochemistry*, **8**(6), 2227–2242 (1969).
Amendments: *Archives Bioch. Biophys.*, **147**(1), 4–7.

Textbooks

Briggs, M. H. and J. Brotherton (1970). *Steroid Biochemistry and Pharmacology*. Academic Press, London and New York.
Djerassi, C. (1963). *Steroid Reactions*. Holden-Day, San Francisco.
Fieser, L. and M. Fieser (1959). *Steroids*. Reinhold, N.Y.
Fried, J. and J. A. Edwards (1972). *Organic Reactions in Steroid Chemistry*, 2 vols. Van Nostrand Reinhold, N.Y.
Hanson, J. R. (1968). *Introduction to Steroid Chemistry*. Pergamon, Oxford.
Kirk, D. N. and M. P. Hartshorn (1968). *Steroid Reaction Mechanisms*. Elsevier, Amsterdam.
Klyne, W. (1965). *The Chemistry of the Steroids*. Methuen, London.
Shoppee, C. W. (1964). *Chemistry of the Steroids*. Butterworths, Washington.

CHAPTER 2

Methodology for steroid hormone studies

I. INTRODUCTION

This chapter will be devoted to an outline of the important methods used for the isolation, identification and quantitation of steroids as they are usually encountered in biological media.

II. SEPARATION OF A STEROID FROM ITS NATURAL ENVIRONMENT

The lengths to which one goes to isolate a particular steroid from the medium in which it occurs depends on what sort of information is being sought from the experiment. If the assay method is sensitive to other substances, one would have to purify to the stage where interference is reduced to an acceptable level. If on the other hand the structure of a new substance is to be established, then a high degree of purity will be required before meaningful data can be obtained.

A. Solvent Extraction

If the substance occurs in a fluid, e.g. urine, plasma or buffer medium, extraction with an immiscible organic solvent is required. This procedure also separates the steroid from water soluble substances. Extraction is usually carried out by shaking the fluid with the solvent in a separating funnel. Several repetitions may be necessary to remove all of the steroid. In extreme cases, when the steroid is not very soluble in the organic solvent, continuous extraction with special equipment may be necessary.

When the sought-after material occurs in a solid medium, e.g. tissue, it is firstly necessary to homogenize in aqueous media followed by extraction with organic solvent. Steroids can also be effectively extracted from solid media with solvents by means of a Soxlet or other type of percolation apparatus. This technique is frequently used for extracting steroids from plant material.

B. Pretreatment for Conjugation

Very often steroids occur in a conjugated form, for example as glucuronides or sulphates (see Figure 10.2), which make them more water soluble and extractions with organic solvents more difficult. If one is not interested in isolating the steroid in this form, various procedures can be used to liberate the free compound. There are commercially available enzyme preparations containing β-glucuronidase which will cleave glucuronides with little or no side reaction. Acid hydrolysis is used for hydrolysis of steroid sulphates. With the latter method, care has to be taken to ensure that artifacts are not formed due to the acid treatment.

C. Countercurrent Distribution

A method which has been effectively used to isolate conjugates is countercurrent distribution. This is an extension of the separatory funnel technique. The apparatus consists of a series of connected tubes where successive extractions of the mixture may occur. The resolving power of the equipment is proportional to the number of tubes and the relative solubilities of the components in the two liquid phases. Each tube is roughly equal to one funnel extraction and a 100 tube arrangement is quite usual. This method can, of course, be used for non-conjugated steroids as well and it is occasionally advantageous to extract by this procedure.

D. Column Chromatography

The solution of the steroid in an organic solvent obtained by any of the above methods can now be subjected effectively to more efficient purification procedures. The volume of the mixture can be reduced by evaporation and the concentrated solution applied to a suitable chromatographic system. Chromatographic separations of steroids may be conveniently divided into two categories based on the physical processes involved. (It is not possible to be too rigid in this classification since there are many situations in which both processes operate.) *Adsorption systems* consist of a solid phase with 'active sites' and a fluid phase, usually a non-polar solvent. *Partition systems* are made up of two immiscible fluid phases which are in contact with each other.

A typical adsorption system is made by passing a solvent such as benzene down a column of alumina. The mixture of steroids is applied to the top of the column and the solvent is then allowed to pass down the column and the fractions are collected below. As the molecules of the mixture move past the solid phase they are pulled onto the surface by charged or polar areas on the alumina. Steroids containing several oxygen functions will be more strongly attracted than those whith none or only one. The predominant factor in this system is that of the hydrogen bond. A relatively strong attraction exists between the hydroxyl hydrogens of a steroid alcohol and the oxygens of the alumina. Ketone and ester groups will be less strongly bound and hydrocarbon residues hardly at all. The result of this differential attraction will be that the components of the mixture will move or be eluted at different rates down the column, thereby effecting the separation.

The countercurrent distribution method mentioned above is a simple type of partitioning system in which, any particular component of the mixture is divided between the two phases according to its solubility in each, which is defined as its 'partition coefficient'. This parameter which is a constant for any given compound in a given mixture of solvents is a true equilibrium constant.

This distribution effect has been incorporated into a number of very efficient methods for separating steroid mixtures. The celite column is an example of such an application. Celite is a very fine, porous form of silica which has the capacity of retaining large volumes of liquid. This is saturated with one phase of the partitioning mixture which becomes the 'stationary phase'. The slurry is packed into a glass column of small diameter relative to its height. The mixture is then applied at the top as a concentrated solution and the other phase of the partitioning mixture is passed down the column becoming the 'mobile phase'. Since the two phases are immiscible, a continuous interface between the two is established for the length of the column: rather like a series of very small countercurrent tubes with each particle of celite acting as container for a drop of stationary phase. As in the case of the adsorption process, the compounds which are more soluble in the 'stationary phase' will move down the column more slowly, thus producing a gradient of mobilities depending upon the partition coefficient of each substance.

In partition systems in general, there is an inverse relationship between sample capacity and resolving power. The counter-current method allows the separation of several grams of mixture while the partition column will handle only a few hundred milligrams but with tremendously increased separating power. Some of the techniques discussed below have even greater powers of separation, but can handle only very small amounts.

E. Paper Chromatography

A partition method which was originally developed for amino acid separations but which has found very wide application in steroids is paper chromatography. Here the matrix of cellulose fibres of the paper serves as the solid support for the stationary phase just as the celite does in the column method. In general, paper chromatography exhibits the characteristics of a partitioning system.

The separations are carried out by applying a solution of the mixture as a small spot at one end of a strip of paper which is, or will be, saturated with stationary phase. This is suspended in a closed glass tank which is saturated with the vapours of both phases. In the ascending method the paper is arranged so that the spot is at the bottom, and this end of the paper is immersed in a container of mobile phase which rises up the paper by capillary action. In the descending method, a trough of mobile phase is placed near the top of the tank and the spotted end of the strip immersed in it. The solvent moves down the paper, again by capillary action.

There are two general categories of paper systems; one type employs non-volatile solvents for the stationary phase and is often called a Zaffaroni system, the other uses volatile solvents and is referred to as a Bush system. Both types have their advantages and their use is governed by the specific problem. The faster running volatile systems seem to have found more widespread use. Paper chromatography is usually limited to samples of less than 50 μg of mixture per spot for effective separation. This method has had extensive application in the analysis and purification of radioactive steroids where very small amounts of steroid are under investigation.

F. Thin-layer Chromatography

With this method the distinction between partition and adsorption processes often disappears and we find cases where both must play a role. Finely-divided silica gel is the medium usually used for steroid work. This is coated in a thin layer as a slurry on glass plates and dried in an oven for a suitable period. The result is a layer of hydrated silica gel, usually of the order of 0.25 mm, supported on a glass plate. Precoated plates are commercially available; these give the most consistent and reliable results.

Separations are carried out by applying a concentrated solution of the mixture near one end of the plate. This is then stood edgewise in a shallow layer of a solvent contained in a closed glass tank. The liquid rises by capillary action past the spot and is allowed to proceed nearly to the top of the plate. In some solvent systems the silica gel will act as an adsorbent in a manner similar to the alumina column mentioned previously with other solvent mixtures. The silica can also act as the supporting phase (e.g. like celite of the partition columns) by trapping part of the solvent mixture and allowing the formation of a stationary phase. It often contains enough moisture which also acts to amplify this effect.

The most outstanding advantage of thin-layer chromatography is the short running-time required. Whereas column and paper methods require many hours, thin-layer plates are usually run in less than one hour. The resolving power for steroids is in most cases comparable to the other methods and the sample capacity is much greater than that of paper. One can further increase this last factor by using plates with thicker layers of silica gel, although this decreases the resolution.

G. Gas–Liquid Chromatography

Partition systems can be constructed between a gas and liquid phase as well as between two liquid phases, giving rise to the method known as gas–liquid chromatography (GLC). A non-volatile liquid on an inert solid support material is used as the stationary phase with a gas such as nitrogen or helium as the mobile phase. The column, either a metal or glass tube, is enclosed in an insulated, heated oven.

Steroids are all crystalline solids with quite low volatility, which means that the oven must be operated at temperatures between 200 and 250°C to provide a sufficient concentration of sample in the vapour phase for successful partitioning. This factor has been a severe restriction on the use of this method for many classes of steroids. The high-melting corticoids, for example, are not easily vaporized under these conditions and more elevated temperatures lead to thermal breakdown of the molecules. The high molecular weight sterols are also not easily chromatographed by this procedure; even when they are reasonably volatile, the time required for passage through the column is excessively long. Some of these problems have been overcome through the use of derivatives which render the substance more volatile.

Despite the above shortcomings, gas–liquid chromatography of a steroid possesses inherent advantages, e.g. the resolving power is probably the greatest of any of the methods thus far mentioned. It is also capable of detecting very small quantities (in the nanogram range) because of the detection systems available with this method. In the last part of this chapter these detectors are discussed in more detail because of their capabilities for quantitative measurement.

H. Radioactive Indicators

In the case of the isolation of known substances, the addition of a labelled tracer to the initial mixture can provide extremely useful information. Not only will this allow close monitoring of the location of the compound, but will also give a measure of the inevitable losses along the way.

I. Chemical Methods

Steroidal ketones react with semicarbazide in a quantitative fashion (see Appendix). Advantage has been taken of this fact to provide a method for separating such ketones from other materials in a mixture. If a modified semi-carbazide is used, where a positively charged nitrogen is present, the derivative becomes water soluble.

$$\begin{array}{c}R' \\ \diagdown \\ C=O \\ \diagup \\ R'\end{array} \quad + \quad NH_2-NH-\overset{\overset{\displaystyle O}{\|}}{C}-\overset{\oplus}{N}R_3 \quad \xrightarrow{} \quad \begin{array}{c}R^1 \\ \diagdown \\ C=N-NH-\overset{\overset{\displaystyle O}{\|}}{C}-\overset{\oplus}{N}R_3 \\ \diagup \\ R^1\end{array}$$
$$X^{\ominus} \qquad\qquad\qquad\qquad X^{\ominus}$$

water insoluble steroids   water soluble

A simple partitioning between water and an organic solvent will result in a separation. The ketone can then be regenerated by reaction with pyruvic acid which displaces it. This modified semicarbazide is known as a Girard Reagent of which there are several types depending on whether the R group is methyl, phenyl, etc.

A separation method which removes 3β-hydroxy-5-ene steroids from solution utilizes the natural sapogenin, digitonin. This molecule has the unique property of forming ethanol insoluble complexes with most steroids containing the above mentioned structural features. The steroid—digitonin complex is filtered off and the steroid released by solution in pyridine which cleaves the complex.

The nature of the complex is not well understood even though it was discovered in the early days of steroid research. Most likely it involves some type of hydrogen bonding in which these two types of molecules fit together in a precise fashion. The formation of digitonin precipitate can also be used to identify the 3β-hydroxy-5-ene structure in an unknown steroid since it is quite specific for this structural type.

III. ESTABLISHING THE IDENTITY OF A STEROID

Identifying a spot on a chromatogram or the crystals from a purified extract is a situation often faced by the researcher in steroid biochemistry. There is now a wide variety of powerful methods, as well as a large body of literature, to aid in this task. The choice of methods will, of course, be governed by such considerations as sample size and available instrumentation.

A. Chromatographic Mobility Measurement

This may be the most general method since it has a very low sample requirement and is within reach of every modern laboratory. The identification of known compounds is particularly straightforward by this technique. One simply compares the movement of the unknown with that of authentic standard in several suitable systems. Obviously, the greater the number and variety of systems, the more certain will be the conclusion. The choice of comparison standards will, of course, require some well-founded guesswork; however, other facets of the problem often narrow the possibilities considerably.

An interesting theory which relates chemical structure to mobility in partition systems, has been developed (Bush, 1961). This allows unknown structures to be elucidated solely on the basis of their behaviour in a series of systems. A variation utilizes predictable changes in mobility which are associated with functional group changes brought about by chemical reaction. The expression which describes this effect is the following:

$$R_m = \log\left(\frac{1}{R_f} - 1\right)$$

R_f is the usual measure of chromatographic mobility, namely the ratio of distance travelled by the compound, to the distance the solvent front travels. According to the theory, the change in R_m (ΔR_m) will be constant for a given structural change irrespective of the rest of the molecule. For example, if we oxidize testosterone to androstenedione, the ΔR_m of this change would be the same as that observed in converting estradiol to estrone. If we now encounter an unknown steroid which exhibits a similar ΔR_m for such a change, we could say with some certainty that it contained a 17β-hydroxyl group. The theory will hold so long as each functional group in the molecule contributes independently to the mobility of the substance. Unfortunately, in many cases functional groups interact with each other making interpretations more difficult. Further details and examples of the use of ΔR_m values are given by Bush (1961).

B. Isotope Dilution

If the material we are seeking to identify is radioactive, it is possible to dilute the tracer with an authentic sample of non-radioactive substance and test the mixture in one or more separation procedures. Crystallization and chromatography are generally used and the specific activity measured after each attempted separation. If the specific activity is reasonably constant after several such tests, one would be reasonably safe in concluding that the tracer and standard are identical. This type of experiment is usually done only after the investigator is fairly sure of the identity so that isotope dilution generally serves as confirmatory evidence.

C. Spectral Properties

There are a number of spectroscopic methods which are used primarily by the organic chemist but which find their way into steroid biochemistry on certain occasions. Some of these techniques can also be used for quantitative measurements because of their precise relationship to the amount of sample present. In this section, these methods are only discussed with regard to their ability to yield information about structural features.

There are several *ultraviolet* absorbing chromophores which occur commonly in steroids. The most important are the ketones conjugated with a double bond, such as the 4-en-3-ones and six-membered aromatic ring systems found in the estrogens. Occasionally, conjugated systems of two double bonds are encountered such as in the vitamin D series. In order to measure the ultraviolet spectrum, the sample must be quite pure or at least free of all other absorbing materials. Relatively small samples are needed for good spectra since only about 1 ml at a concentration of 10^{-3} to 10^{-5} M is needed.

Absorption spectra of steroids in the *infrared* region can reveal a good deal about the nature of the molecule. This is the area in the energy spectrum where the bond bending and stretching frequencies of organic compounds occur. In the case of steroids a number of functional groups show characteristics bands almost independent in frequency of the rest of the molecule. In addition, there is an area of the spectrum, rich in bands which are characteristic of the entire molecule. This area, known as the 'fingerprint region', is almost impossible to interpret; however, it is useful for identification by comparison with authentic spectra. For infrared measurements, samples of around 1 mg are needed, although with special equipment, this can be somewhat reduced. Here, as in the previous method, reasonable sample purity is required for simple interpretation. Infrared spectroscopy has seldom been used for quantitation in biochemical experiments because of the high sample requirements and sensitivity to impurities; its main use has been in elucidating new structures.

Nuclear magnetic resonance spectroscopy (n.m.r.) differs from the previous two methods in that energy other than light is involved. The method is based upon the principle that certain atoms when placed in a high strength, oscillating magnetic field, produce radiofrequency signals which can be monitored. The only substance in this category which is of interest to the steroid biochemist is hydrogen. However, since every steroid contains many hydrogen atoms this has become a very useful tool in analysing structures.

If all of the hydrogen atoms in a steroid produced the same signal, the method would be obviously of limited value. The observation that the electronic environment (that is the types of bonds) in the vicinity of a particular atom will influence its signal, has made this a very subtle method for determining steroid structures. A discussion of these effects is beyond the scope of this book and further details may be sought in one of the many books on n.m.r.; suffice it to say that this technique has revolutionized structural analyses of steroids. N.m.r. is also capable of detecting hydrogen bonding and a few studies of this important effect in biological systems have been reported.

A method akin to n.m.r., known as *electron spin resonance* (e.s.r.) has the capability of detecting free radicals, or unpaired electrons in solution. This has been applied with interesting results in the study of electron transport mechanisms in biological media.

Mass spectroscopy represents a totally different type of measurement, in that energy transitions are not being monitored. The sample is vaporized and ionized *in vacuo* thereby disintegrating the molecule into a number of charged particles. These are passed into a spectrometer which records the precise mass and relative numbers of each fragment. Under carefully controlled conditions, it is possible to get a molecular ion peak representing the ionized but unfragmented molecule. This allows measurement of the molecular weight with great precision, which in turn allows the carbon, hydrogen and oxygen content to be determined obviating the need for combustion analysis.

For the steroid biochemist one of the valuable features of mass spectroscopy is the small sample requirement. When a gas chromatograph is coupled with a mass spectrometer it is possible to analyse the individual compounds as they appear at the end of the column provided there is sufficient time between peaks. Compounds labelled with deuterium can also be analysed by this method since most instruments can readily distinguish molecules differing by one mass unit.

D. Chemical Reaction

The identification of a substance may be aided by studying its chemical reactivity. In a biological problem, a reaction between a steroid and a reagent is usually observed by a change in chromatographic mobility (see above) or by the production of a typical colour. Alternatively, in certain cases where there is sufficient sample the reaction product may be isolated and its spectral properties determined. If the structure of the product can be thus established, then the identity of the sample can be determined by analogy with other reactions.

Colour reactions are most often used for measuring the quantities of steroids in a sample and those reactions will be discussed in subsection IV. There are, however, some colour tests which serve primarily for identification purposes. The degree of specificity as well as the sensitivity varies considerably, since some reagents react with most steroids while others give positive reactions with only one structure.

Steroidal ketones will react with *2,4-dinitrophenylhydrazine* (see Appendix) to give bright red or orange-coloured derivatives. The absorption maximum of the product is indicative of the type of ketone present. For example, a saturated 3-ketone will give a maximum at 367 nm while the corresponding compound with a double bond at position 4 will exhibit a 392 nm maximum. This test requires a pure sample since many substances interfere; therefore its application to biological samples is limited.

Steroids containing reactive groups will reduce *phosphomolybdic acid* (PMA) to the metal. This test is usually carried out on paper or thin-layer chromatograms, where a dark blue spot is obtained. The reagent is not very specific although differences in intensity and speed of development are observed with various functional groups. The common 5-ene-3β-hydroxy group gives a fast intense test while the ketonic non-hydroxylated steroids react slowly. This reagent has moderate sensitivity, again varying with the substance, and is used widely in conjunction with thin layer chromatography.

A reagent similar to PMA but using phosphotungstic acid is *Folin–Ciocalteau Reagent*. This is specific for phenols, hence most of the estrogens react positively; however, it cannot readily distinguish between the various examples in this class. The sensitivity is comparable to PMA.

An example of a highly specific colour test is the *Kägi–Miescher Reaction*. A steroid containing a secondary 17α-hydroxyl group gives a positive test while other hydroxy steroids (even the 17β-) will not react. The first part of the test is a dehydration and migration of the adjacent methyl group.

The colour is then generated by adding bromine to the acidified solution.

The five-membered unsaturated lactone ring of the cardenolides can be detected by means of the *Legal colour reaction*. A solution of the substance in pyridine containing sodium nitroprusside is made alkaline producing a deep red colour if a cardenolide is present. An interesting feature is that the bufadienolides, which have a six-membered doubly-unsaturated lactone ring, do not react.

It has been observed that solutions of steroids in concentrated sulphuric acid give characteristic adsorption spectra in the 220—600 nm range. The underlying reactions(s) for this phenomenon is not known, however sufficient data has been accumulated to make this a useful method for identifying small samples of known compounds. The method, unfortunately, is sensitive to a variety of little understood factors which limits its use as a quantitative tool although a useful feature is its fairly low sample size requirement.

IV. MEASURING THE AMOUNTS OF STEROID IN A BIOLOGICAL SYSTEM

Assaying biological materials for the presence and quantity of various steroids is of importance not only to the research worker but also to the clinician. The endocrinological status of a patient can often be diagnosed with the help of various steroid estimations. For the latter application, the method must be rapid, simple and not involve very expensive equipment. On the other hand, the person engaged in research can utilize a more involved procedure since, in general, it will not be necessary to assay vast numbers of samples. The general objectives of any assay are precision, accuracy and sensitivity.

A. Spectral Band Intensities

These methods depend upon the interaction of light energy with the compound to be assayed. The ultraviolet absorptions of several types of structures (see previous section) are directly proportional to the amount of substance present. Beer's Law states that:

$$\text{Absorbance} = \left(\frac{\text{intensity of incident light}}{\text{intensity of emergent light}} \right)$$

where: Absorbance = cell length (l) x molar concn. (c) x specific absorbance (k).

The absorbance (commonly and less desirably called the optical density) is the amount of energy absorbed by the substance and is the parameter measured by the instrument. The product of the concentration and the path length through which the light travels is the amount of substance interacting with the light. The specific absorbance (also known as the *absorption coefficient* or the *extinction coefficient*) is the proportionality constant relating the other quantities; its magnitude is characteristic of a particular chromophoric group.

The molar absorbance (or molecular extinction coeff.) = k x molecular weight. As mentioned earlier (Subsection III) certain steroids can be detected at quite low levels by ultra-violet light. Unfortunately, this method is not always useful for clinical assay since the sample must be free of interfering substances of which there are usually an abundance. There are a number of reagents which produce chromophores with various steroids and whose light absorption can be estimated quantitatively with reasonable sensitivity and accuracy. In many cases the chemical nature of the chromophore is not known, however the results are still quite useful.

Table 2.1.
Spectrophotometric methods of steroid determinations*

Assay	Compounds	Application
Porter-Silber Assay (modified method: Silber and Porter, 1957)	17,20-dihydroxy-; 20-oxosteroids	urine
Appleby et al., (1955)	17-hydroxycorticosteroids**	urine
Norymberski et al., (1953)	17-oxogenic steroids***	urine
Gray et al., (1969)	17-oxogenic steroids***	
Zimmermann Assay (modifications: Zimmermann, 1955)	17-oxosteroids	urine
Mattingly (1962)	11-hydroxycorticosteroids	plasma
Brown et al., (1968) (Kober reaction)	estrogens (estriol in pregnancy urine)	urine

*See Loraine and Bell (1971) for details of these and similar assays.
**Measures numerous steroids including 17α-hydroxyprogesterone, pregnanetriol, 11-deoxy-cortisol, cortisol, cortisone, cortol and cortolone (steroids possessing C-17 side-chains: $>COH.CO.CH_2OH$, $>COH.CHOH.CH_2OH$, $>COH.CHOH.CH_3$ and $>COH.CO.CH_3$).
***Also measures many steroids (those possessing C-17 side-chains: $>COH.CO.CH_2OH$, $>COH.CHOH.CH_2OH$ and $>COH.CHOH.CH_3$).

Solutions of certain steroids in strong acid not only produce absorption spectra as mentioned above, but also give very intense fluorescence spectra. The solution is irradiated with light of a certain wavelength, usually the 436 nm mercury line for steroids. The molecules absorb light energy and are transformed to an excited state. They then undergo a second transition back to the ground state and emit a quantum of energy at a longer wavelength. By this method one can measure amounts of some steroids of the order of a microgram or less. Since this is a sensitive, but not a specific method, very pure samples and reagents are required for accurate, reproducible results. Special precautions are also often required to prevent high blanks from contaminated glassware.

Strong bases can also promote intense fluorescence, particularly with steroids containing the 4-en-3-one system. This can be carried out in solution or on paper strips by spraying with sodium hydroxide solution. The strips can be passed through a spectrofluorometer by means of a special scanning attachment. The location and intensities of fluorescent spots are recorded on a strip chart. This method has been used successfully for steroids in plasma, with samples containing about 1 μg of steroid.

Many of the original methods, and also some of the recent modifications based on absorption of light by chromophores, estimate groups of steroids (see Table 2.1) rather than individual compounds. In a modern steroid biochemistry laboratory many methods are now available (see below) for the determination of individual steroids; the group methods are, however, still important diagnostic tools. This is especially true for the corticosteroids which are found (as metabolites) in large amounts in urine and also for urinary estriol during pregnancy. The Mattingly procedure for estimating 11-hydroxycorticosteroids (mainly cortisol) in plasma is also extensively used. Methods for assaying ovarian and testis function on the other hand depend much more on determination of individual steroids (e.g. estradiol, progesterone and testosterone) in plasma.

B. Double Isotope Derivatives

The *double isotope derivative assay method* was one of the first assays to be developed using radioisotopes which could measure small quantities of steroids in biological fluids. In this procedure the sample (S) is mixed with a tracer amount of labelled steroid (T) giving a mixture (ST) of lower specific activity (SA_{ST}). The mixture is then quantitatively converted to a suitable derivative using a reagent (R) labelled with a different isotope of known specific activity (SA_R).

$$S + T \longrightarrow ST$$
$$ST + R \longrightarrow ST-R$$

Since ST and R combine in a precise proportion, and since the isotopes can be independently counted, it is possible to calculate the specific activity of the steroid (SA_{ST}) and hence the amount that was in the original sample.

$$\frac{\text{Moles R}}{\text{Moles ST}} = \frac{1}{1}$$

$$\frac{SA_R}{SA_{ST}} = \frac{\dfrac{\text{dpm R}}{\text{moles R}}}{\dfrac{\text{dpm ST}}{\text{moles ST}}} = \frac{\text{dpm R}}{\text{dpm ST}}$$

In most cases the mass of the tracer is so small compared to the sample that it can be ignored in the calculation. This method has sufficient sensitivity for the measurement of many physiological steroid levels; however, it is considerably more time consuming than the saturation analysis technique described below. Table 2.2 lists some of the steroids which have been assayed by the double isotope derivative method.

Table 2.2.
Double isotope derivative method

Compound	Reagent	Sensitivity (ng) = 10^{-9} g	Applications
Aldosterone	Acetic anhydride	1	Urine, plasma
Aldosterone	Pipsan	1	Plasma
Cortisone	Acetic anhydride	50	Plasma
Digitoxin	Acetic anhydride	10	Plasma, urine, stool
Testosterone	Thiosemicarbazide	20	Plasma
Testosterone	Acetic anhydride	8.7	Plasma
Estrone	Pipsyl chloride	1	Plasma

C. Saturation Analysis Techniques

Radioimmunoassay (RIA) competitive protein binding analysis (CPB) and radio-ligand receptor assays (RLA) are all examples of saturation analysis which depends on the reversible binding of the compound being assayed (the ligand) with specific proteins. All these methods have been applied to steroid analysis and are now the main methods used both in the research and clinical laboratory. Historically this technique developed from Yalow and Berson's method of radio-immunoassay for plasma insulin using insulin antibodies and Ekins' work on the assay of thyroxine using thyroxine-binding globulin.

There are several proteins which occur in plasma and preferentially bind certain steroids (see chapter 14). These proteins have been used extensively for CPB analyses of steroids. In many cases CPB has now been superseded by the more sensitive radioimmunoassays. Steroids themselves are not antigenic so it is necessary first to couple the steroid covalently to a large protein such as albumin. This complex is injected into animals over a period of several months producing antibodies against this antigen which have a high binding affinity for the original steroid molecule used. The specificity of the antibodies formed depend very much on how and where the albumin is coupled to the steroid molecule.

In target organs protein receptors exist which exhibit high affinity and specificity for their hormones (see chapter 14). Theoretically these receptors are ideally suitable for use in hormone assays. They have the important advantage over radioimmunoassay that the specificity is directed toward the biologically active region of the hormone rather than to some immunologically active portion which may have a dubious, if any, involvement with the expression of hormonal activity. As far as steroid hormone receptors are concerned, they occur in such small quantities in biological tissues, that they have not yet been generally developed for use in assay methods. One exception is the uterine cytosol which has been used for the assay of estradiol; radioimmunoassay is, however, used in preference because of its higher sensitivity. Receptor assays for other hormones, especially the protein hormones, are being rapidly developed (see Sönksen, 1974).

For the saturation analysis of a steroid hormone the requirements are:

a) The radioactive steroid (S^*).
b) Binding protein (P) e.g. antibody (or antiserum containing the antibody) raised against the antigen, or specific plasma binding protein.
c) Sample to be assayed containing an unknown amount of non-radioactive steroid (S).
d) Samples of standard, known amounts of non-radioactive steroid.

The sample to be assayed for steroid (S) is added to a known amount of radioactive hormone (S^*) and binding protein (P) of limited capacity. S and S^* compete for the binding sites on the protein. Thus, the less hormone (S) there is in the sample undergoing assay, then the more S^* is bound to the protein and vice versa. After its formation, the steroid—protein complex (i.e. the bound steroid: $S.P + S^*.P$) is separated from the free hormone ($S + S^*$), and the radioactivity in the bound and/or free form determined. The amount of steroid in the assay sample is determined from a standard curve, constructed by simultaneously performing the radioassay on standard samples containing known amounts of unlabelled and labelled hormone. This standard curve may be a plot of percentage bound or percentage free or free/bound against the total amount of steroid used.

The bound and unbound steroid can be separated from each other by a variety of procedures. One favoured method is absorption of the free steroid onto dextran-coated charcoal; after centrifugation the amount of bound steroid can be determined in the supernatant. Alternatively the steroid—protein complex can be precipitated by the addition of ammonium sulphate solution.

None of the steroid antibodies formed so far are absolutely specific for one steroid; they all show some cross reaction with structurally similar compounds. Naturally occurring steroid binding proteins are similarly not absolutely specific. It is necessary therefore with both RIA and CPB methods to purify biological extracts by chromatography before assay, if good specificity is required. If large amounts of the steroid being assayed are present in the samples and it has previously been determined that cross-reacting substances are present only in relatively small quantities, then it is possible to carry out assays on relatively crude extracts without chromatography. Because of the simplicity of saturation analysis techniques, many samples can be determined at the same time. Automatic apparatus is also being developed to deal with the large number of analyses often carried out. One of the most important aspects of saturation analysis, especially radioimmunoassay, is the high sensitivity of the method; all of the hormonal steroids can be determined (see Table 2.2) using small amounts of plasma. Under suitable conditions RIA can detect steroids in amounts as low as 1—2 pg/ml. The normal working range for assay of steroids is usually 10—200 pg/ml.

One of the disadvantages of steroid RIA is that the radioactive isotope used is tritium which requires long counting times especially when high sensitivity is

Table 2.3.
Steroids Assayed by Radioimmunoassay*

Steroid	Sex	Normal value (ng/100 ml plasma)	Approximate plasma volume required	Special conditions
Progesterone	♂	22.6 ± 9.7	1.0 ml	
	♀	26.5 ± 19.2		follicular phase,
		828 ± 634		luteal phase
Testosterone	♂	590 ± 149	0.3—3.0 ml	
	♀	32 ± 7		
Estradiol	♂	18.1 ± 1.80 (pg/ml)	1.0—5.0 ml	
		21.4 ± 2.62 (pg/ml)		follicular phase,
		68.5 4.70 (pg/ml)		luteal phase
Aldosterone		1.35	5.0 ml	normal Na diet, supine position
		12.2 ± 7.4		ambulant position

*Data from review by Skelley, Brown and Besch (1973)

required (at high sensitivity the mass of tritiated steroid added is of the same order as the mass of the steroid being assayed and therefore the amount added is kept as low as possible). If a γ-emitting isotope (e.g. ^{125}I) could be introduced into the steroid molecule the sensitivity would be increased because ^{125}I gives about 25 times the detectable counting rate given by 4 atoms of ^3H. The use of γ-labelled steroids would give radioimmunoassay the added advantage of being easier and less expensive to perform. Present results from RIA of steroids labelled with a γ-emitter indicate that the specificity of the assay is less than with tritiated steroids, but further development of suitable derivatives may eliminate these initial difficulties.

D. Gas—Liquid Chromatography (GLC) and Mass Spectrometry Detection Systems

The value of GLC in steroid analysis depends mainly on the sensitivity of the detection systems used. The most widely used is the flame ionization detector. In this technique the column effluent is mixed with hydrogen and burned between highly charged electrodes. The current generated by the flame is measured by an electrometer and can be recorded on paper. The size of the current is directly proportional to the amount of material in the column effluent. The result is the appearance of a peak on the chart whenever a compound emerges from the column. This type of detector is capable of measuring samples containing less than 1 μg of steroid. It is responsive to any substance which can burn, necessitating preliminary removal of extraneous substances from the sample.

The electron capture detector is based on the reaction of certain substances with a stream of electrons generated by the detector. The advantage of this system lies in its greater sensitivity compared with the flame detector. Measurements in the nanogram range are common and in some cases even smaller amounts can be detected. Unfortunately, only a small number of steroids can be assayed with this detector, hence it has found limited application.

GLC has been mainly used in research laboratories because of the expensive equipment required and the necessity of a highly skilled operator. Table 2.4 gives a few examples of types of steroid analyses possible with GLC.

Recently there have been an increasing number of reports of the use of gas—liquid chromatography combined with mass spectrometry (GCMS) for the

Table 2.4.
Steroid Analysis by Gas Chromatography

Compound	Sensitivity (μg)	Application
Estrone	5	Urine
Estradiol	5	Urine
Estriol	5	Urine
Progesterone	0.005	Plasma
Testosterone	0.01	Plasma, urine

quantitative measurements of steroids in biological fluids. This is achieved by the use of derivatives selectively detected by GCMS and giving spectra containing characteristic ions in relatively high abundance. High sensitivity has been claimed and Aldercreutz has predicted that measurement of femtogram (10^{-15} g) quantities will be possible soon (see Brooks and Middleditch in Heftman, 1973).

E. Bioassay

This type of measurement is based on the effects of specific compounds or classes of compounds on a biological system, usually a laboratory animal. The method can be used to follow the isolation of a compound from its source as in the separation of cardiac glycosides from plants or toad venom. It is more often used to quantitate the amount of steroid present in a tissue or fluid.

In some instances bioassay can be used to advantage over the physical and chemical methods discussed above. For example, purification is not usually necessary since only the hormone will produce a particular biological effect. On the other hand, precision is usually very low since the test animals can vary greatly in their response. The use of statistical methods can reduce this source of error to some extent.

Steroid bioassay is quickly falling into the category of out-dated classical methods as more rapid and precise methods based on physical principles are being developed. Table 2.5 lists a few of the well-known assays and their applications.

Table 2.5.
Several Examples of Steroid Bioassays

Assay or Common Name	Substance(s) Measured	Species Used	Sensitivity (μg)
Allen−Doisy Test	Estrogens	Rat, mouse	10^{-3}
Pincus Method	Progesterone	Rabbit	250
Electrolyte Test	Deoxycorticosterone	Rat, mouse	1
Capon's Comb Test	Testosterone	Chicken	150
−−−	Cardiac glycosides	Cat, pigeon	−−−

V. REFERENCES

Chromatography

Neher, R. (1964). *Steroid Chromatography*. Elsevier.
Bush, I. E. (1961). *The Chromatography of Steroids*. Pergamon Press.

Countercurrent Distribution

Weisiger, J. R. (1954). In Mitchell, Holthoff, Proshauer and Weissburger (Eds), *Organic Analysis*, Vol. 2. Interscience, pp. 277−326.

Gas Chromatography

Eik Nes, E. B. and E. C. Horning (1968). *Gas Phase Chromatography of Steroids.* Springer-Verlag.

Spectral Analyses

Appleby, J. I., G. Gibson, J. K. Norymberski and R. D. Stubbs (1955). Indirect analysis of corticosteroids. The determination of 17-hydroxycorticosteroids. *Biochem. J.* 60, 453–467.

Brown, J. B., C. Macnaughtan, M. A. Smith and B. Smyth (1968). Further observations on the Kober colour and Ittrich fluorescence reactions in the measurement of oestriol, oestrone and oestradiol. *J. Endocr.* 40, 175–188; also 42, 5–15.

Engel, L. L. (Ed.) (1963). *Physical Properties of the Steroid Hormones.* Macmillan Co.

Gray, C. H., D. N. Baron, R. V. Brooks and V. H. T. James (1969). A critical appraisal of a method of estimating urinary 17-oxosteroids and total 17-oxogenic steroids. *The Lancet* 1, 124–127.

Hobkirk, R. and A. Metcalfe-Gibson (1963). *Standard Methods of Clinical Chemistry,* Vol. 4. Academic Press, pp. 65–83.

Mattingly, D. (1962). A simple fluorimetric method for the estimation of free 11-hydroxycorticoids in human plasma. *J. Clin. Path.* 15, 374–9.

Norymberski, J. K., R. D. Stubbs and H. F. West (1953). Assessment of adrenocortical activity by assay of 17-ketogenic steroids in urine. *The Lancet* 1, 1276–1281.

Silber, R. H. and C. C. Porter (1957). Determination of 17,21-Dihydroxy-20-Ketosteroids in Urine and Plasma. In *Methods of Biochem. Anal.* 4, 139–169.

Zimmermann, W. (1955). *Hoppe-Seyler's Zeitschrift physiol. chem.* 300, 141.

Immunoassay—Protein Binding

Abraham, G. E. (1974). Radioimmunoassay of Steroids in Biological Fluids. *Clin. Biochem.* 1, 193–201.

Hayes, R. L., F. A. Goswitz, B. E. P. Murphy (Eds) (1968). Radioisotopes in Medicine: In Vitro Studies. *U.S. Atomic Energy Comm. Symposium Series No. 13.*

Kirkham, K. E. and W. M. Hunter (Eds) (1971). *Radioimmunoassay Methods.* Churchill Livingstone, Edinburgh and London.

Midgley, A. R., G. D. Niswender, U. L. Gay and L. E. Reichert (1971). Use of Antibodies for Characterization of Gonadotropins and Steroids. *Recent Progr. in Hormone Res.* 27, pp. 235–301.

Odell, W. D. and W. H. Daughaday (Eds) (1971) *Principles of competitive Protein-Binding Assays.* Lippincott Co., Philadelphia & Toronto.

Sönksen, P. H. (Ed) (1974) *Radioimmunoassay and Saturation Analysis.* British Medical Bulletin, *30*, No. 1.

Skelley, D. S., L. P. Brown and P. K. Besch (1973) Radioimmunoassay. *Clin. Chem.* **19**, 146.

Wide, L. (1969). Radioimmunoassays Employing Immuno-Sorbents. *Acta Endocr. Kbh. Supple.*, **142**, 207.

Double Isotope Derivatives

Whitehead, J. K. and H. G. Dean (1968) The Isotope Derivative Method in Biochemical Analysis. In *Methods of Biochemical Analysis*, Vol. 16, Interscience.

Bioassay

Loraine, J. A. and E. T. Bell (1971). *Hormone Assays and Their Clinical Applications*, 3rd ed. E. & S. Livingstone Ltd. Edinburgh and London.

Dorfman, R. I. (1962). Methods in Hormone Research. *Bioassay*, Vol. II, Academic Press.

General

Heftman, E. (Ed) (1973). *Modern Methods of Steroid Analysis*. Academic Press.

CHAPTER 3

Methods for endocrine tissue investigations

I. INTRODUCTION

There are many ways of investigating tissue secretions and molecular mechanisms, each of them having their own advantages and limitations. The choice must depend on the questions being asked. For example, perfusion of a whole organ will give valuable information about the total products secreted and can be used to study control by external stimuli. However, this type of study will not yield information on the synthesis of specific substances by the different cell types present or about the molecular mechanisms of control processes within the different cell types present. Very often a combination of techniques is required. For example, after administration of a hormone to the whole animal, tissues can be isolated and subfractionated to determine the characteristics of the response in a specific cell type or subcellular fraction.

The various possibilities will now be summarized and some of the advantages and disadvantages of the available methods will be discussed. The various approaches have been divided into the following:

1. Whole body studies
2. Organ systems
3. Tissues and cells
4. Subcellular fractions

More detailed accounts can be found in excellent comprehensive reviews edited by Diczfalusy (1971), O'Malley and Hardman (1974) and Dorfman (1975), which bring together details of most if not all the available methods for hormone research.

II. WHOLE BODY STUDIES

Results of studies based on the measurement of substances in body fluids (i.e. blood, urine, faeces, etc.) will reflect both secretion by specific organs and metabolism by other tissues. The classical studies of isolation and purification of substances from urine and plasma extracts, from intact animals and after removal of specific organs, led to the discovery of the source and structure of many of the hormones. In present-day biochemical and clinical studies, analysis of body fluids is used mainly to assess the nature and rate of secretion of hormones from the glands producing them.

Secretion Rates. The rate at which a metabolite of a steroid hormone is secreted in urine can be used to assess the rate of secretion of the hormone and hence provides an estimate of the endocrine gland function. For example the secretion rates of specific metabolites of cortisol (usually tetrahydrocortisol or tetrahydrocortisone) are used to assess adrenal cortical function. The method that is generally used involves the administration of a ^{14}C- or ^{3}H-labelled hormone and measurement of the specific activity of the hormone metabolite in a 24—48 h urine sample. The **secretion rate** of the hormone (in mg/24—48 h) is then equal to:

$$\frac{\text{dose administered (in counts/min)}}{\text{specific activity of metabolite (counts/min/mg)}}$$

The method is based on the principle of isotope dilution and depends on the complete mixing of the isotopically labelled hormone with the endogenous hormone. It is essential that the metabolite is formed exclusively from the hormone and that all of the radioactivity is recovered in the 24—48 h urine (see Loraine and Bell, 1971, Jenkins, 1968, and Cope, 1964, for further discussion of this method).

The *Metabolic Clearance Rate* (MCR) is a very useful parameter relating the secretion rate to the plasma concentration. It has the dimensions of volume divided by time and may be defined as:

$$\text{MCR} = \frac{\text{Secretion rate}}{i}$$

where i = plasma hormone concentration.

In the *steady state*, the amount of steroid secreted will be equal to that entering the circulation, i.e. the production rate will equal the secretion rate. A steady state can be achieved for metabolic studies by continuous infusion of the substance under investigation. It is assumed that the continuous infusion of a radioactive compound simulates the secretion of the gland. The ratio of the rate of infusion of radioactive steroid to the final concentration of radioactive hormone will then be equal to the ratio of the hormonal secretion rate to the non-isotopic steroid plasma concentration. This ratio in both cases is the MCR.

In practice the MCR's of progesterone and aldosterone are found to be very high (2500—5000 litres plasma/day) compared with cortisol and corticosterone (200—300 litres plasma/day). Estrone and estradiol have intermediate values (1400—2000 litres plasma/day).

These values reflect the rate at which these steroids are cleared from the blood i.e. the higher the MCR, the more quickly is the hormone removed from the circulation. Thus the MCR is a measure of efficiency; it is the volume of blood that is completely and irreversibly cleared of the hormone per unit time. A practical demonstration of physiological factors affecting MCR is given in the guinea pig. In this animal during pregnancy the progesterone concentration rises after the 15th day of pregnancy. This rise is accompanied by a fall in MCR which is caused by the raised concentrations of specific binding proteins in blood which have a high affinity for progesterone. Thus the rate at which progesterone is cleared from the blood is decreased.

The theory of the steady state and the practical applications and pitfalls of MCR measurements have been extensively discussed and will not be dealt with further here. Excellent reviews have been published by Tait (1963), Lieberman and Gurpide (1966), Balikian et al., (1968) and Baird et al., (1969). It is probable that the most reliable estimates of blood production rates are obtained following evaluation of the blood values.

III ORGAN SYSTEMS

A. Whole Organs

One of the disadvantages of measurements of substances in peripheral plasma and urine is that it is possible that the substances being studied do not originate from one source and/or different precursors may form the same metabolite(s). The relative ease with which it is now possible to catheterize vascular vessels has made it possible to perfuse specific organs in situ with whole blood and directly study the secretion products and effect of regulatory agents. This type of approach has been particularly successful with liver, adrenal gland, ovarian and testis tissues (Douglas et al., 1961; Eik-Nes, 1971). It also has the added advantage that substances secreted by an organ are in higher concentrations in the venous effluent blood than in the peripheral blood, making identification easier. The demonstration of the higher concentration in venous blood is of course one of the prerequisites for proving secretion of a substance by a gland.

The collection of venous blood requires surgical interference with the animal which precludes long term studies, although indwelling catheters have been used. One possible way round this problem is to transplant the organ to a more accessible place. Such a transplantation technique has been utilized for studies on the sheep ovary by McCracken, Baird and Goding (1971) in which the ovary (together with the uterus) was transplanted to the neck of the sheep. This preparation allows direct access to both the arterial and venous sides of the ovarian circulation, repeatedly, in the conscious animal (Figure 3.1). Thus the secretion and factors controlling the ovary can be studied under more physiological conditions than are normally available. The results from a similar technique for transplanting the sheep adrenal have also provided valuable information (Blair-West et al., 1970; Wright et al., 1972).

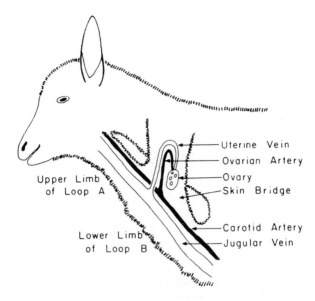

Figure 3.1 Diagram of ovarian autotransplant showing anastomosis of ovarian vascular pedicle with vessels in jugulocarotid skin loop (prepared three months previously). From McCracken and Baird (1969). Reproduced by permission of Meredith Corporation, New York.

Another perfusion system which has been used particularly by Diczfalusy and coworkers, involves perfusion of the foeto-placental unit (Diczfalusy, 1969) (Figure 3.2). The foetus is placed in an artificial amniotic fluid. The placenta (connected by an intact umbilical circulation to the foetus) is placed in a separate vessel containing oxygenated fresh blood. The system shown can be used for perfusion of the whole unit or the simultaneous but separate perfusion of the foetus and placenta. Using this system, it is possible to maintain a foetal—placental circulation at 37°C for 90—150 min and to introduce labelled precursors and collect the products secreted. In addition, the products retained within the individual organs can be later extracted and identified.

B. Quartered or Sliced Tissues

Many studies have been carried out by incubating *in vitro* quartered or sliced organs. Care has to be taken with these preparations to ensure good oxygenation of the tissues, i.e. it is important that slices are not more than 1 mm thick although of course this increases the number of cut or damaged cells. The quartered glands moreover have the disadvantage that the cells within the tissue fragments have limited accessiblity to components of the incubation medium and to O_2. It is clear that the processes for providing nutrients to cells within tissue fragments incubated *in vitro* (as well as those for removing their cellular products), differ markedly from those operating *in vivo*. However many useful studies have been carried out with

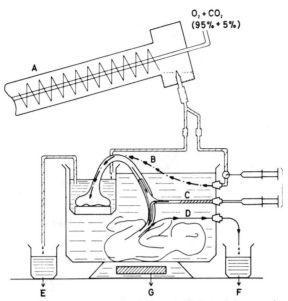

$O_2 + CO_2$
$(95\% + 5\%)$

Figure 3.2 System for the *in vitro* perfusion of the complete foeto-placental unit at midpregnancy. (From Lerner and Diczfalusy, 1968.) A = oxygenator, B = placental perfusion via an umbilical artery, C = T-tube in an umbilical vein for foetal perfusion, D = catheter in the other umbilical vein to collect foetal perfusate, E = perfusate from the 'maternal' side, F = container with foetal perfusate, G = heater. Reproduced by permission of *Excerpta Medica*, Amsterdam.

these preparations and they do in general react to trophic hormone stimulation with increased steroidogenesis (albeit relatively poorly).

One main disadvantage of the normal static *in vitro* incubation is that it is often found that the accumulated products inhibit their own further production. This difficulty can be overcome by using the *superfusion* system in which the incubation medium is continuously infused and withdrawn. In such a continuous-flow incubation technique whereby the incubation products are continuously withdrawn for analysis, some of the principles developed for *in vivo* metabolic studies may be applied. Conventional static incubation procedures suffer serious limitations when kinetic data are required. For example, quantitative data on the relative importance of various biosynthetic or metabolic pathways in a steroidogenic tissue cannot be obtained in static incubations with the usual single analysis following addition of a trace quantity of precursor at the start of the incubation. The biosynthetic pathway may be biased towards the contribution of a precursor added in sufficient quantity to ensure that the specific activity of precursor and product remain virtually constant during the incubation, and moreover, some biochemical or metabolic pathways may be selectively inhibited. The development of the superfusion system arose from such considerations and three laboratories independently evolved procedures for this technique (Orti *et al.*, 1965; Tait *et al.*, 1967; Saffran *et al.*, 1967). The basis of the apparatus is the same for all systems that have been developed and comprises a small incubation vessel connected to a carefully controlled pumping system on one side and to an outflow system on the other side. Further details on the fundamentals and applications of the system to problems related to the control of adrenal steroidogenic function have been reviewed (Saffran *et al.*, 1971; Tait and Schulster, 1974).

C. Organ Culture

The techniques of tissue and organ culture have also been used to examine the characteristics of endocrine tissue metabolism. These methods differ from the slice and quartered gland techniques in that tissue fragments are incubated under sterile conditions over a period of days or weeks, and thus long term studies are possible. However, they have the disadvantage that tissues tend to dedifferentiate on cultivation *in vitro* and their biochemical characteristics may be quite unlike the original tissue. For example pathways of steroid biosynthesis quantitatively change during tissue and organ culture.

IV. TISSUES AND CELLS

The techniques described so far have dealt with the whole gland and have not taken into consideration the fact that many different cell types are present in each gland. It is of course important to know what products are produced by the total gland, but is is equally important to know what the contributions are of the individual cell types, if we are to understand the molecular mechanisms which take place.

In the ovary the different tissue types, e.g. stromal, interstitial and granulosa tissue, have been separated and their characteristics with respect to steroidogenesis and trophic hormone stimulation are discussed in Chapters 7 and 13. Granulosa cells and tissue have for example been extensively studied (Channing, 1970) and have been successfully grown in cell culture. Rat testis can be separated by wet dissection into seminiferous tubules and interstitial tissue (Christensen and Mason, 1965) and still retain their responsiveness to trophic hormone stimulation (see Chapter 13). The technique consists of pulling out the tubules from the total testis tissue with fine forceps. The interstitial tissue remains after removal of all the tubules. Wet dissection of testes from other species is difficult with this technique because of their different structures. Interstitial tissue can also be separated from seminiferous tubules by microdissection of freeze-dried slices of total testis (van Doorn *et al.*, 1974). Tissue from the glomerulosa, fasciculata and reticularis zones of the adrenal gland can be obtained using the 'Glick Technique' (Grunbaum *et al.*, 1956). The gland is frozen to $- 15^{\circ}$C and a cylinder of tissue is bored from the frozen gland. The cylinder of tissue is mounted on a microtome and slices are cut. Every third or fourth slice is removed for histological examination and the remainder are added to individual incubation tubes. By this means it is possible to localize the site of adrenal steroid biosynthesis and of trophic hormone action and the different zones of the foetal and adult adrenal gland (Cooke, 1970; Griffiths and Cameron, 1970).

A wide variety of tumour cells have been developed that retain their hormone responsiveness and thus have proved of great value as model systems for investigations into the mechanism of action of different hormones. Sato and coworkers have cultivated mouse adrenal tumours (Buonassissi *et al.,* 1962) that have provided valuable information on the control of steroidogenesis and a recent volume of *Methods in Enzymology* (O'Malley and Hardman, 1974) details endocrine tissue cells that have been exploited by many laboratories in studies into hormonal modes of action. Some tumour cells have provided a powerful tool for investigations into the mechanism of steroid action and for example much valuable information on glucocorticoid mechanism of action has derived from the use of hepatoma cells (see Chapter 16). Moreover the use of mutants, deficient in particular aspects of the control system, offer a useful approach for further biochemical investigations.

A recent development involves the preparation of isolated cell suspensions from normal (as opposed to tumour) tissue. Although work with tumour cells has proved of great value it is subject to the limitation that the control systems in these cells are likely to differ considerably from those in normal cells. Suspensions of normal cells have been prepared using a variety of disaggregation procedures (Halkerston, 1968; Kloppenborg *et al.,* 1968; Haning *et al.,* 1970; Sayers *et al.,* 1971, 1973; Richardson and Schulster, 1972; Moyle and Ramachandran, 1973), and employ enzymes such as collagenase and trypsin to disrupt the molecules binding the cells together in the intact tissue. The prime advantages of the isolated cell system are threefold. Firstly, the cells can be prepared from glands from a number of different animals and studies performed on aliquots from this pool of cells, thereby eliminating the biological variation between animals and greatly increasing the accuracy of the data. Secondly, cell types may be separated, purified and studies on discrete cell-types undertaken (e.g. adrenal glomerulosa cells), and important advances in this area have been made recently (Tait *et al.,* 1974). Thirdly, in suspension, each and every cell had direct access to medium components and O_2 and its products are readily released into the medium — with the consequence that the magnitude and rapidity of the response to trophic hormonal stimulation closely approaches that observed using *in vivo* techniques. A further refinement has been to develop a superfusion system for isolated cell suspensions in order to combine the advantages of these techniques for dynamic studies into the characteristics of the control of isolated normal cells (Schulster, 1973).

V. SUBCELLULAR FRACTIONS

In order to understand the molecular mechanism within the cell one must resort to breaking open the cell. Differential centrifugation is extensively used to separate the cell components after homogenization. The nuclei sediment at quite low speeds ($300\,g$), then the mitochondria at higher speeds ($10,000\,g$) and the microsomal fraction at still higher speeds ($100,000\,g$). The soluble fraction containing free ribosomes remains as the supernatant. It is very difficult to obtain pure cell fractions containing only nuclei, mitochondria or microsomes (ribosomes plus endoplasmic reticulum) and particularly difficult to prepare pure plasma membranes (De Pierre and Karnovsky, 1973). It is therefore essential to employ good enzyme markers whose exact localizations within the cell are well extablished. By this means the purity of the sub-cellular fractions obtained can be ascertained. Unfortunately most broken cell preparations no longer react to hormonal stimulation, presumably because of the disruption of the intracellular machinery and the breakdown of the delicate structure of the plasma membrane where most protein hormone responses are initiated. If the hormone response by cells is to be studied intracellularly then it is usual to stimulate the intact cells *in vivo* or *in vitro* and then determine the intracellular events which have taken place, by for example isolation of intracellular receptors or studying changes in enzymic activity.

VI. REFERENCES (*denotes review or book)

*Baird, E. T., R. Horton, C. Longcope, and J. F. Tait (1969). Steroid dynamics under steady state conditions. *Recent Progress in Horm. Res.,* 25, 611–664.

Balikian, H. M., A. H. Brodie, S. L. Dale, J. C. Melby and J. F. Tait (1968). Effect of posture on the metabolic clearance rate, plasma concentration and blood production rate of aldosterone in man. *J. Clin. Endoc. Metab.,* 25, 1630–1640.

Blair-West, J. R., A. Brodie, J. P. Coghlan, D. A. Denton, C. Flood, J. R. Goding, B. A. Scoggins, J. F. Tait, S. A. S. Tait, E. M. Wintour and R. D. Wright (1970). Studies on the biosynthesis of aldosterone using the sheep adrenal transplant. *J. Endocrinol.,* 46, 453–476.

Buonassissi, V., G. Sato and A. I. Tchen, (1962). Hormone producing cultures of adrenal and pituitary origin. *Proc. Nat. Acad. Sci., (U.S.),* 48, 1184–1190.

*Channing, C. P. (1970). Influences of the *in vivo* and *in vitro* hormonal environment upon luteinization of granulosa cells in tissue culture. *Recent Progress in Horm. Res.,* 26, 589–622.

Christensen, A. K. and N. R. Mason (1965). Comparative ability of seminiferous tubules and interstitial tissue of rat testes to synthesize androgens from progesterone-4-^{14}C *in vitro. Endocrinology,* 76, 646–656.

*Cooke, B. A. (1970). Biosynthesis of dehydroepiandrosterone sulphate in human foetal adrenal glands: Pathways, localization and development in enzymes. Symposium on Reproductive Endocrinology, held in Edinburgh 1969, *Proc. Royal Soc. Medicine.* Livingstone, Edinburgh, 84–94.

Cope, C. L. (1964). Measurement of aldosterone secretion rates. In E. E. Baulieu and P. Robel, (eds), *Aldosterone, a symposium.* Blackwell, Oxford. p. 73.

*De Pierre, J. W. and M. L. Karnovsky (1973). Plasma membranes of mammalian cells. A review of methods for their characterization and isolation. *J. Cell Biol.,* 56, 275–303.

*Diczfalusy, E. (1969). In *"The Foeto-Placental Unit".* A. Pecile and C. Finzi (Eds). Proceedings of an International Symposium, Milan, September 1968. *Excerpta Medica International Congress Series No. 183,* pp. 65–109.

*Diczfalusy, E. (Ed.) (1971). In vitro methods in Reproductive Cell Biology (Karolinska Symposium on Research Methods in Reproductive Endocrinology). Supplement No. 153. *Acta Endocrinologica.*

*Dorfman, R. I. (Ed.) (1975). Steroid Hormones. In S. A. Berson and R. S. Yalow

(General Eds), *Methods in Investigative and Diagnostic Endocrinology*, Vol. 3, North-Holland Publ. Co., Amsterdam and New York.

Douglas, W. W., and R. P. Rubin (1961). The role of calcium in the secretory response of the adrenal medulla to acetylcholine. *J. Physiol. (Lond.)*, **159**, 40—57.

*Eik-Nes, K. B. (1971). Production and secretion of testicular steroids. *Recent Progress in Horm. Res.*, **27**, 517—535.

*Griffiths, K., and E. H. D. Cameron (1970). Steroid Biosynthetic Pathways in the Human Adrenal. In M. H. Briggs (Ed.), *Advances in Steroid Biochemistry and Pharmacology*, Vol. 2. Academic Press, London and New York. pp. 223—265.

Grunbaum, B. W., F. R. Geary and D. Glick (1956). Studies in histochemistry XLIII. The design and use of improved apparatus for the preparation and freeze-drying of fresh-frozen sections of tissue. *J. Histochem. Cytochem.*, **4**, 555.

Halkerston, I. D. K. (1968). Heterogeneity of the response of adrenal cortex tissue slices to adrenocorticotrophin. In K. W. McKerns, (ed.), Functions of the Adrenal Cortex, Vol. 1. pp. 399—461. Appleton-Century-Crofts, New York.

Haning, R., S. A. S. Tait and J. F. Tait (1970). In vitro effects of ACTH, angiotensins, serotonin and potassium on steroid output and conversion of corticosterone to aldosterone by isolated adrenal cells. *Endocrinology*, **87**, 1147—1167.

*Jenkins, J. S. (1968). *An Introduction to Biochemical Aspects of the Adrenal Cortex*. Edward Arnold Limited, London.

Kloppenborg, P. W. C., D. P. Island, G. W. Liddle, A. M. Michelakis and W. E. Nicholson (1968). A method of preparing adrenal cell suspensions and its applicability to the *in vitro* study of adrenal metabolism. *Endocrinology*, **82**, 1053—1058.

Lerner, U., and E. Diczfalusy (1968). A new method for the *in vitro* perfusion of the human foeto-placental unit. In A. Pecile and G. B. Carruthers, (Eds), *Abstracts, International Symposium on Foeto-placental Unit, Milan, 1968*, Excerpta Medica, Amsterdam. International Congress Series No. 170, p. 19.

*Lieberman, S., and E. Gurpide (1966). Isotopic Dilution Methods for the Estimation of Rates of Secretion of the Steroid Hormones. In G. Pincus, T. Nakao and J. F. Tait, (Eds), *Steroid Dynamics*. Academic Press, New York. pp. 531—547.

*Loraine, J. A., and E. T. Bell (1971). *Hormone assays and their clinical applications*, 3rd ed. Livingstone Ltd, Edinburgh/London.

McCracken, J. A., and D. T. Baird (1969). In K. W. McKerns, (Ed.), *The Gonads*, Appleton-Century-Crofts, New York. Chap. 7, p. 175.

*McCracken, J. A., D. T. Baird and J. R. Goding (1971). Factors affecting the secretion of steroids from the transplanted ovary in the sheep. *Recent Progress in Horm. Res.*, **27**, 537—582.

Moyle, W. R., and J. Ramachandran (1973). Effect of LH on steroidogenesis and cyclic AMP accumulation in rat Leydig cell preparations and mouse tumour Leydig cells. *Endocrinology*, **93**, 127—134.

O'Malley, B. W., and J. G. Hardman (Eds) (1974). Hormones and Cyclic Nucleotides. *Methods in Enzymology*, Vol. 39. Academic Press, New York.

Orti, E., R. K. Barker, J. T. Lanman and N. Brasch (1965). Simple method for *in vitro* metabolic studies with continuous flow incubation. *J. Lab. Med.*, **66**, 973—979.

Richardson, M. C., and D. Schulster (1972). Corticosteroidogenesis in isolated adrenal cells: Effect of adrenocorticotrophic hormone, adenosine 3', 5'-monophospate and [1-24]adrenocorticotrophic hormone diazotized to polyacrylamide. *J. Endocrinol.*, 55, 127—139.

Saffran, M., P. Ford, E. K. Mathews, M. Kraml and L. Garbaczewska (1967). An automated method for following the production of corticosteroids by adrenal tissue *in vitro*. *Can. J. Biochem.*, 45, 1901—1907.

Saffran, M., E. K. Mathews and F. Pearlmutter (1971). Analysis of the response to ACTH by rat adrenal in a flowing system. *Recent Progress in Horm. Res.*, 27, 607—630.

Sayers, G., R. L. Swallows and N. D. Giordano (1971). An improved technique for the preparation of isolated rat adrenal cells: a sensitive accurate and specific method for the assay of ACTH. *Endocrinology*, 88, 1063—1068.

Sayers, G., R. J. Beall, S. Seelig and K. Cummins (1973). Assay of ACTH: isolated adrenal cortex cells. In A. Brodish and E. S. Redgate, (Eds), *Brain-pituitary-adrenal interrelationships* Karger, Basel. pp. 16—35.

Schulster, D. (1973). Regulation of steroidogenesis by ACTH in a superfusion system for isolated adrenal cells. *Endocrinology*, 93, 700—704.

*Tait, J. F. (1963). Review: The use of isotopic steroids for the measurement of production rates *in vitro*. *J. Clin. Endocr. Metab.*, 23, 1285.

*Tait, S. A. S., and D. Schulster (1974). Superfusion techniques for assessment of steroid hormone production in endocrine tissue and isolated cells (adrenal). In B. W. O'Malley and J. G. Hardman, (Eds), *Methods in Enzymology: Hormones and cyclic nucleotides*, Vol. 89, part D. Academic Press, New York.

Tait, S. A. S., J. F. Tait, M. Okamoto and C. Flood (1967). Production of steroids by *in vitro* superfusion of endocrine tissue. I. Apparatus and a suitable analytical method for adrenal steroid output. *Endocrinology*, 81, 1213—1225.

Tait, J. F., S. A. S. Tait, R. P. Gould and S. R. Mee (1974). The properties of adrenal zona glomerulosa cells after purification by gravitational sedimentation. *Proc. Royal Soc. Lond.*, 185, 375—407.

Van Doorn, L. G., H. W. A. de Bruijn, H. Galjaard and H. J. van der Molen (1974). Intercellular transport of steroids in the infused rabbit testis. *Biology of Reprod.*, 10, 47—53.

*Wright, R. D., J. R. Blair-West and J. P. Coghlan (1972). The structure and function of adrenal autotransplants. *Aust. J. Exp. Biol. Med. Sci.*, 50, 873—892.

CHAPTER 4

Biosynthesis of steroid hormones

I. INTRODUCTION

Each of the steroid secreting endocrine organs can produce almost any of the steroid hormones. The testis secretes not only androgens but also estrogens and corticosteroids, while the ovary manufactures not only progesterone and estrogens but androgens as well. The adrenal cortex secretes predominantly adrenocortical steroids but it is also capable of yielding progesterone, androgens and estrogens. The pathways in Figure 4.1 apply equally to the testis, ovary and adrenal. The placenta is an incomplete organ incapable of *de novo* steroid synthesis, but nevertheless has the capacity to produce androgens in addition to progesterone and estrogens. As with all generalizations there are exceptions and of course some steroids are secreted solely by highly specialized tissues. As an example, aldosterone, the hormone responsible for sodium retention, is synthesized by the cells in the outer layer of the adrenal cortex, the zona glomerulosa, and there has been no report to date on the production of aldosterone by any tissue other than this. Specific hormones such as this are however metabolic end-products and it would appear that the specificity of their production lies in only a few unique enzymic conversions from systemically available or locally synthesized precursors.

Secretion of steroids not usually associated with a particular gland — such as androgens from the adrenal or ovary — may normally not be clinically apparent. However, there are numerous disease conditions, such as that existing in the polycystic ovary or the adrenogenital syndrome, where aberrations from the common biosynthetic routes may give rise to relatively large amounts of these atypical steroids.

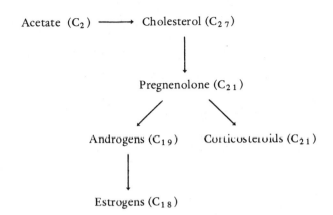

Figure 4.1   Outline   for   the   biosynthesis   of   the steroid hormones.

During mammalian embryonic development, the adrenal cortex and the gonads arise from adjacent regions of the uro-genital ridge. In the normal adult each of these endocrine organs secretes distinctive patterns of steroid hormones, but how they assume differing biosynthetic abilities having had a more or less common origin is still a matter for speculation. Although present knowledge points to differences of detail for the biosynthesis of steroids in the various endocrine glands, the overall picture is of a single, coherent biogenetic pathway. The subcellular localization of the enzymes and the individual enzymes themselves, appear to be similar for all steroid-forming endocrine glands. For this reason the biosynthesis of steroids is described by reference to endocrine organs in general and their production by individual tissues considered only where the differences merit emphasis.

The bare essentials of the biosynthesis of the biologically important steroid hormones can be summarized as shown in Figure 4.1. Each of these steps will now be considered individually.

II. ACETATE $(C_2) \rightarrow$ CHOLESTEROL (C_{27})

The details of this pathway have been reviewed by Clayton (1965) and this aspect of the subject has been adequately covered by several general biochemistry textbooks. For this reason only an outline of the current ideas will be given here. Most of the work has been done using enzyme extracts from both liver and yeast and in 1964 Block and Lynen were independently awarded a Nobel prize for their studies in this field. Other workers who have provided notable contributions to our understanding in this area are Cornforth and Popjack.

It is clear that cholesterol with 27 carbon atoms is a relatively complex molecule and obviously its synthesis from the simple acetate molecule involves many intricate enzymic steps.

Among the first important studies was the demonstration that squalene and

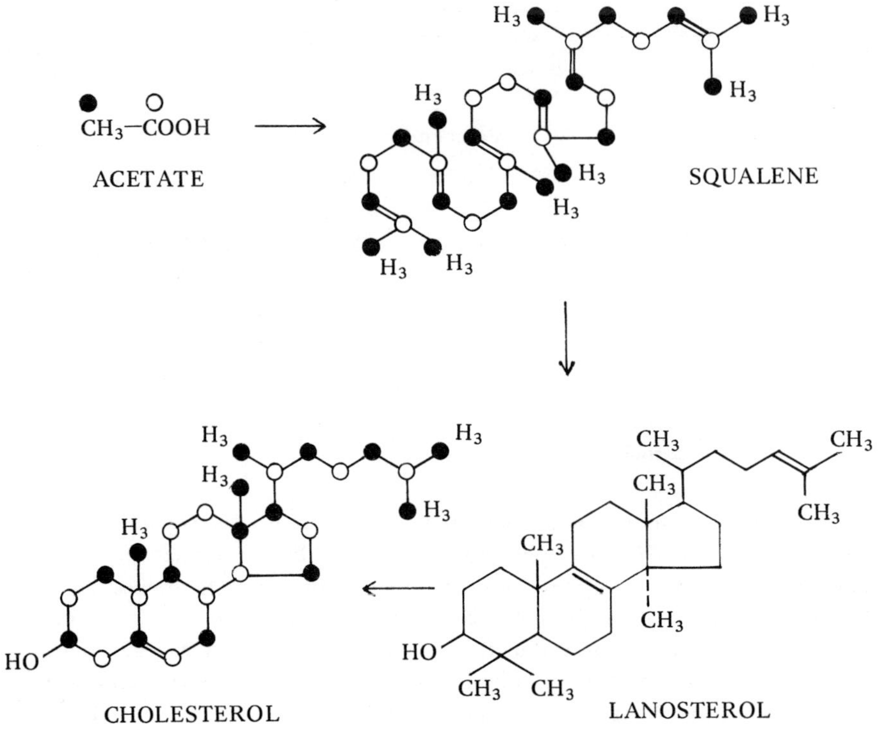

Figure 4.2 Outline for the biosynthesis of cholesterol.

lanosterol were derived from acetate and were precursors of cholesterol both *in vivo* and *in vitro* in the rat. Following the use of radioactive acetate, the biosynthesis of radioactive squalene and cholesterol was demonstrated. Furthermore the total degradation of these compounds, after isolation and purification, delineated the origin of each C atom from either the methyl or carbonyl C atom of the labelled acetate molecule. The experimental results obtained both by Bloch and by Cornforth and Popjack showed the pattern of labelling to be more complex than just a straightforward regular arrangement. Since these results were in total agreement with the postulated arrangement, they provided convincing evidence for the intermediary role of squalene and the percursor role of acetate.

The distribution of radioactivity in squalene and cholesterol after incubating rat liver in the presence of acetate labelled with ^{14}C, either in the methyl (●) or the carbonyl (○) group is shown in Figure 4.2. Moreover the involvement of lanosterol as an intermediate on the pathway from squalene to cholesterol has been established both by biosynthesis of lanosterol from labelled acetate and by its conversion into cholesterol both *in vitro*, using rat liver, and *in vivo*.

The detailed biosynthesis of squalene has now been elucidated and shown to involve mevalonic acid and isopentenyl pyrophosphate according to the scheme shown in Figure 4.3. The initial enzyme reaction involves acetyl-coenzyme A as

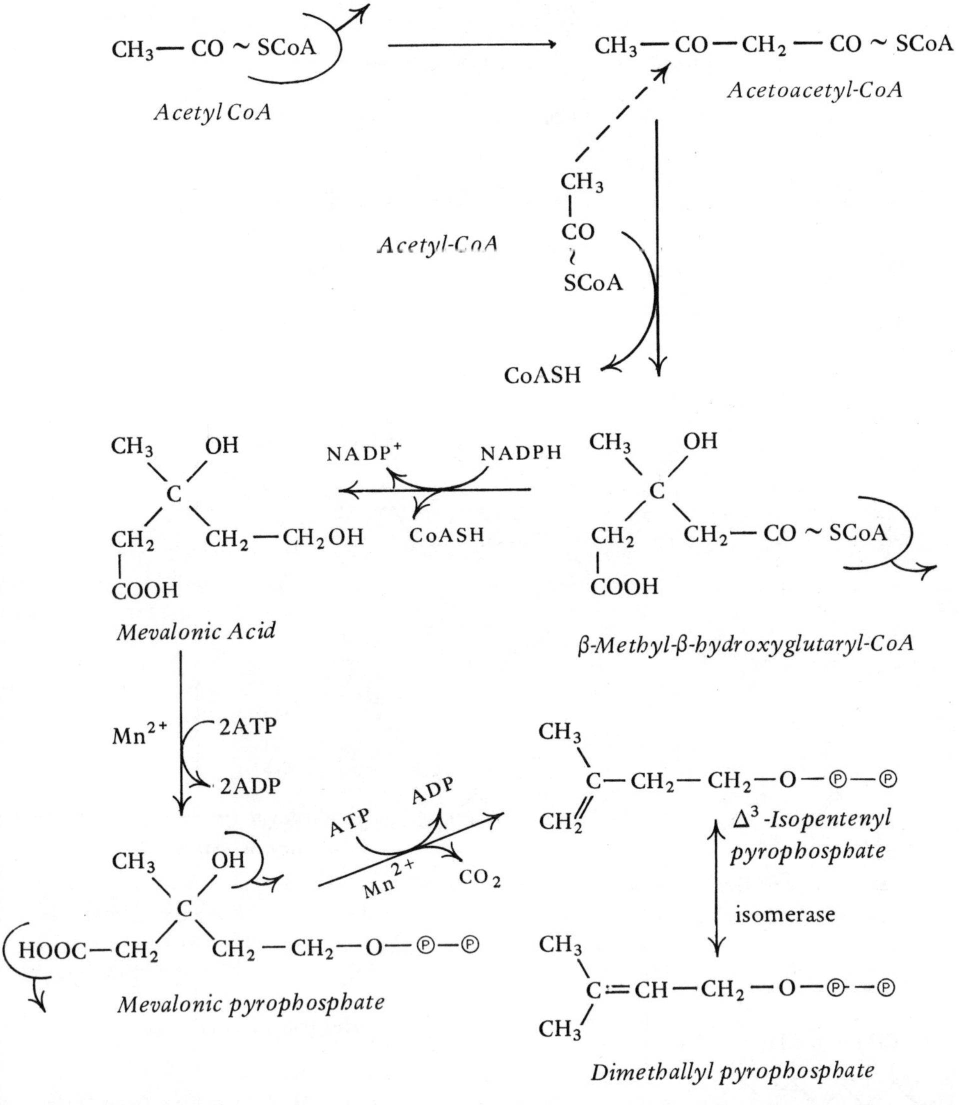

Figure 4.3 Simplified scheme for the biosynthesis of mevalonate and other precursors of cholesterol.

substrate which may be readily generated by glycolysis or by the breakdown of fatty acids or proteins.

β-Methyl-β-hydroxyglutaryl-CoA is produced first and this is reduced by NADPH to mevalonate — a compound that appears to function solely as an intermediate in steroid and terpenoid biosynthesis. Elimination of CO_2 and the elements of water is effected following the ulitization of ATP in an activation step to form mevalonic pyrophosphate. The products of this first sequence of enzymic conversions are Δ^3-isopentenyl pyrophosphate and dimethallyl pyrophosphate which are

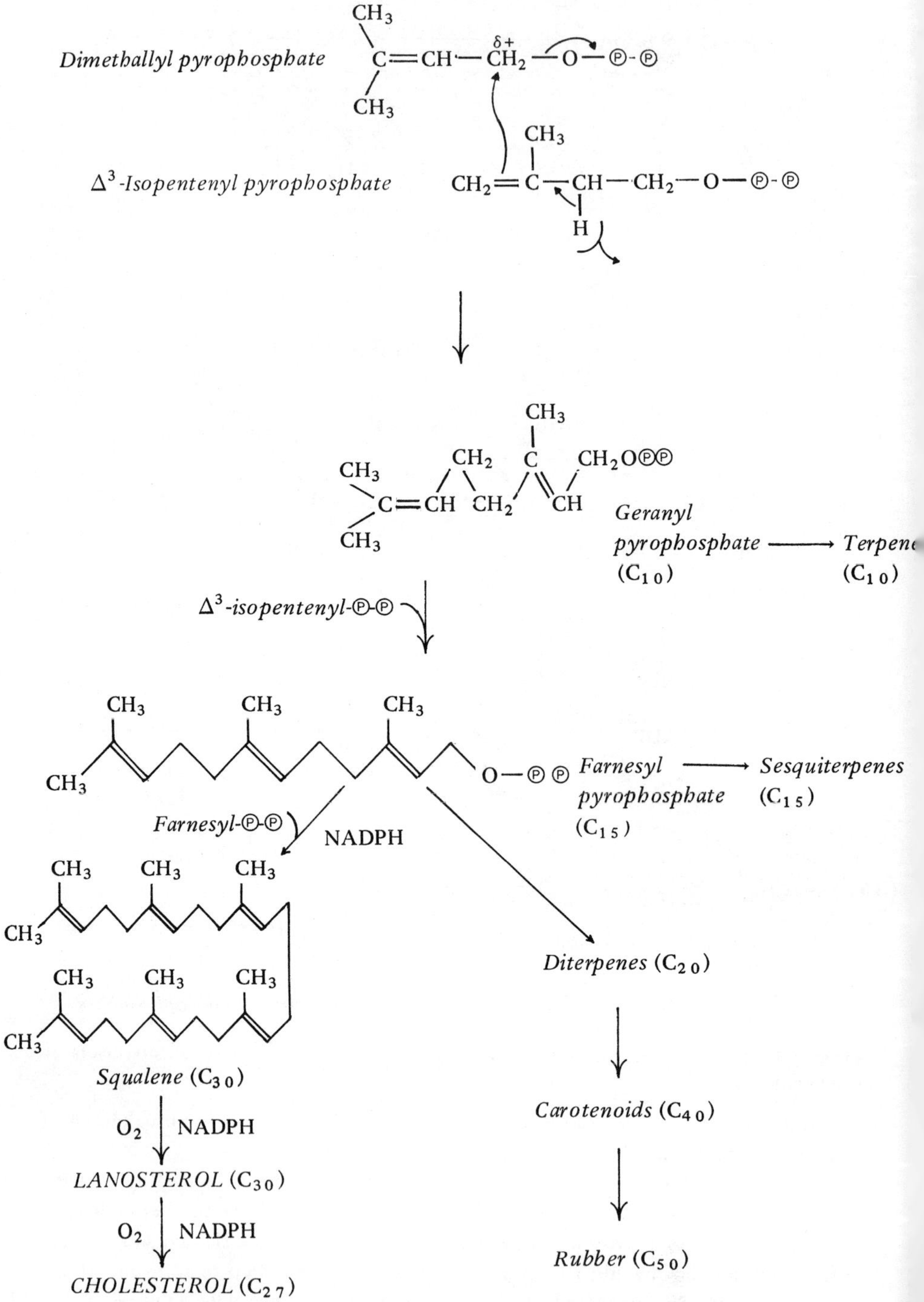

Figure 4.4 Biosynthesis of cholesterol and the terpenes from isoprenoid precursors.

interconvertible by the action of an isomerase. No randomization of the methyl groups occurs during this isomerization. These two isomers then become the basic building blocks for the synthesis of long chain unsaturated hydrocarbons. Head-to-tail enzymic condensations occur to form molecules containing 10, 15, 20, 30, etc. C atoms, as shown in Figure 4.4. The two C_5 isomers condense to form firstly geranyl pyrophosphate (C_{10}; a precursor of the monoterpenes) and subsequently farnesyl pyrophosphate, (C_{15}; a precursor of the sesquiterpenes). Each addition occurs at the terminal electrophilic C atom with the loss of the pyrophosphate residue and a hydrogen atom, as depicted in Figure 4.4. Two molecules of farnesyl pyrophosphate then condense to form the triterpene molecule, squalene.

The final steps in the biosynthesis involve the cyclization of squalene via an expoxide intermediate, for which molecular oxygen is utilized. This cyclization of a long chain unsaturated hydrocarbon molecule into the characteristic steroid structure of four adjoining rings is really quite an extraordinary process and cannot at present be adequately explained. It is presumed that the enzyme responsible, squalene cyclohydroxylase, imposes a specific type of conformation on the squalene, thereby facilitating the electron transfers necessary for the cyclization to lanosterol, a C_{30} steroid. During the further conversion of lanosterol, the two methyl groups at C-4 and the α-methyl group at C-14 are lost, yielding ultimately the C_{27} steroid cholesterol. This conversion also involves a shift in the ring double-bond from C-8 to C-5, and the saturation of the double bond in the side-chain at C-24 (see Figure 4.2). Various intermediates have been implicated in this process; the more important appear to be zymosterol ($8,24$-(5α)-cholestadien-3β-ol) and then desmosterol ($5,24$-cholestadien-3β-ol). Further details of these biosynthetic pathways are given in Mahler and Cordes (1971).

III. CHOLESTEROL (C_{27}) → PREGNENOLONE (C_{21})

There is considerable evidence to suggest that the steroidogenic pituitary hormones such as ACTH and LH exert their controlling influence by directly affecting the conversion of cholesterol to pregnenolone (3β-hydroxy-5-pregnen-20-one) — see Chapters 11, 12 and 13. Consequently, many workers regard this conversion as a control point for steroid biosynthesis, and since the investigation of a rate-limiting step is of obvious importance to the further understanding of hormonal control mechanisms, considerable interest has been directed towards elucidating the details of this conversion. The key role of pregnenolone as a precursor for the synthesis of other steroid hormones may be observed by reference to Figure 4.5.

The details of pregnenolone synthesis from cholesterol are shown in Figure 4.6 and it is currently believed to involve firstly oxidation of cholesterol to an enzyme bound dihydroxy-derivative of cholesterol, via the 22R-hydroxy-derivative.

The normal products isolated after cholesterol conversion by this cleavage system — sometimes referred to as a $20\alpha,22$-C_{27}-*desmolase* or *lyase* — are

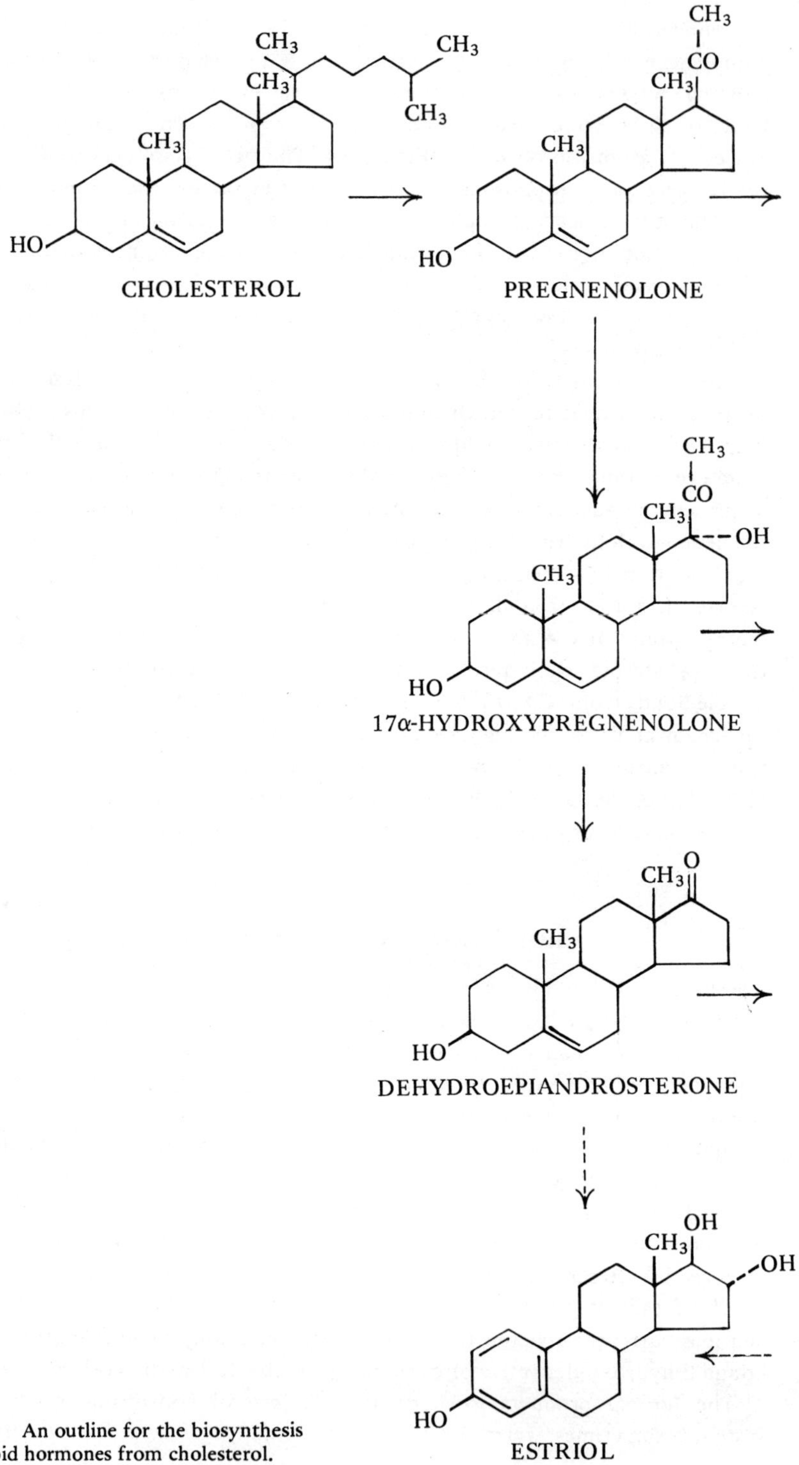

Figure 4.5 An outline for the biosynthesis of the steroid hormones from cholesterol.

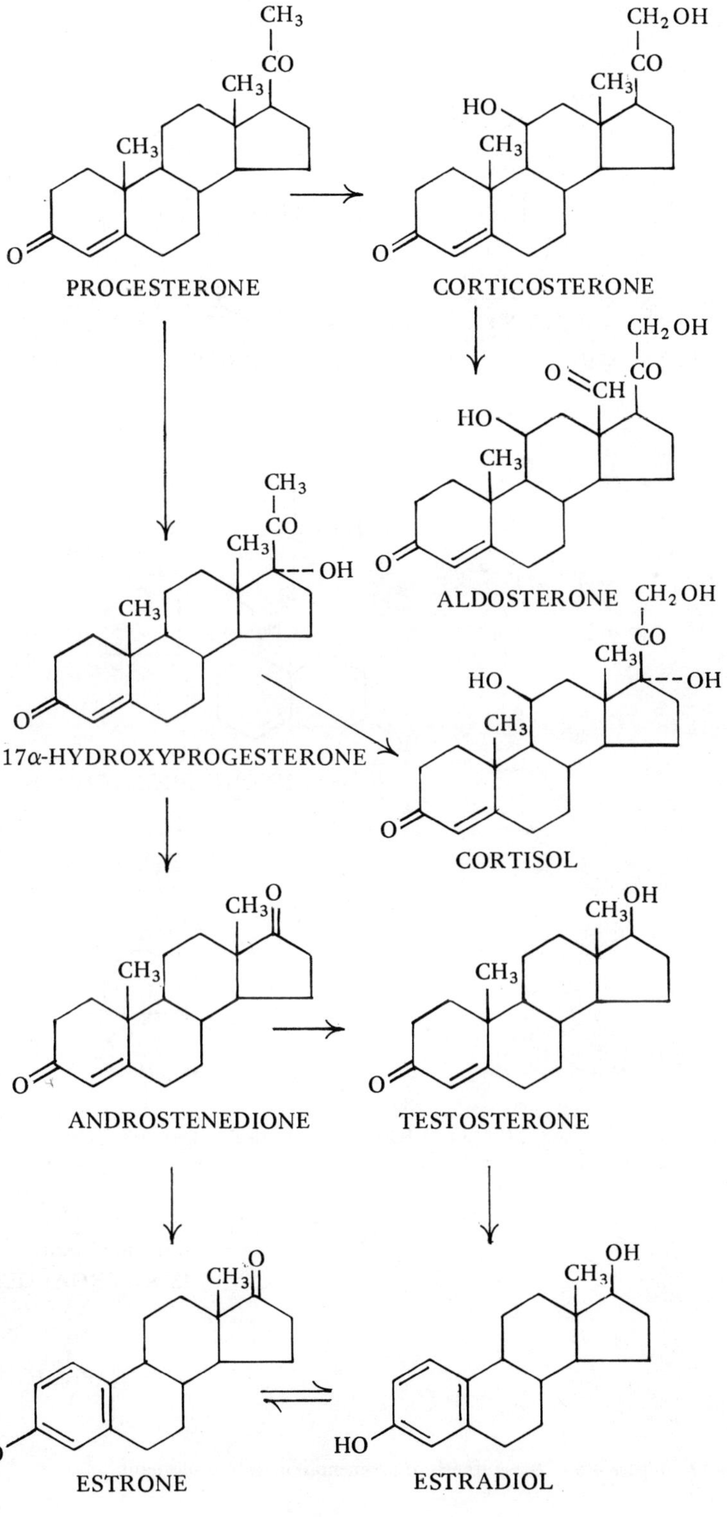
CH3
CO
CH3
CH3
O
PROGESTERONE
CH2OH
CO
CH3
HO
CH3
O
CORTICOSTERONE
CH2OH
O
CH
CO
HO
CH3
O
ALDOSTERONE
CH3
CO
CH3
OH
CH3
O
17α-HYDROXYPROGESTERONE
CH2OH
CO
CH3
HO
OH
CH3
O
CORTISOL
CH3
O
CH3
O
ANDROSTENEDIONE
CH3
OH
CH3
O
TESTOSTERONE
CH3
O
HO
ESTRONE
OH
CH3
HO
ESTRADIOL

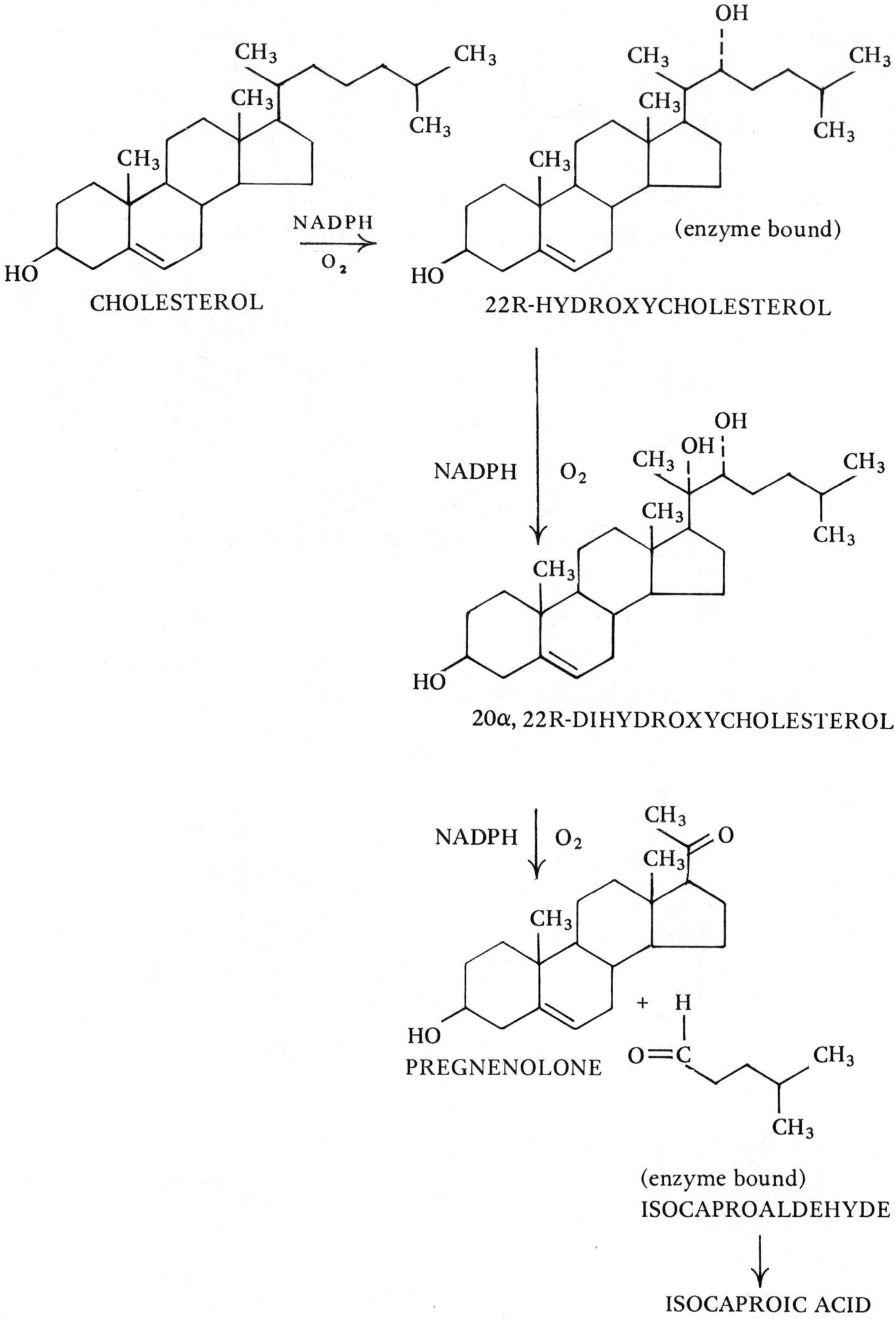

Figure 4.6 Biosynthesis of pregnenolone from cholesterol.

pregnenolone and isocaproic acid. The other intermediates have been isolated as radioactive products when [^{14}C]cholesterol is used as a substrate. Moreover, when these intermediates are radioactively labelled and used as precursors, they can also be shown to act as substrates for the desmolase system. However, only very minute quantities of these intermediates are detectable in the reaction mixture unless large amounts of trapping agents, such as sterols, or inhibitors, such as pregnenolone or progesterone, are added. It is believed that the desmolase (or cleavage enzyme) exists in the cell as a highly organized complex, with the basic rate-limiting step being the initial oxygenation of cholesterol to 22R-hydroxycholesterol. It is important to note that each of the enzymic steps involved in the conversion of cholesterol to pregnenolone has a requirement for oxygen and reduced NADP$^+$ as a cofactor. Adequate oxygenation and availability of NADPH must therefore play an important role in this, the suggested control point of steroid biosynthesis. In this context the characteristic capillary, vascular system of steroidogenic glands such as the adrenal cortex (confer Chapter 6) would appear to be important in providing an adequate supply of oxygenated blood directly to each cell in the tissue.

The C-17 side-chain of cholesterol was originally reported to be removed as isocaproic acid, but it has now been shown that isocaproaldehyde is initially formed and that this is subsequently oxidized. Cell-free extracts have been used, with non-labelled isocaproaldehyde as a trapping agent, to demonstrate this point, as well as purified extracts which have lost the ability to oxidize the aldehyde to the acid. Again the inability to detect the aldehyde in the absence of the trapping agent suggests that this lipophilic aldehyde remains bound to the desmolase complex and is oxidized in this bound form to the acid.

The exact details of this crucial step in steroid biosynthesis are still far from clear, although the recent work of Burstein and Gut (1973) has provided elaborate kinetic analyses supporting the scheme shown in Figure 4.6. These workers have demonstrated that this sequence occurs at a considerably higher rate than alternative sequences involving other hydroxylated intermediates. Nevertheless it is possible that the true intermediates in the biosynthesis of pregnenolone from cholesterol are not isolatable, side-chain hydroxylated derivatives at all, but rather that they are transient, reactive species of unknown structures (see Hochberg et al., 1973). Consistent with this concept is the suggestion (Simpson and Boyd, 1967) that cholesterol and oxygen complex with the desmolase enzyme and that the side-chain is then cleaved by an unspecified concerted process. Our precise understanding of this aspect of steroidogenesis must await future experimentation.

IV. PREGNENOLONE (C_{21}) → PROGESTERONE AND CORTICOSTEROIDS (C_{21})

There are a large number of different C_{21} steroids found in biological systems, and their biosynthesis is of a complex nature. Nevertheless several features stand out, from which a simplified scheme may be constructed. Pregnenolone appears to be the precursor of all the other C_{21} steroids, and from pregnenolone the biosynthetic route follows two alternative pathways depending upon the product. The route

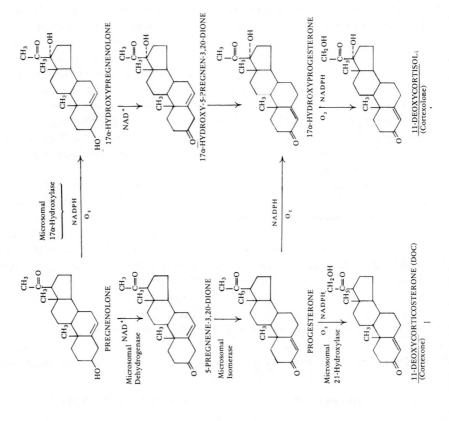

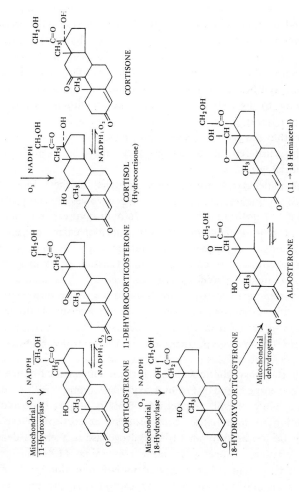

Figure 4.7 The major biosynthetic pathways for the mineralo- and glucocorticoids in the human.

passes either via progesterone and 11-deoxycorticosterone to corticosterone and ultimately to aldosterone, or via 17α-hydroxyprogesterone and 11-deoxycortisol to yield cortisol (see Figure 4.7). While the ovary and the foeto-placental unit are the major sites for the synthesis of progesterone, which is secreted as such, the endocrine gland responsible for the production of the corticosteroids under normal circumstances is the adrenal cortex.

After homogenization and fractionation of adrenal tissue, some of the enzymes involved in corticosteroidogenesis have been located within the mitochondria, while others have been found in the microsomal or cytoplasmic fraction. The disposition of the various enzymes involved suggests that the complete biosynthesis of these corticoids involves the transport of certain of the intermediates in the scheme, across the mitochondrial membrane as shown in Figure 4.8. From this scheme it may be seen that pregnenolone synthesized within the mitochondria must first cross the mitochondrial membrane to the enzymes situated extramitochondrially, before its further metabolism can occur. Conversely both 11-deoxycortisol and 11-deoxycorticosterone are synthesized by cytoplasmic enzymes, and must penetrate the membrane before the final corticosteroid products may be formed by the appropriate mitochondrial enzymes.

The details of the molecular transformations involved in these biosynthetic pathways are outlined in Figure 4.7. An initial step involves hydroxylation of pregnenolone at the 17-position to form 17α-hydroxypregnenolone. This 17α-hydroxylase has a requirement for NADPH and molecular oxygen. Both pregnenolene and 17α-hydroxypregnenolone, subsequently follow a similar sequence of enzymic reactions. The conversion of pregnenolone to progesterone involves firstly an NAD$^+$-linked dehydrogenase followed by an isomerase. It was previously believed that these two steps were brought about by one enzyme, it being suggested that the isomerization occurred spontaneously. However, the isomerase has now been separated from the dehydrogenase. This conversion, as well as the analogous one of 17α-hydroxypregnenolone to 17α-hydroxyprogesterone, is irreversible.

The next enzyme in the biosynthetic sequence is the microsomal 21-hydroxylase that converts progesterone and 17α-hydroxyprogesterone to 11-deoxy-corticosterone and 11-deoxycortisol, respectively. This is followed by hydroxylation at the 11-position to form either corticosterone or cortisol. These latter compounds may then be oxidized by an 11β-dehydrogenase to yield 11-dehydro-corticosterone and cortisone respectively, both containing 11-ketone groups. Aldosterone, noted for its potent enhancement of sodium retention by the kidney (Chapter 15), contains an aldehyde function at position C-18, which is able to undergo acetal formation with the 11β-hydroxyl group. The pathway of aldo-sterone biosynthesis is not yet clearly defined. The essential step is 18-hydroxyl-ation, and progesterone, 11-deoxycorticosterone and corticosterone can all be hydroxylated in this position, thereby serving as potential precursors for aldo-sterone. Both corticosterone and 18-hydroxycorticosterone have been suggested as the immediate precursors of aldosterone, while some studies have shown that progesterone may be an even more significant intermediate. However, despite some

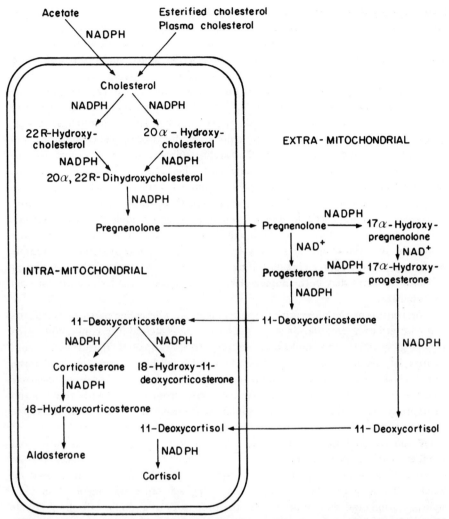

Figure 4.8 Biosynthesis of corticosteroids. The intracellular locations of enzymes for steroid conversions in the adrenal. (For further details see Simpson, E. R., and J. I. Mason (1976). Reprinted with permission from Schulster (1974), in M. H. Briggs and G. A. Christie (Eds) *Adv. Steroid Bioch. Pharm.*, **4**, 233–295. Copyright Academic Press Inc. (London) Ltd.)

controversy, recent reports support the scheme outlined in Figure 4.7, whereby aldosterone is formed via 18-hydroxycorticosterone by a mitochondrial dehydrogenase system (Coghlan and Blair-West, 1967). Unlike the other corticosteroids, aldosterone biosynthesis is restricted exclusively to the zona glomerulosa cells of the adrenal cortex. Studies on the secretion and metabolism of 18-hydroxy-11-deoxycorticosterone (the most abundant mineralocorticoid secreted by the adrenal cortex of the rat) have been reviewed (Melby *et al.*, 1972) and this steroid may also act as a precursor of aldosterone (Grekin *et al.*, 1973).

The biosynthetic scheme as outlined in Figure 4.7 relates to the sequence of events predominating in man. However, this is not a rigid scheme and in different species others may pertain. For example, it is well established that progesterone may be hydroxylated in a variety of different positions, although there appear to be limitations on the sequence of the hydroxylation steps, such as a restriction preventing 17α-hydroxylation from following 21-hydroxylation. There are therefore alternative sequences possible for the hydroxylations at C-17, C-21 and C-11 other than those shown in Figure 4.7. Moreover, hydroxylation can precede reduction by the NAD-linked dehydrogenase since it has been established that 21-hydroxypregnenolone can act as a precursor for 11-deoxycorticosterone and corticosterone, and similarly 17α,21-dihydroxypregnenolone can give rise to 11-deoxycortisol. Nevertheless the simplified scheme presented accounts for the quantitatively most significant biosynthetic routes for the principal corticosteroids produced by the adrenal cortex. In the human these corticosteroids are cortisol, cortisone, 11-deoxycortisol, 11-deoxycorticosterone, 11-dehydrocorticosterone, corticosterone and aldosterone. Although these steroids are also produced by other mammals, the relative quantities vary from species to species, the rat for example producing predominantly corticosterone but virtually no cortisol, whereas current evidence indicates that in the human gland the secretion of the latter corticosteroid predominates.

One feature of the biosynthetic route (Figure 4.7) deserving particular emphasis is the variety of hydroxylation steps involved in these steroid interconversions, each involving NADPH and molecular oxygen. It now appears that these various hydroxylations at positions 17-, 21-, 11- and 18-, all have a common mechanism and involve a cytochrome system and scheme known as *reversed electron transport*. Our knowledge of this system stems from studies with the 17- and 21-hydroxylases of the adrenal microsomal fraction and the 11- and 18-hydroxylase systems of the adrenal mitochondria. It was firstly shown that in the presence of $^{18}O_2$ and tritiated steroid substrates, the ^{18}O atom appears in both the steroid product and in the water molecules, and that the oxygen replaces tritium stereospecifically at the particular C atom attacked. Then it was discovered by Estabrook that a carbon monoxide combining substance was involved in C-21 hydroxylation, and shortly afterwards the properties of a similar carbon monoxide combining substance obtained from a liver microsomal fraction were examined by Omura and Sato who named this substance *cytochrome P-450*, because it showed a strong absorption band at 450 nm when combined with carbon monoxide (Figure 4.9). The role of cytochrome P-450 in the biosynthesis of adrenocorticoids and the purification of this cytochrome has been surveyed (Hall, 1973; Simpson and Mason, 1975).

The carbon monoxide difference spectra and other characteristics of the P-450 cytochrome are the same, whether it is obtained from steroid degrading tissues such as the kidney or liver, or from steroid synthesizing tissues such as the adrenal cortex. It is therefore believed that this cytochrome is widely distributed in all tissues rich in steroid hydroxylases. Moreover, the P-450 cytochrome system is of general importance in the body and functions to hydroxylate a large number of molecules (e.g. many different drugs) prior to their elimination from the body. The steroid

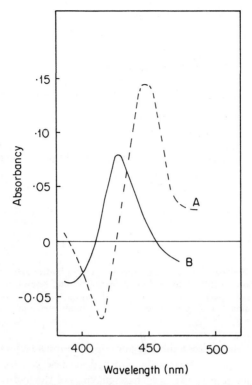

Figure 4.9 Difference spectra of carbon monoxide treated mitochondria (A) and reference mitochondria (B). The difference spectrum changes after bubbling carbon monoxide through the solution in the sample cuvette, from that with a maximum at 430 nm to that with a maximum at 450 nm.

hydroxylase system has the characteristics of a mixed function oxidase since two substrates — NADPH and the steroid — are oxidized. The system has been extensively studied using adrenal mitochondria, and the components of this mixed function oxidase have been shown to include:

a) a flavoprotein dehydrogenase (Fp) specific for NADPH, (also known as adrenodoxin reductase).

b) a protein known as adrenodoxin, containing non-haem iron (NHFe-P), also called iron—sulphur protein (ISP).

c) a small submitochondrial particle containing the P-450 cytochrome. Electron transport in adrenal mitochondria during steroid hydroxylation is believed to follow the pathway:

$$NADPH \longrightarrow F_p \longrightarrow NHFe\text{-}P \longrightarrow \text{Cytochrome} \xrightarrow{2H^+} \begin{array}{cc} \text{H-Steroid} & \text{HO-Steroid} \\ & \\ O_2 & H_2O \end{array}$$

P-450

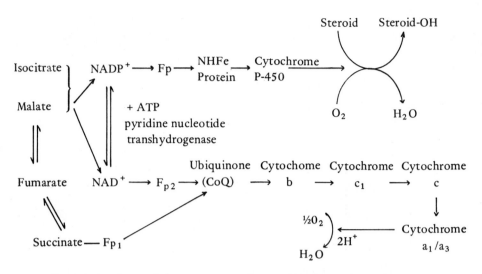

Figure 4.10 Reversed electron transport for steroid hydroxylation. The mixed function oxidase (P-450 chain) is linked to the normal respiratory chain via a transhydrogenase. NAD^+: nicotinamide adenine dinucleotide. $NADP^+$: nicotinamide adenine dinucleotide phosphate. Fp: flavoprotein. NHFe protein: non-haem iron protein.

It has also been shown that the enzymes of the normal respiratory chain and an energy-controlled pyridine nucleotide transhydrogenase can function together in the transport of electrons to the oxygenase enzymes of the hydroxylating pathway. The mixed function oxidase responsible for steroid hydroxylation is believed to be linked to the normal respiratory chain as shown in Figure 4.10.

The citric acid cycle intermediates, such as isocitrate, malate or succinate can function as hydrogen donors for the transport of electrons down the normal respiratory chain via the flavoproteins Fp_1 or Fp_2 and the usual cytochrome system, leading ultimately to the reduction of molecular oxygen. It has been known since 1954 that these same citric acid cycle intermediates can readily support mitochondrial hydroxylation reactions, but not until recently has the mechanism for this been described. It is thought to involve firstly a reversal of electron transport through the energy requiring pyridine nucleotide transhydrogenase to produce NADPH. The flavoprotein Fp (also called adrenodoxin reductase) functions as an NADPH reductase and electrons are then passed on through the non-haem iron protein (NHFe-P; adrenodoxin) to the cytochrome P-450, and finally allows the oxidase to effect the concomitant hydroxylation of the steroid molecule and the reduction of oxygen to water.

Although the precise details of the actual hydroxylation mechanism are not yet fully known, it is possible to summarize the reaction of cytochrome P-450 with the steroid intermediates as shown in Figure 4.11. This scheme indicates that oxidation of reduced P-450 is largely dependent upon the presence of steroid substrate which conforms with recent experimental findings.

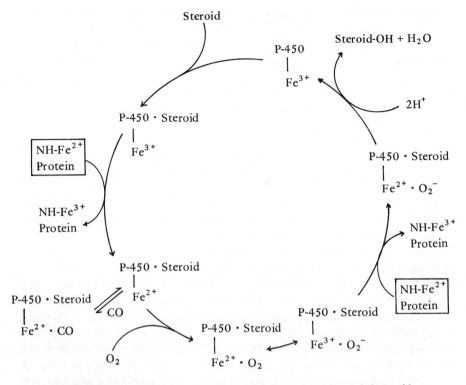

Figure 4.11 Cytochrome P-450 oxygenase cycle and coupled steroid hydroxylation. Two molecules of non-haem iron protein (NH—Fe^{2+} protein) are oxidized during each steroid hydroxylation step.

V. BIOSYNTHESIS OF C$_{19}$ STEROIDS : ANDROGENS (C$_{21}$ → C$_{19}$)

Early studies on the biosynthesis of androgens established that acetate can act as a precursor for a variety of C$_{19}$ steroids. Following *in vivo* administration of radioactive compounds such as acetate, cholesterol and progesterone, several C$_{19}$ steroids have been isolated in the urine including dehydroepiandrosterone and androsterone. Perfusion of the isolated intact gland has proved a valuable technique in studying many aspects of steroid biochemistry and using for example perfused canine, equine and human testis, conversion of acetate to testosterone and 4-androstene-3,17-dione has been shown. Moreover, numerous reports over the past twenty years have documented the conversion of progesterone to 17α-hydroxy-progesterone and thence to androstenedione by both testicular and ovarian tissue. This observation has been extended to adrenal tissue and an accepted pathway of androgen elaboration is as follows:

$$\text{progesterone} \rightarrow \begin{array}{c}\text{17α-hydroxy-}\\\text{progesterone}\end{array} \rightarrow \begin{array}{c}\text{4-androstene-}\\\text{3,17-dione}\end{array} \rightleftharpoons \text{testosterone}$$

Similar studies to those described above have established that pregnenolone and 17α-hydroxypregnenolone can also act as precursors for the C_{19} steroids. Dehydroepiandrosterone has been isolated following the *in vivo* administration of both pregnenolone and 17α-hydroxypregnenolone. Furthermore incubations of a variety of homogenized endocrine tissues with these radioactively labelled C_{21} steroids have resulted in the isolation of radioactive dehydroepiandrosterone, testosterone and androstenedione. It is clear that another important pathway for androgen biosynthesis is:

$$\text{pregnenolone} \rightarrow \begin{array}{c} \text{17α-hydroxy-} \\ \text{pregnenolone} \end{array} \rightarrow \begin{array}{c} \text{dehydroepi-} \\ \text{androsterone} \end{array} \rightarrow \begin{array}{c} \text{4-androstene-} \\ \text{3,17-dione} \end{array} \rightleftharpoons \text{testosterone}$$

Altogether, six different routes for androgen biosynthesis have been postulated (Dorfman and Ungar, 1965), but many of these remain theoretical and unsubstantiated. It is however clear that in the testis, testosterone is made chiefly via the 4-ene-3-ketonic intermediates such as progesterone and 17α-hydroxyprogesterone, while the contribution of alternative pathways is minimal in the normal tissue. It has also been demonstrated that the enzymes involved in this former route — the 17α-hydroxylase, the 17α-hydroxyprogesterone side-chain cleavage system (or $C_{17} - C_{20}$ lyase) and the 17β-hydroxysteroid dehydrogenase activities — all reside in the testicular microsomal fraction and that NADPH is an essential cofactor for these enzymic conversions. In addition, both the 17α-hydroxylase and the $C_{17} - C_{20}$ lyase have a requirement for molecular oxygen. However, whereas the 17α-hydroxylase incorporates molecular oxygen into progesterone directly to form 17α-hydroxyprogesterone, in the case of the subsequent side-chain cleavage, although molecular oxygen is required it is not incorporated into either the immediate steroid product androstenedione, or the subsequent product testosterone. The details of this conversion have been studied by incubating testicular tissue with progesterone and 17α-hydroxyprogesterone under an $^{18}O_2$-enriched atmosphere, when it was established that the oxygen atoms at C-17 in both androstenedione and testosterone originate from the 17α-hydroxyl group of the precursor (Figure 4.12).

The detailed mechanism involved in splitting the C-20,21 side-chain from the 17α-hydroxylated C_{21} steroids to yield the C_{19} androgens still remains to be clarified. One postulate invokes hydration of the 20-ketone to form an intermediate containing two hydroxyl functions at the C-20 position. This unstable intermediate may then undergo side-chain scission by loss of a proton from one of these 20-hydroxyl groups and subsequent electronic rearrangement, to yield acetate and a 17-ketone.

The adrenal cortex is responsible for the production of 11-oxygenated androgens. Two routes are known for their synthesis. Corticosteroids such as cortisol and 21-deoxycortisol can undergo side-chain cleavage between C-17 and C-20, to yield 11β-hydroxyandrostenedione. This in turn can be oxidized to an 11-ketone (adrenosterone). In addition, C_{19} steroids such as androstenedione, testosterone

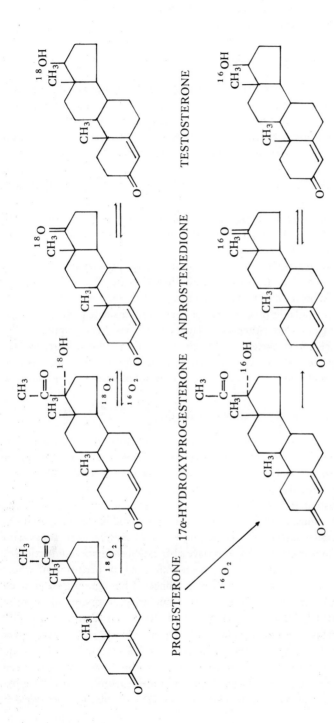

Figure 4.12 Origin of the oxygen function at C-17 in C_{19} steroids. Incubation of testicular tissue with progesterone under an atmosphere enriched with $^{18}O_2$ gives rise to 17α-hydroxyprogesterone labelled in the 17α-hydroxyl group. This precursor incubated in either $^{16}O_2$ or $^{18}O_2$ atmosphere yields C_{19} steroids labelled in the oxygen atom at the C-17 function. These experiments demonstrate that this oxygen derives from the C-17 side-chain of 17α-hydroxyprogesterone (cf. Nakano et al., 1967. Bioch. Biophys. Acta, **137**, 335).

and dehydroepiandrosterone, may themselves be hydroxylated at the 11-position, with the formation of a variety of 11-oxygenated C_{19} steroids.

VI. BIOSYNTHESIS OF C_{18} STEROIDS: ESTROGENS ($C_{19} \to C_{18}$)

The term estrogen describes all substances which bring about secondary female sex changes, characterized by estrus, vaginal cornification and uterine weight alterations. The classic biologically active estrogens in the human, estrone, estradiol and estriol are all C_{18} steroids with an aromatic A-ring. A great variety of chemical molecules exhibit an estrogenic character and the only reasonably constant feature of these molecules is the presence of an aromatic or phenolic ring structure. Even the synthetic estrogens such as hexestrol, methylstilbestrol and 17α-ethynylestradiol, which are effective by oral administration, contain phenolic residues. In recent years twenty or more different C_{18} steroids have been isolated from human urine and although these compounds have little or no biological activity they are nevertheless usually referred to as 'estrogens'.

The biosynthesis of estrogens involves a lengthy series of enzymic steps from acetate through cholesterol to C_{19} steroids and hence to the C_{18} estrogens. The details of the former steps have been described in the earlier sections of this chapter and ample evidence is available that this route constitutes a single pathway for the biosynthesis of estrogens. No other postulated route has been supported by experimental evidence. Nevertheless, although it has been shown that acetate, cholesterol, progesterone and C_{19} steroids can each give rise to estrogens, it is very difficult to prove beyond doubt that these compounds are obligatory intermediates.

A. Acetate, Cholesterol and C_{21} Steroids $\to$ Estrogens

Among the first experiments of relevance in this field were those of Heard and his coworkers in which the isolation of radioactive estrone from the urine of pregnant mares was accomplished after the injection of radioactive acetate. The *in vivo* biogenesis of estrone from acetate was thereby established.

Early work on testicular tissue both *in vitro*, using cell-free homogenates and testicular slices, and using 'in situ' perfusion techniques readily demonstrated the conversion of radioactive acetate to estrone and estradiol. Similar techniques with slices and cell-free homogenates of ovaries have also established the production of estrogens from acetate, and this has again been confirmed by perfusion of whole ovaries with radioactive acetate. The follicular linings of human ovaries obtained after *in vivo* stimulation with ovine follicle-stimulating hormone, have been incubated *in vitro* with [^{14}C]acetate demonstrated (Ryan and Smith, 1965). This latter study illustrates the great value and sensitivity of radioactive tracer techniques provided that exact criteria for radiochemical purity are maintained and reliable purification procedures are adhered to. Among other tissues that have been examined, perhaps the most prolific producer of steroids from [^{14}C]acetate has proved to be the corpus luteum which after *in vitro* incubation has yielded progesterone, 17α-hydroxyprogesterone, androstenedione, estrone and estradiol as well as many other intermediate steroids.

The *in vivo* and *in vitro* conversion of acetate to estrogens has been amply demonstrated and it is concluded that acetate is a precursor of estrogens as well as of cholesterol and the neutral C_{21} and C_{19} steroids.

The production of estrogens from cholesterol has now been demonstrated both *in vivo* in the pregnant woman and *in vitro* using the human ovary (previously stimulated *in vivo* with follicle-stimulating hormone) as well as in numerous studies using testis homogenate from various species. Earlier sections of this chapter have described those experiments demonstrating the conversion of cholesterol to C_{21} and C_{19} steroid intermediates of estrogen biosynthesis, and the ability of cholesterol to act as a precursor for the synthesis of estrogens is reasonably well documented.

One of the problems associated with studying cholesterol metabolism arises from the very low solubility of this lipid in aqueous media. The resulting difficulties in transporting the radioactive precursor to the enzymic sites within the tissue, coupled with the relatively large amounts of endogenous cholesterol present in all endocrine tissues, have limited the ability of investigators to provide data proving its ability to act as a precursor to estrogens.

Several reports appeared in 1956 documenting the conversion of progesterone to 17α-hydroxyprogesterone and thence to androstenedione by ovary and testis. It was already known at this time that androstenedione may be aromatized to estrogens in these tissues and this led to the proposition of a biosynthetic route from progesterone to estrogens; this idea was soon confirmed by the isolation of radioactive estrogens following the *in vivo* administration of labelled progesterone to the human. A similar conversion was demonstrated *in vitro* (see Ryan and Smith, 1965) using human ovaries previously stimulated *in vivo* by follicle stimulating hormone. These workers found that the yield of estrogens from progesterone was 10% compared with 0.1% from cholesterol and 0.02% from acetate. It can be seen from these results that the yield of estrogens increased as the number of intermediate enzymic steps decreased and this provided additional evidence for the involvement of both cholesterol and progesterone as obligatory intermediates in the biosynthesis of estrogens by the ovary. Both progesterone and pregnenolone have been shown to act as precursors of estrone and estradiol in the human ovary, and 17α-hydroxyprogesterone is also known to be converted to estradiol by the dog ovary both *in vivo* and *in vitro*. Furthermore, the biosynthesis of estriol from 16α-hydroxyprogesterone by minced sow ovary has been demonstrated and it has been suggested that this represents a direct pathway for estriol formation.

Although the functional significance of adrenal estrogens is obscure, significant quantities of estrone (but no estradiol) have been found in adrenal venous plasma collected from the human and from sheep with a transplanted adrenal gland, and under abnormal conditions, such as carcinoma, the adrenal has been found to serve as a source of estrogens.

In general there appears to be evidence from many sources that the C_{21} steroids progesterone and pregnenolone as well as their 17-hydroxylated derivatives can act as precursors in the biosynthesis of estrogens. (Confer Figure 4.5 for the overall features of these biosynthetic pathways).

B. Aromatization of C_{19} Steroids → Estrogens

Zondek first suggested, in 1934, that androgens are the biosynthetic precursors of estrogens, but not until the studies of Heard and coworkers twenty years later was proof obtained for the *in vivo* conversion of [^{14}C]testosterone to [^{14}C]estrone using a pregnant mare. This was followed by *in vitro* studies with human ovarian slices to demonstrate a similar aromatization, and efficient conditions for this *in vitro* ovarian conversion have been described by Ryan and Smith (1965).

Androstenedione, dehydroepiandrosterone and testosterone have been shown to be aromatized to estrogens by different tissues from several species including the ovary, corpus luteum, testis and adrenal cortex. The details of the enzymic reactions involved in the aromatization of C_{19} steroids to C_{18} steroids were first approached by the studies of Meyer. After incubation with bovine adrenal homogenates, 19-hydroxyandrostenedione was identified as a product of androstenedione; realizing the significance of the 19-hydroxylated androgen as an aromatization intermediate, Meyer looked for and isolated estrone and estradiol following the incubation of 19-hydroxyandrostenedione with slices of human placenta. Follicular fluid and adrenals of cows also converted 19-hydroxyandrostenedione into estrone.

A microsomal enzyme system, first obtained from human placenta by Ryan, is capable of aromatizing androstenedione to estrone in yields exceeding 50% and the use of this system has greatly facilitated further studies on this mechanism. It has been shown that this aromatizing enzyme system is localized in the microsomal fraction and requires oxygen and NADPH. After incubation with this placental enzyme system, Ryan found that 19-hydroxyandrostenedione gave a greater yield of estrone than did androstenedione. Furthermore placental microsomes incubated with [^{14}C]androstenedione produced a small amount of [^{14}C]19-hydroxy-androstenedione, which was converted to estrone after reincubation with the same microsomal system. Similarly dehydroepiandrosterone was shown to be aromatized to a lesser extent than 19-hydroxydehydroepiandrosterone. The kinetic studies of Wilcox and Engel have shown that the 19-hydroxylated derivative is an obligatory intermediate in the conversion of androstenedione to estrone and estradiol by human placental microsomes.

The role of the 19-hydroxylated derivative as an intermediate in the aromatization reaction has been convincingly established and moreover, it is agreed that 19-nortestosterone, 19-norandrostenedione, 1,4-androstadiene-3,17-dione and 17α-hydroxy-1,4-androstadien-3-one are all less rapidly aromatized than either androstenedione or 19-hydroxyandrostenedione. However, since placental microsomes incubated with 19-oxo-androstenedione yield the same amount of estrone as that obtained following incubation with 19-hydroxyandrostenedione, it is highly likely that 19-oxo-androstenedione is an intermediate in the aromatization reaction (see Figure 4.13).

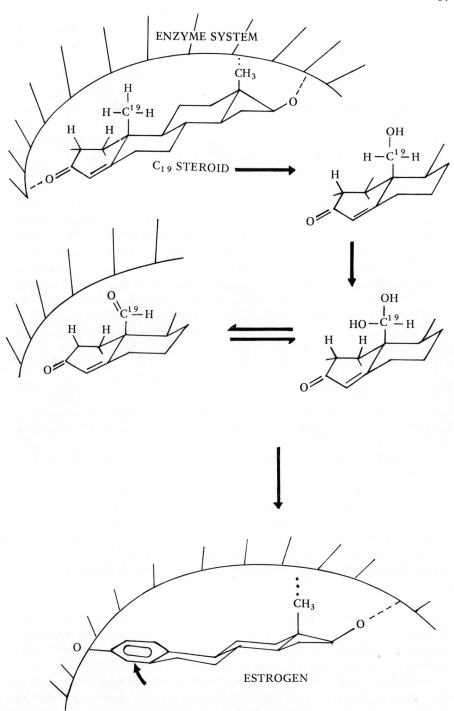

Figure 4.13   Mechanism of aromatization of C_{19} steroids.

Deeper understanding of the aromatization mechanism requires a knowledge of the form in which the angular 19-methyl group is eliminated, and recent studies have shown that it may be liberated in the form of either formic acid or formaldehyde depending upon the precise experimental incubation conditions used. The stereochemistry of the reaction has been established using samples of androstenedione labelled predominantly at either 1α- or 1β-positions with tritium. When these two samples were incubated with human placental microsomes, the [1α-^{3}H]substrate was converted to [^{3}H]estrone, whereas the estrone derived from the [1β-^{3}H]substrate contained only insignificant amounts of tritium.

The details of the aromatization mechanism have now been largely elucidated and detailed by Osawa (1973). Figure 4.13 provides a schematic summary of the process. The steroid substrate presents its β-side to the active site of the aromatase enzyme and one of the three hydrogen atoms at the C-19 position becomes hydroxylated giving rise to a 19-hydroxy-4-en-3-one steroid. This is then followed by a second hydroxylation yielding the 19,19-dihydroxysteroid which may reversibly dehydrate to the 19-oxosteroid. Either or both of these intermediates may then undergo a concerted conformational change with a simultaneous breaking of the C10-C19, C1-H1β and C2-H2β bonds. The latter bond is cleaved by an enolization mechanism which is irreversible since it involves a conformational flip. This process may itself occasion the release of the newly-formed estrogen from the enzyme active site.

C. The Foeto-placental Unit

The biosynthesis of steroids has been described thus far largely by reference to tissues other than the placenta, although this organ is a prolific source of progesterone and estrogens during pregnancy. The manner in which these steroids are elaborated by the placenta differs in several important aspects from the biosynthetic route in other endocrine tissues.

Placental tissue appears to be almost incapable of synthesizing cholesterol from either acetate or mevalonate. Levitz and coworkers using perfused placentae could demonstrate only a minimal formation from acetate and none from mevalonate. Moreover, less than 0.005% conversion of acetate to cholesterol was obtained using tissue minces, and it is now believed that the placenta, being unable to synthesize the steroid nucleus, must use previously made steroid precursors for the elaboration of further steroids.

Progesterone is generated at the rate of about 250 mg/day during late pregnancy and this synthesis has been shown to continue in the absence of a living foetus, maternal ovaries or maternal adrenals. It is now clear that this large amount of progesterone is formed by the placenta to a very great extent, and it is believed to be derived from circulating pregnenolone and cholesterol.

Pregnenolone is distributed in umbilical cord blood mainly as the 3-sulphate. The placenta can use pregnenolone sulphate circulating from the foetus to synthesize pregnenolone and progesterone, which can then be secreted back into the circulation that returns to the foetus. There is also abundant evidence that cholesterol can act as an efficient precursor of both pregnenolone and progesterone in the placenta. A maternal source of precursor is indicated, as progesterone production continues unimpaired even in the absence of a living foetus, and since the quantity of cholesterol distributed in normal adult blood greatly exceeds that of pregnenolone, maternally produced cholesterol is probably the main progesterone precursor.

Careful investigation using a variety of techniques has failed to demonstrate the conversion of radioactive progesterone into estrogens by the perfused intact foeto-placental unit. Moreover, although the *in vitro* conversion of progesterone to androstenedione by human placenta has been reported, the yields obtained were very low. It appears, therefore, that even if the placenta or foeto-placental unit does produce small amounts of estrogens from progesterone, this pathway does not constitute a quantitatively significant route in this tissue.

Although the placenta is poor or deficient in several important enzymes, such as those necessary for the *de novo* synthesis of cholesterol or for the conversion of C_{21} to C_{19} steroids, it nevertheless has considerable capacity to aromatize C_{19} precursors to estrogens. This ability is limited during the first twelve weeks of pregnancy, but increases progressively thereafter and parallels the increase in urinary estrogens. In contrast to the situation in the placenta, Solomon has shown that the foetus can synthesize the steroid nucleus directly from acetate. Furthermore the foetus can provide dehydroepiandrosterone either by *de novo* synthesis from acetate or by using circulating pregnenolone as a precursor. The formation of dehydroepiandrosterone in sulphated form probably occurs in the foetal adrenal whilst 16α-hydroxylation is performed by the foetal liver. Simmer and coworkers have calculated that the foetus might make available to the placenta about 75 mg of dehydroepiandrosterone sulphate per day, and possibly even a greater supply of 16-hydroxydehydroepiandrosterone is indicated by the much higher concentrations of this compound and its sulphate, found in plasma from cord artery as opposed to that from cord vein. This means that during pregnancy all of the placental estrogen production can be accounted for in terms of these C_{19} steroid precursors.

It is evident that a complex interplay exists between the placenta and maternal and foetal circulation for the biosynthesis of estrogens in pregnancy. The co-ordination between the foetus and placenta in this context is indicated by the distribution of some of the enzymes involved, shown in Table 4.1.

The unified concept currently envisaged for the synthesis of steroids by the foeto-placental unit is depicted in Figure 4.14. The 3β-hydroxysteroids reaching the placenta via the material and foetal circulation are rapidly converted into the corresponding α,β-unsaturated ketone. Thus, pregnenolone and 17α-hydroxypregnenolone, yield progesterone and 17α-hydroxyprogesterone, while dehydroepiandrosterone and 16α-hydroxydehydroepiandrosterone yield androstenedione and 16α-hydroxyandrostenedione. This is preceded by placental hydrolysis to the free steroid if the 3β-hydroxysteroids are circulating as sulphates (e.g. dehydroepiandrosterone sulphate). Progesterone and 17α-hydroxyprogesterone are not further metabolized by the placenta, but secreted directly to the maternal and foetal circulation. The foetus then metabolizes the steroids it receives from the

Table 4.1.
Enzyme Activities in the Placenta and Foetus

Enzyme System	Examples	Placenta	Foetus
3β-Hydroxy-Dehydrogenase	pregnenolone $\rightarrow$ progesterone	High	Low
Aromatization	$C_{19} \rightarrow C_{18}$	High	Low
Sulphatase	DHA Sulphate $\rightarrow$ DHA	High	Low
Sulphokinase	DHA $\rightarrow$ DHA Sulphate	Low	High
16α-Hydroxylase	DHA $\rightarrow$ 16α-OH-DHA	Low	High
17α-Hydroxylase	Pregnenolone $\rightarrow$ 17α-OH-pregnenolone	Low	High
17,20-Desmolase	$C_{21} \rightarrow C_{19}$	Low	High
Steroid Synthesis from Acetate	Acetate $\rightarrow$ Cholesterol	Low	High

placenta and by extensive sulphurylation, hydroxylation and desmolase reactions produces dehydroepiandrosterone and its 16α-hydroxylated and sulphated derivatives, which supplement the *de novo* synthesis of these steroids by the foetus. These C_{19} steroids are then transferred to the placenta where they are aromatized to estrogens.

In the non-pregnant female, estriol is derived primarily by 16-hydroxylation of estrone and estradiol. During pregnancy, however, the production of estriol increases greatly and becomes quantitatively the most significant estrogen pro-

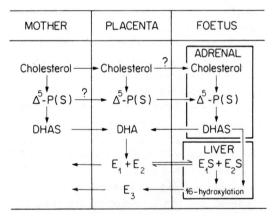

Figure 4.14 Biosynthesis of estrogens from dehydro-epiandrosterone sulphate in the foeto-placental unit. Δ^5-P(S) = pregnenolone or pregnenolone sulphate. DHA = dehydroepiandrosterone. DHAS = dehydro-epiandrosterone sulphate. E_1 = estrone. E_2 = estradiol-17β. E_3 = estriol. E_1S = estrone sulphate. E_2S = estradiol-17β sulphate. E_3S = estriol sulphate. Reprinted with permission from Cooke, B. A. (1970), in Symposium on Reproductive Endocrinology. *Proc. Royal Soc. Medicine*, Livingstone, Edinburgh, 84—94.

duced. It is believed that this increased synthesis arises largely by increased foetal production of 16α-hydroxylated neutral steroids which are converted directly to estriol. In addition, some estrone formed in the placenta may be transferred to the foetal compartment where it is 16α-hydroxylated and then returned to the placenta for conversion to estriol. Further details of the steroidogenic functioning of the foeto-placental unit are given in Chapter 9.

VII. REFERENCES (*denotes a review or book)

*Abraham, G. E. and A. D. Tait (1971). Ovarian metabolism of steroid hormones. A chart in the series *Research in Reproduction*, R. G. Edwards (Ed.), Vol. 3, No. 5. International Planned Parenthood Fedn., London.

*Bloch, K. (1965). The biological synthesis of cholesterol. *Science, N.Y.*, **150**, 19–28.

Breuer, H. (1962). Metabolism of the natural estrogens. *Vitamins and Hormones*, **20**, 285–335.

*Burstein, S. and M. Gut (1973). Conversion of cholesterol to pregnenolone. In R. O. Scow (Ed.), *Endocrinology*. Excerpta Med., Amsterdam Int. Congress, Series No. 273, p. 808.

*Clayton, R. B. (1965). Biosynthesis of sterols, steroids and terpenoids I. Biogenesis of cholesterol and the functional steps in terpenoid biosynthesis. II. Phytosterols terpenes and the physiologically active steroids. *Quart. Revs. Chem. Soc.*, **19**, 168.

*Coghlan, J. P. and J. R. Blair-West (1967). Aldosterone. In *Hormones in Blood*, C. H. Gray and A. L. Bacharach (Eds), 2nd edn. Academic Press, London, pp. 391–488.

*Cornforth, J. W. (1968). Terpenoid biosynthesis. *Chem. in Britain*, 102–106.

*Diczfalusy, E. (1969). Steroid metabolism in the foeto-placental unit. In A. Pecile and C. Finzi (Eds), *The Fetoplacental Unit*. Excerpta Med. Foundn., Amsterdam, pp. 65–109.

*Dorfman, R. I. and D. C. Sharma (1965). An outline of the biosynthesis of corticosteroids and androgens. *Steroids*, **6**, 229.

*Dorfman, R. I and F. Ungar, (1965). *Metabolism of Steroid Hormones*, Academic Press, New York.

*Grant, J. K. (1968). The biosynthesis of adrenocortical steroids. *J. Endocrinol.*, **41**, 111–135.

Grekin, R. J., S. L. Dale and J. C. Melby (1973). The role of 18-hydroxy-11-deoxycorticosterone as a precursor in human adrenal tissue in vitro. *J. Clin. End. Metab.*, **37**, 261–264.

*Griffiths, K. and E. H. D. Cameron (1970). Steroid biosynthetic pathways in the human adrenal. In M. H. Briggs (Ed.), *Advances in Steroid Biochem. Pharmacol.* Vol. 2, pp. 223–265.

*Hall, P. F. (1973). The role of cytochrome P-450 in the biosynthesis of adrenocortical steroids. In R. O. Scow (Ed.), *Endocrinology*. Excerpta Med., Int. Congress Series No. 273, p. 820.

*Hochberg, R. B., P. D. McDonald and S. Lieberman (1973). Transient reactive intermediates in the biosynthesis of pregnenolone from cholesterol. In R. O. Scow (Ed.), *Endocrinology.* Excerpta Med., Int. Congress Series No. 273, p. 808.

*Mahler, H. R. and E. H. Cordes (1971). In *Biological Chemistry*, 2nd edn. Harper & Row, New York and London. pp. 738—755.

*Melby, J. C., S. L. Dale, R. J. Grekin, R. Gaunt and T. E. Wilson (1972). 18-hydroxy-11-deoxycorticosterone (18-OH-DOC) secretion in experimental and human hypertension. *Rec. Prog. Horm. Res.,* **28**, 287—351.

*Mitchell, F. L. (1967). Steroid metabolism in the fetoplacental unit and in early childhood. *Vitamins & Hormones*, **25**, 191—269.

*Oakey, R. E. (1970). Steroid metabolism in the foeto-placental unit. In M. H. Briggs (Ed.), *Advances in Steroid Biochem. and Pharmacol.* Vol. 2. Academic Press.

*Osawa, Y. (1973). Mechanism of aromatization. In R. O. Scow (Ed.), *Endocrinology.* Excerpta Med., Int. Congress Series No. 273, p. 814.

*Ryan, K. T. J. and O. W. Smith (1965). Biogenesis of steroid hormones in the human ovary. *Recent Prog. Horm. Res.,* **21**, 367—409.

Shikita, M. and P. F. Hall (1973). Cytochrome P-450 from bovine adrenocortical mitochondria: an enzyme for the side-chain cleavage of cholesterol. I. Purification and properties; II. Subunit structure. *J. Biol. Chem.,* **248**, 5598—5604 and 5605—5609.

*Solomon, S., C. E. Bird, W. Ling, M. Iwamiya and P. C. M. Young (1967). Formation and metabolism of steroids in the fetus and placenta. *Rec. Prog. Horm. Res.,* **23**, 297—347.

Simpson, E. R. and G. S. Boyd (1967). The cholesterol side-chain cleavage system of bovine adrenal cortex. *Europ. J. Biochem.,* **2**, 275.

Simpson, E. R. and J. I. Mason (1976). Molecular aspects of steroid biosynthesis in the adrenal. In G. N. Gill (Ed.), *Int. Encyclopaedia of Pharmacol and Therapeutics.* Pergamon Press. *In press.*

*Tamaoki, B. I. and M. Shikita (1966). Biosynthesis of steroids in testicular tissue in vitro. In G. Pincus, T. Nakao and J. F. Tait (Eds.), *Steroid Dynamics.* Academic Press, New York. pp. 493—530.

SECTION II

Endocrine Glands and other Tissues Regulating Steroid Hormone Levels

CHAPTER 5

Pituitary gland and hypothalamus

I. INTRODUCTION

The pituitary or *hypophysis* is an ovoid gland – in man about 1 cm in diameter and situated centrally within the head at the base of the brain. It is connected to the brain by the pituitary stalk through which runs the portal blood system, and it has been referred to as a 'master' endocrine gland. It was so designated because of its close communication – via the hypothalamus – with the brain, and because the peptide and protein hormones released from the pituitary regulate the cellular metabolism of so many (but not all) other endocrine tissues. The gland comprises several distinct regions, each characterized by different cell types responsible for particular hormonal secretions. The anatomical description of these areas is complex and since the structure varies considerably from species to species, an accurate morphological description is difficult. A simplified general structure of the pituitary gland and its adjacent hypothalamic region is shown in Figure 5.1. Hypophysectomy comprises the removal of the pituitary gland, although the median eminence, the infundibular stem and most of the pars tuberalis are usually left intact. Many valuable endocrinological studies have been performed using hypophysectomized animals. Although they are susceptible to infection and cannot withstand stress, such animals will, with care, live until old age and they exhibit the

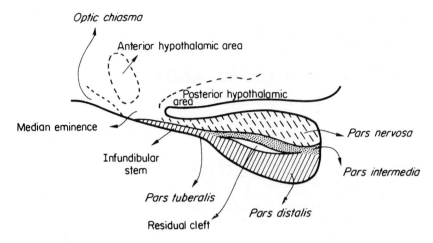

Figure 5.1 General structure of pituitary gland and adjacent hypothalamic regions.

following effects:

a) decreased food intake and consequent loss of weight;
b) general decrease or cessation of growth;
c) atrophy of the gonads and adrenal cortex with a decay in steroid hormone production by all of these tissues;
d) atrophy of the thyroid and a considerable decline in metabolic rate.

II. STRUCTURE OF THE PITUITARY GLAND

The pituitary gland consists of an anterior lobe — the *adenohypophysis*, and a posterior lobe — the *neurohypophysis* (Table 5.1). These two lobes are of quite different embryological origin. Those regions which are derived from the embryonic forebrain are known as the neurohypophysis and include the *pars nervosa, infundibular stem* and the *median eminence*. The adenohypophysis on the other hand has its embryological origin in epithelial cells derived from embryonic buccal (mouth) ectoderm (Rathke's pouch) and may be subdivided into the *pars distalis, pars tuberalis* and the *pars intermedia*. The latter is obvious in some species as a region quite distinct from that of the *pars distalis* and separated from it by a narrow cleft. The relative positions of the adenohypophysis and neurohypophysis vary considerably from species to species and the terms anterior and posterior lobes are therefore somewhat inaccurate descriptions, although they remain in common usage.

The adenohypophysis is very vascular and all the various cell types identified within it are adequately supplied with blood via an extensive capillary system. The neurohypophysis contains nerve-fibres originating in the hypothalamus and form the hypothalamo-hypophyseal tract. The nerve terminals in the neurohypophysis meet with the capillary blood system, and are the storage site of neurosecretory granules which have been conveyed along the nerve fibres from the hypothalamus.

Table 5.1

Anatomical Subdivisions of the Pituitary Gland

Pituitary Gland

Adenohypophysis			Neurohypophysis		
Pars distalis	Pars tuberalis	Pars intermedia	Pars nervosa	Infundibular stem	Median eminence

Anterior lobe   Posterior lobe   Hypophyseal stalk

A. Cell Types of the Adenohypophysis

Seven different cell types have been distinguished in the adenohypophysis of several mammals by staining techniques and the use of fluorescent antibodies. Seven adenohypophysial hormones are known and it is now considered highly likely that each hormone is the product of a separate cell type. These cells have been characterized by their general morphology, the size and composition of their granules and their ultrastructure, as well as by their location in the gland and their responses to cyclical and experimentally induced changes such as pregnancy, lactation, adrenalectomy, thyroidectomy or castration. In several species, including man, two types of acidophilic cell, four types of mucoid cell and one type of chromophobe have been distinguished (Table 5.2). The cytology of the adenohypophysis has been reviewed by Purves (1966) and the ultrastructural features of some of these cell types are shown in Figure 5.2.

1. Acidophils stain with acid dyes (e.g. eosin Y and B, orange G) that react with positively charged proteins. The granules in these cells do not stain for glycoprotein and are thought to comprise only protein. *Somatotrophs* are the most abundant of this class of cells. Labelling studies utilizing fluorescent antibody have demonstrated that they secrete growth hormone (GH; somatotrophin). *Lactotrophs* (or *mammotrophs*) form the minor proportion of acidophilic cells. Although earlier studies were unable to distinguish a prolactin separate and distinct from growth hormone in the human, it has now been substantiated that in many species (including the human) these cells secrete prolactin (LTH; luteotrophic hormone). The *lactotrophs* increase greatly in number during late pregnancy and during lactation.

2. Mucoid cells (Basophils) stain with basic dyes that colour, among other structures, negatively charged proteins. The granules within these cells respond positively to tests for glycoprotein. Thus the *gonadotrophs, thyrotrophs* and most *pars intermedia* cells stain magenta after preliminary oxidation with periodic acid, followed by Schiff's reagent (a test for polysaccharides). Different methods of staining with basophilic dyes and for differentiation between various glycoproteins, reveal the several, different cell types within this class.

3. Thyrotrophs vary considerably in size and shape and are the origin of thyroid stimulating hormone (TSH; thyrotrophin). *Gonadotrophs* are small,

Table 5.2.
Cell Types for Adenohypophyseal Hormones

| Hormone | CELL TYPE | | | Diam. of granules (nm) (Rat)* |
	General name	Functional name	Localization	
Growth Hormone (GH; Somatotrophin)	Acidophil	Somatotroph	pars distalis	350—400
Prolactin (LTH; Luteotrophin)	Acidophil	Lactotroph	pars distalis	600—900
Thyroid-stimulating hormone (TSH)	Basophil	Thyrotroph	pars distalis	150—200
Follicle-stimulating hormone (FSH)	Basophil	Folliculotroph	pars distalis	200—250
Luteinizing hormone (LH; Interstitial cell-stimulating hormone, ICSH)	Basophil	Luteotroph (Interstitiotroph)	pars distalis	200
Melanocyte-stimulating hormone (MSH; Intermedin)	Basophil	Melanotroph	pars intermedia (intermediate zone in man)	
Adrenocorticotrophic hormone (ACTH)	Neutrophil	Corticotroph	pars distalis (intermediate zone in man)	100—200

*From: Farquhar, M. G., 1971. Processing of secretary products by cells of the anterior pituitary gland. In H. Heller and K. Lederis, (Eds). *Memoirs of Soc. End., 19. Subcellular organization and Function in Endocrine Tissues.* Cambridge Univ. Press. pp. 79—122.

lightly-granulated cells located mainly within acidophil-rich regions of the gland. In some species *folliculotrophs* specializing in secretion of follicle-stimulating hormone (FSH) and *luteotrophs* (*interstitiotrophs*) which secrete luteinizing hormone (LH; also known as interstitial cell-stimulating hormone, ICSH), have been distinguished. *Thyrotrophs* and *gonadotrophs* both stain with the periodic acid—Schiff reagent, although in some species (e.g. the rat) they are distinguishable by means of the little understood dye aldehyde-fuchsin, which selectively stains the *thyrotrophs* (although this is not true for all species studied, by any means). The *thyrotrophs* and *gonadotrophs* are most readily distinguishable when seen by electron microscopy, the former tending to have the more angular profile and possessing, in all species so far examined, the smallest secretory granules (see Figure 5.2).

4. *Melanotrophs* are present in the *pars intermedia* and are the most abundant and clearly visible of the basophils. They are responsible for the secretion of melanocyte-stimulating hormone (MSH; also called intermedin). In some mammals (including man) however there is no discrete *pars intermedia*, and in these species MSH is found widely distributed in the *pars distalis*. In man a region of the *pars distalis* adjacent to the neural lobe differs in cell population from the rest of the *pars distalis*; this region has been called

the 'intermediate zone' and contains only *melanotrophs* and *corticotrophs* (see below).

5. *Chromophobes* show no distinctive staining properties and their granules are only weakly coloured, if at all, by any staining method. They are irregularly shaped cells that uniquely enlarge in size and increase in number after adrenalectomy. It has been shown that one week after adrenalectomy in

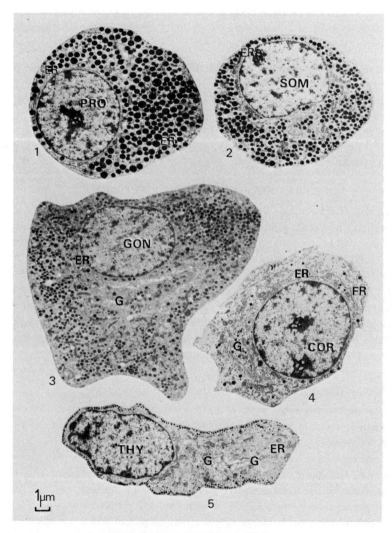

Figure 5.2 Some cell types from the pars distalis in the rabbit. 1, prolactin cell; 2, somatotroph; 3, gonadotroph; 4, corticotroph; 5, thyrotroph. ER, endoplasmic reticulum; FR, free ribosomes; G, Golgi area. (Reproduced with permission of copyright owners from Foster C. L. (1971). In "Memoirs of Soc. End. 19. Subcellular organization and Function in Endocrine Tissues". Heller, H. and Lederis K. (Eds.) Cambridge Univ. Press. p. 128)

the rat these cells increase from about 0.15 per cent to about 1.5 per cent of the total cell content of the pituitary. These cells are now accepted as *corticotrophs* responsible for the secretion of adrenocorticotrophic hormone (ACTH; corticotrophin).

Some immunocytologic observations have suggested that cells containing ACTH also reside in the *pars intermedia*. However, removal of the adenohypophysis or neurohypophysis and measurements of plasma ACTH and corticosterone after various procedures, have recently indicated that the *pars intermedia* and *pars nervosa* do not secrete functionally significant amounts of ACTH (Greer *et al.*, 1975).

The sizes of the granules in these different pituitary cell types are given in Table 5.2. Although there is some variation in size in different mammalian species, the size graduation: *lactotroph > somatotroph > gonadotroph > corticotroph > thyrotroph* — seems to be preserved. Valuable references on the pituitary include a general text by Harris and Donovan (1966), a more recent book devoted to the rat pituitary by Costoff (1973) and a comprehensive text edited by Knobil and Sawyer (1974).

III. HORMONES OF THE PITUITARY

The six well characterized hormones of the anterior pituitary are given in Table 5.3. The pituitary hormones directly involved in regulating the steroidogenic function of endocrine tissues are adrenocorticotrophin (ACTH), prolactin (luteotrophic hormone, LTH), and the gonadotrophins: follicle-stimulating hormone (FSH) and luteinizing hormone (LH) (also referred to as interstitial cell-stimulating hormone (ICSH) when it is acting in the male). For completeness the mammalian neurohypophyseal hormones, oxytocin and vasopression and the intermediate lobe hormone melanocyte-stimulating hormone (MSH) are also shown in Table 5.3. Various other pituitary hormones such as the fat mobilizing lipotrophins have been identified but little is known of their biological role.

A. Adrenocorticotrophin (ACTH)

This is a single chain polypeptide hormone containing 39 amino acid residues and is the smallest adenohypophyseal hormone, (Porcine and human ACTH have molecular weights of 4567 and 4541, respectively.) The complete structure of ACTH derived from several species is shown in Figure 5.3 and the synthesis of human ACTH (among others) has been achieved. The first 24 amino acid residues are the same for the hormones derived from the human, sheep, pig and cow. It is only in amino acid residues 25—33 that species differences are apparent, and since the synthetic polypeptide comprising the first 24 amino acids from the N-terminal end of ACTH (i.e. 1—24 ACTH) has full biological activity, it is not surprising that the activities of the different animal hormones are all very similar to that of human ACTH.

Melanocyte-stimulating hormone (MSH) has a structure closely related to that of ACTH and exists in the pituitary in two forms, designated as α-MSH and β-MSH.

ACTH, α-MSH and the different β-MSH molecules found in various species all have a common sequence of seven amino acids as well as similar amino acid residues at other positions, as indicated in Figure 5.3.

Recently 'Big ACTH' has been identified in plasma and in pituitary extracts (Yalow and Berson, 1973). This is a more acidic molecule than ACTH itself and although the precise size of 'Big ACTH' has not yet been estimated it is believed to be larger than human growth hormone (191 amino acid residues) and to approach that of serum albumin. A component that markedly resembles ACTH can be released from 'Big ACTH' and it is possible that this latter may be the storage form of ACTH within the corticotroph cell (similar to the function of proinsulin as the macromolecular precursor form of insulin in the pancreas: Chance *et al.*, 1968).

The main physiological action of ACTH is on the adrenal cortex and the adrenal responds to ACTH in a variety of ways.

a) Adrenal corticosteroid formation and content is stimulated.

b) Blood-flow rate through the gland is increased.

c) There is a trophic effect and adrenal weight is increased.

d) Adrenal phosphate turnover and the hydrolysis of cholesterol esters is accelerated.

e) Glycogenolysis and glucose oxidation in the adrenal is stimulated.

f) Adrenal content of ascorbic acid, lipid and cholesterol is decreased.

The corticosteroidogenic effect of ACTH is very rapid and *in vitro* studies have demonstrated that within 3 min of ACTH addition, adrenocortical cells have achieved their maximal rate of corticosteroid synthesis (see Chapter 11). On this basis the steroidogenic activity of ACTH must be considered as one of the most important and primary effects. Degradative studies on the ACTH molecule and the use of synthetic analogues have demonstrated that elimination of much of the C-terminal sequence does not markedly reduce the steroidogenic activity (Table 5.4). It is clear that the C-terminal sequence is unimportant for the steroidogenic effect of ACTH, and Hofmann *et al.* (1970) have deduced that major sites for binding to adrenocortical cells (see Chapter 11.IV) are located in amino acid residues at positions 11–20 in the ACTH molecule. Moreover the sequence lys-lys-arg-arg (positions 15–18) is considered to be an important binding site for the hormone, while the biologically active site of the ACTH molecule is attributed to the N-terminal sequence (positions 4–10) which is believed to contain the full complement of amino acids involved in the activation of adrenal cell receptors for ACTH (Schwyzer *et al.*, 1971; Seelig *et al.*, 1971).

The secretion of ACTH from the pituitary occurs in a pulsatile manner and measurements of plasma ACTH concentrations throughout the day have shown frequent peaking of these values which are paralleled by frequent peaking of the plasma 17-hydroxycorticosteroids in these subjects. The pattern of these secretions is shown in the following chapter (Figure 6.5). Although a circadian rhythmn in normal subjects is not clearly discernible, nevertheless plasma ACTH concentrations are usually lowest towards midnight. Normal subjects infrequently have plasma ACTH concentrations above 100 pg/ml in the morning and these usually fall in the

Table 5.3.

Some of the Important Pituitary Hormones

Origin	Pituitary Hormone	Molecular nature	Number of amino acid residues	Mol.Wt.	Site of Action	Effects
Anterior lobe	Adrenocorticotrophic hormone (ACTH)	single chain polypeptide	39	4,541 (human)	Adrenal cortex	corticosteroid synthesis; adreno-cortical growth
	Growth hormone (GH)	single chain protein	199	21,500 (human)	Entire organism	general growth
	Prolactin (Luteotrophic hormone, LTH)	protein	199	23,000	Corpus luteum; Mammary gland	progesterone synthesis
	Follicle-stimulating hormone (FSH)	glycoprotein 2 peptide chains 7% carbohydrate 5% sialic acid	α 89−96 β 155	29,000	Ovarian follicles; Testes seminiferous tubules	estrogen synthesis; follicular growth; spermatogenesis
	Luteinizing hormone (LH) (= Interstitial cell-stimulating hormone, ICSH)	glycoprotein 2 peptide chains	α 89−96 β 119	28,000	Ovarian follicle; Testes Leydig cells	estrogen synthesis; formation of corpus luteum; androgen synthesis
	Thyroid stimulating hormone (TSH)	glycoprotein 2 peptide chains 8% carbohydrate 1% sialic acid	α 96 β 113	28,000	Thyroid	thyroid hormone synthesis

Posterior lobe	Oxytocin	cyclic peptide	9	1,007	Uterus; Mammary gland	contraction
	Arginine Vasopressin* (phe^3-arg^8-oxytocin; Antidiuretic hormone, ADH)	cyclic peptide	9	1,084	Kidney tubule	water reabsorption
Intermediate lobe	Melanocyte-stimulating hormone: α-MSH	polypeptide	13		Skin	synthesis and dispersion of melanin pigment
	β-MSH	polypeptide	22	2,661 (human)		
			18	2,134 (sheep, pig, etc)		

*For all mammals except the pig, which has lysine vasopressin (phe^3-lys^8-oxytocin.) For further details on the structures of the pituitary hormones see Wallis, M. (1975). The molecular evolution of pituitary hormones. *Biol. Rev.*, **50**, 35–98.

84

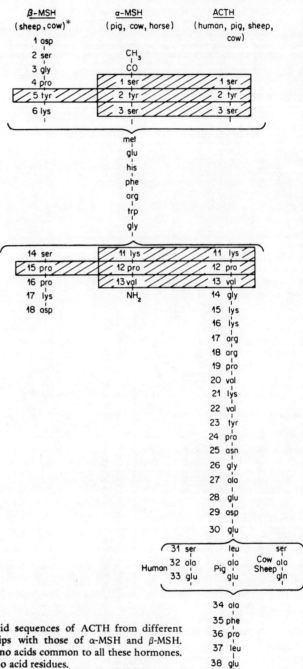

Figure 5.3 The amino acid sequences of ACTH from different species and the relationships with those of α-MSH and β-MSH. Shaded regions indicate amino acids common to all these hormones. *Human β-MSH has 22 amino acid residues.

Ref. Dayhoff, M. O. (1972). Atlas of protein sequence and structure. Vol. 5 and 1973 Vol. 5, Suppl. 1. *Nat. Biomed. Res. Foundn.*, Washington, USA; and Wallis, M. (1975). The Molecular Evolution of Pituitary Hormones. *Biol. Rev.*, 50, 35–98.

Table 5.4
Adrenal Steroidogenic activity of ACTH Peptides of Various Chain Lengths

ACTH analogue	STEROIDOGENIC POTENCY	
	IN VITRO[+]	IN VIVO[*]
	Molar ratios	*Int. Units/μ mole*
natural (1—39)ACTH	100	474
synthetic (1—26)ACTH	—	390
synthetic (1—24)ACTH	140	390
synthetic (1—23)ACTH	—	247
synthetic (1—19)ACTH)	—	110
synthetic [Lys^{17},Lys^{18}] (1—18)ACTH amide	0.05	—
synthetic (1—17)ACTH	—	11.2
synthetic (1—16)ACTH amide	0.05	—
synthetic (1—16)ACTH	—	0.4
synthetic (1—10)ACTH	3.7×10^{-5}	0.003
synthetic (4—10)ACTH	7.5×10^{-5}	—
synthetic (5—24)ACTH	0.03	—

Various polypeptides incorporating the first few amino acids from the N-terminal end of ACTH compared with ACTH in their ability to stimulate adrenal steroidogenesis.(*) From: Ramachandran, J., and C. H. Li (1967). Structure activity relationships of the adrenocorticotropins and melanotropins: the synthetic approach. *Adv. in Enzymology*, 29, 391—477.

(+)From: Seelig, S., and G. Sayers (1973). Isolated adrenal cortex cells: ACTH agonists, partial agonists, antagonists; cyclic AMP and corticosterone production. *Arch. Bioch. Biophys.*, 154, 230—239. Molar potencies [given relative to (1—39)ACTH]

$$= \frac{\text{molar concentration of (1—39)ACTH for half maximal steroidogenic response}}{\text{molar concentration of ACTH analogue for half maximal steroidogenic response}} \times 100$$

late evening. Very ill hospital patients do sometimes have plasma concentrations above 200 pg/ml in the morning.

B. Gonadotrophins

Two glycoproteins, originating from the anterior lobe of the pituitary, affect gonadal activity and function. These are *follicle-stimulating hormone* (FSH) and *luteinizing hormone* (LH). *Interstitial cell-stimulating hormone* (ICSH) was the name which was originally given to this latter glycoprotein when derived from male pituitaries. It has now been shown to be identical with the LH derived from females of that particular species. The term LH is applied when the hormone acts in either the male or female. Structurally these are the most complex macromolecular hormones produced by the pituitary and these glycoproteins contain two long polypeptide chains each covalently linked to a relatively small carbohydrate prosthetic group. Each polypeptide chain contains about 100 amino acid residues and the two chains in each hormone may be dissociated from one another by denaturing conditions — indicating that they are linked by non-covalent bonds. Sequence analysis has shown that the α-chains of FSH and LH are very similar and possibly identical, whereas the β-chains and the carbohydrate groups of the two hormones are quite different. FSH has a molecular weight of 29,000 and contains 5% sialic acid, which is essential for its biological activity as indicated by its inactivation by neuraminidase. LH has a molecular weight of about 38,000 and is thought to be a globular glycoprotein stabilized by cystine disulphide bridges (Ward *et al.*, 1973).

In any individual there are large changes in plasma LH and FSH levels over short time periods. Recent studies have shown that these fluctuations are due to a rapid pulsatile release of these pituitary hormones (similar to that described for ACTH — see Figure 6.5) with an oscillatory period of about an hour. This has now been demonstrated for many different mammals, but was originally observed in monkeys (Dierschke *et al.*, 1970) and humans (Dolais *et al.*, 1970). The recent observation of a pulsatile release of LH in the domestic fowl (Wilson and Sharp, 1975) suggests that this is a general neuroendocrine control mechanism and applies not only to mammals.

Three gonadotrophins of non-pituitary origin also exist. *Human menopausal gonadotrophin* (hMG) exhibits biological activities similar to both FSH and LH, and has been extracted from the urine of menopausal women. It has a molecular weight of 31,000 and contains about 30% carbohydrate. *Human chorionic gonadotrophin* (hCG) is a glycoprotein of molecular weight 30,000 and contains about 20% carbohydrate. It is produced by the placenta and is evident in pregnant women's urine within one week of conception. Predominantly it has LH-like activity, but also has FSH-like activity at high concentrations. A gonadotrophin (PMS) derived from *pregnant mare's serum* originates from the uterine endometrium. This has a molecular weight of 23,000 and contains about 30% carbohydrate, although this may be due to the presence of carbohydrate impurities. The major gonadotrophic effect of PMS is like that of FSH, with a minor LH-action.

The biological effects of the gonadotrophins on steroidogenesis by the ovary and testis, as well as on follicular development, the estrous cycle and spermatogenesis are detailed in Chapters 7, 8 and 13.

C. Prolactin (Luteotrophic hormone, LTH)

Prolactin is a single chain polypeptide hormone. The molecular weight of pure ovine prolactin is 23,000 and contains 199 amino acid residues. The sequences of the hormones derived from sheep and cow have been determined and found to be homologous with that of growth hormone (GH). It is a relatively stable protein but may be inactivated by a variety of chemical procedures. Human pituitaries have a great deal of prolactin activity, but some of this is attributable to human growth hormone which also exhibits lactogenic activity. Recent work (Greenwood, 1972) however, shows the existence of a human prolactin distinct from human growth hormone.

The biological function of prolactin varies with different species. It is widely distributed among the vertebrates and in mammals functions primarily as a lactogenic hormone affecting mammary gland growth and milk formation and secretion. In rodents it is involved together with LH and FSH in the production of progesterone by the corpus luteum. However, in non-mammalian vertebrates it has other important effects. For example in pigeons, prolactin stimulates crop sac 'milk' secretion and in tadpoles it inhibits tail resorption and excretion of urea. In many lower animals it exhibits general metabolic effects similar to those of growth hormone. Although prolactin is found in both sexes, its function in the male is undetermined.

D. Placental lactogenic hormone (PL)

This is a protein hormone with lactogenic and slight growth-promoting activity that has been extracted from human and monkey placentae. Large amounts are secreted during the later part of pregnancy. Human PL shows a strong structural similarity to human GH — approximately 85% of the amino acid residues are identical.

IV. BLOOD SUPPLY TO THE PITUITARY

The adenohypophysis and the neurohypophysis are supplied by quite separate blood systems and appear to be functionally distinct. An extensive and specialized vascular pathway for the supply of blood to the pituitary gland arises from the hypophyseal arteries. These arteries branch into two sets of capillary networks i) upwards into the hypothalamus and ii) downwards into the pituitary itself. Blood is therefore supplied to the gland both directly from the arterial system and also from a hypophyseal — hypothalamic portal system (Figure 5.4). It has been demonstrated by Harris that these portal vessels must remain intact for the regulation of pituitary hormone secretion. Long portal vessels originating in the median eminence and short portal vessels originating in the pituitary stalk have been observed, both types terminating in the adenohypophysis.

There is a limited amount of detailed data concerning the flow of blood through the pituitary for any species but the rat. Extensive studies have however been made of the pituitary blood flow in this animal (Porter *et al.*, 1973). It has been calculated that the long portal vessels in the rat carry about 70% of the blood to the anterior pituitary and that the short portal vessels carry the remaining 30%. In man, monkey and sheep, it has been estimated that the short portal vessels carry about 10—20% of the blood to the anterior pituitary.

It appears that the blood flowing through the short portal vessels is inadequate for the metabolic requirements of the whole pituitary gland; stopping the flow of blood through the long portal vessels leads to necrosis of 70—90% of the anterior pituitary. Despite this, however, it is still theoretically possible that even a small flow of blood via the short portal vessels might carry enough hormonally active molecules from the *infundibular stem* to affect anterior pituitary function. Relatively large quantities of vasopressin are secreted from the *infundibular stem* and the short portal vessels could provide a possible route for the transport of vasopressin (and perhaps other regulatory molecules) from the *infundibular stem* to the anterior pituitary. That this is most unlikely is evident from the elegant studies of Porter *et al.* (1973), in which it was shown that removal of the *infundibular stem*

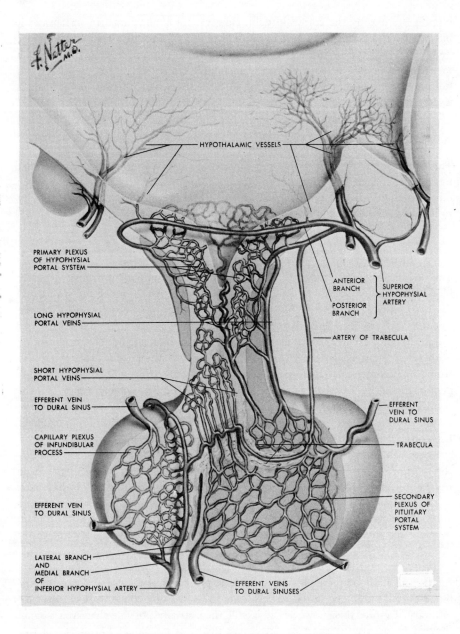

Figure 5.4   Scheme of hypophysial-portal circulation. The sinusoids of the anterior lobe receive their blood supply from the hypophysial portal vessels, which arise from the capillary beds within the median eminence (above) and enter the *infundibular stem* (below). In the anterior lobe (right) they form a secondary plexus of the pituitary portal system. The releasing or inhibiting factors of the hypothalamus or the median eminence enter the pituitary circulation at the primary plexus of the hypophysial portal system which runs from the median eminence via the *infundibular stem* to the *pars distalis* (anterior pituitary lobe). (Copyright: The Ciba Collection of Medical Illustrations by Frank H. Netter, M.D.)

and *pars intermedia* from surgically-stressed rats had no effect on the high corticosterone secretion rate if the *pars distalis* remained intact; on the other hand transection of the pituitary stalk (leaving the short portal vessels intact) led to a marked decrease in corticosterone secretion rate. It was concluded that any factor (e.g. CRH) that is required for maintaining the high ACTH secretion rates observed in surgically stressed rats, is transported to the anterior pituitary via the long portal vessels in the pituitary stalk.

V. RELEASING AND RELEASE-INHIBITING HORMONES

The various secretory cells of the adenohypophysis are now believed to be regulated by the hypothalamus via hormones originating from the median eminence and carried in the blood through the capillaries of the hypophyseal — hypothalamic portal system. This system is composed of an exceedingly well-developed network of fine capillaries originating in the region of the median eminence, where the capillaries are contiguous with the terminals of hypothalamic nerve fibres. Blood from this capillary network flows through the pituitary stalk into the adeno-hypophysis within which it is distributed via a second capillary system. Each cell-type in the adenohypophysis is currently believed to be regulated by factors which can be extracted from median eminence tissue and are now referred to as releasing-hormones and release-inhibiting hormones. Several such hormones have been described (Table 5.5), and the remarkable advances in this rapidly expanding field have been reviewed (Burgus and Guillemin, 1970; Schally *et al.*, 1973; Reichlin, 1973).

The molecular structures of some polypeptides that specifically stimulate or inhibit release of adenohypophyseal hormones have been identified and found to comprise relatively few amino acid residues. Some of these polypeptides have been synthesized. The tripeptide structure thyrotrophin releasing hormone (TRH) and the decapeptide structure of LH- and FSH-releasing hormone (LH-RH/FSH-RH) is depicted in Figure 5.5. Because natural LH-RH and the synthetic decapeptide both possess major FSH-RH (as well as LH-RH) activity in the human

Table 5.5.

Hypothalamic neurohormones controlling the release of adenohypophyseal hormones

Hypothalamic hormone	Abbreviation of hormone (or factor)
Corticotrophin (ACTH)-releasing hormone	CRH (or CRF)
Follicle-stimulating hormone (FSH)-releasing hormone	FSH-RH (or FSH-RF)
Gonadotrophin releasing hormone	GnRH (or LH-RH/FSH-RH)
Growth hormone (GH)-releasing hormone	GH-RH (or GH-RF)
Growth hormone (GH)-release-inhibiting hormone	GH-RIH (or GIF)
Luteinizing hormone (LH)-releasing hormone	LH-RH (or LH-RF)
Melanocyte-stimulating hormone (MSH)-releasing hormone	MRH (or MRF)
Melanocyte-stimulating hormone (MSH) release-inhibiting hormone	MRIH (or MIF)
Prolactin release-inhibiting hormone	PRIH (or PIF)
Prolactin releasing hormone	PRH (or PRF)
Thyrotrophin (TSH) releasing hormone	TRH (or TRF)

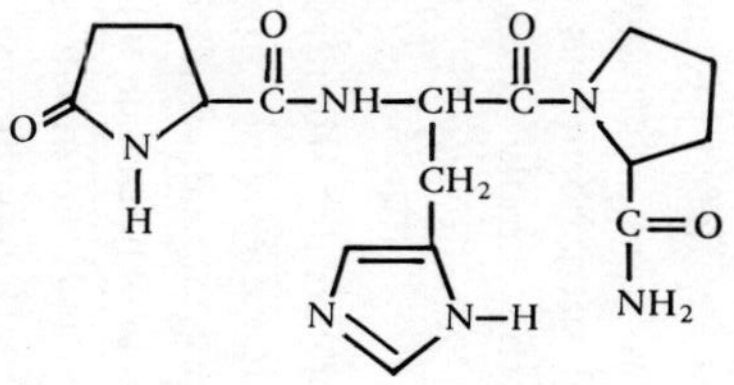

(pyro)Glu–His–Pro–NH_2

a) Structure of thyrotrophin-releasing hormone (TRH).

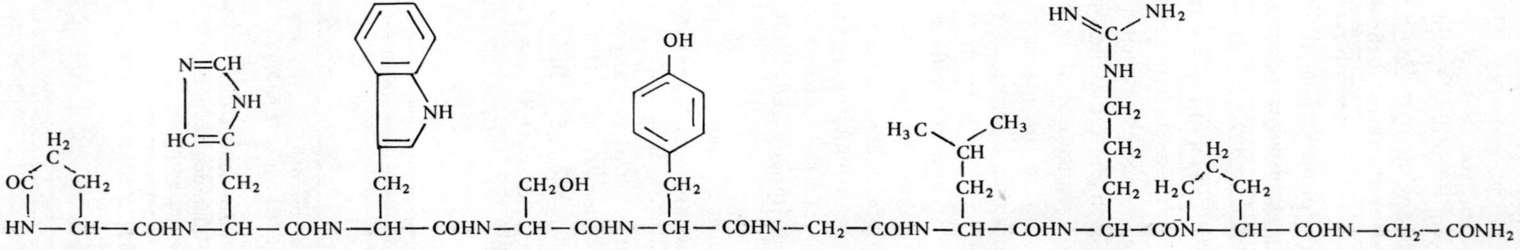

(Pyro)Glu —— His —— Trp —— Ser —— Tyr —— Gly —— Leu —— Arg —— Pro —— Gly —— NH_2

b) Structure of LH- and FSH-releasing hormone (LH–RH/FSH–RH), also known as Gonadotrophin releasing hormone (GnRH)

Figure 5.5 Structures of some hypothalamic releasing hormones.

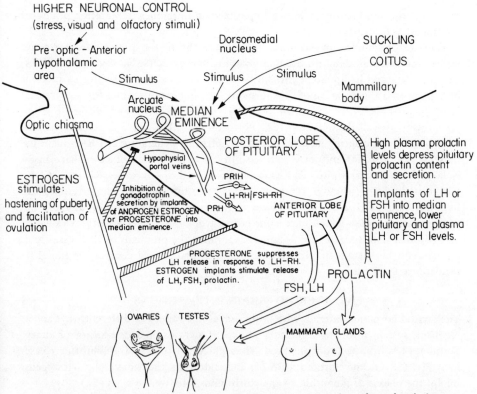

HIGHER NEURONAL CONTROL
(stress, visual and olfactory stimuli)

Pre-optic - Anterior
hypothalamic
area

Dorsomedial
nucleus

SUCKLING
or
COITUS

Stimulus   Stimulus   Stimulus

Arcuate
nucleus   MEDIAN
EMINENCE

Mammillary
body

Optic chiasma

POSTERIOR LOBE
OF PITUITARY

Hypophysial
portal veins

High plasma prolactin
levels depress pituitary
prolactin content
and secretion.

PRIH

ESTROGENS
stimulate:

Inhibition of
gonadotrophin
secretion by implants
of ANDROGEN ESTROGEN
or PROGESTERONE into
median eminence.

LH-RH/FSH-RH

PRH

ANTERIOR LOBE
OF PITUITARY

Implants of LH or
FSH into median
eminence, lower
pituitary and plasma
LH or FSH levels.

hastening of puberty
and facilitation of
ovulation

PROGESTERONE suppresses
LH release in response to LH-RH.
ESTROGEN implants stimulate release
of LH, FSH, prolactin.

PROLACTIN

FSH, LH

OVARIES   TESTES

MAMMARY GLANDS

Figure 5.6   Outline of mechanisms controlling gonadotrophin release from the pituitary. Based mainly on data obtained in the rat. For further details see: Edwards, R. G. (Ed.) (1971). *Research in Reproduction*, Vol. 3, No. 1. International Planned Parenthood Federation, Lower Regent Street, London. (Hypothalamic Map, prepared by Arimura, A., and A. Findlay.) For abbreviations see Table 5.5.

and the rat, it has been suggested (Schally *et al.*, 1973) that only one hormone, termed LH-RH/FSH-RH, may effect the release of both LH and FSH from the anterior pituitary. Although this concept is supported by considerable physiological and biochemical data, demonstrating that the FSH-RH activity is intrinsic to the LH-RH molecule, the possibility remains at present that a separate unidentified hormone exists in the hypothalamus which only, or predominantly, releases FSH. An overall scheme for the regulation of gonadotrophin release is shown in Figure 5.6.

A two-way system — via both stimulatory and inhibitory factors — for hypothalamic control of at least three pituitary hormones, has been recognized. The requirement for hypothalamic inhibitors (as well as stimulators) of GH, MSH and prolactin is reasonable because of the noted lack of products from their target cells which exert any negative feedback effect on the synthesis of these pituitary hormones. On the other hand ACTH, LH, FSH and TSH all stimulate their target cells to produce hormones (corticosteroids, androgens, estrogens, progestogens and thyroxine) which are carried through the blood system to exert a negative feedback effect on the production of either hypothalamic hormones or anterior pituitary hormones, or both.

Corticotrophin-releasing hormone (CRH) was the first hypothalamic hormone whose activity was demonstrated in hypothalmic extracts. However, difficulties with its assay and its apparent instability under the conditions used for extraction have hampered the isolation of this hormone in sufficient quantities for a structural analysis. Although the existence of CRH, in addition to and different from vasopressin, is well documented (e.g. Porter *et al.*, 1973), very little progress has been made in elucidating its structure. Early efforts to characterize CRH sought its presence in posterior pituitary extracts. In the past, various factors have been isolated from posterior pituitary tissue and designated α_1-CRF, α_2-CRF and β-CRF, but it is doubtful whether there is any relationship between the physiological hypothalamic CRH and any of these neurohypophyseal factors or any of the vasopressin analogues which have some corticotrophin-releasing activity. A valuable text (Brodish and Redgate, 1973) appraises some of the problems of CRH assay and provides further details of the releasing-hormone and steroid control systems that regulate ACTH secretion.

VI. STEROID—BRAIN INTERACTIONS

The steroid hormones interact with brain tissues in a variety of different ways and a feedback system involving inhibitory effects of steroids on secretions of pituitary hormones has been well documented. Thus, glucocorticosteroids inhibit the release of ACTH (Sayers and Portanova, 1974) and androgens, estrogens and progestogens inhibit the release of the pituitary gonadotrophins (McEwen *et al.*, 1972).

Within the hypothalamus there appears to be an extensive system of neurons involved in the synthesis of pituitary releasing hormones (Subsection V) and perhaps other factors essential for pituitary function. Present experimental evidence suggests that the feedback action of the adrenal and gonadal steroid hormones is mediated, at least in part, through this neuronal system. Such a neurohormonal feedback system is implicated by studies on the feedback inhibitory or stimulatory effect of the sex-steroids on the LH-RH/FSH-RH producing neurons located in the hypophysiotrophic area, and neurons sensitive to the sex-steroids have been located in the pre-optic hypothalamic area (Flerko, 1973). A similar system is believed to operate for the negative feedback effect of glucocorticoids on ACTH secretion (Brodish and Redgate, 1973) although the complexities of this system do not allow for simple analysis and much uncertainty remains in this field.

A wide variety of techniques have been employed in this field (for review, see McEwen *et al.*, 1972) and include:

A. Pituitary Grafts

Transplanting pituitary tissue into different brain regions of hypophysectomized rats and examination of the histological and functional state of such grafts after several weeks, enabled Halász and co-workers to define that brain region in which grafts retained a normal histology. This region they termed the 'hypophysiotrophic area' and concluded that neurons in this region contain factors necessary for the normal secretion of anterior pituitary hormones.

B. Electrolytic Lesions

The content of releasing hormones in the median eminence has been measured after placing lesions in different areas of the hypothalamus. Using this technique it has been found that CRH-producing neurons are not localized, but diffuse within the medial basal hypothalamus. However, there are problems associated with this technique and the use of some electrodes can not only induce an inflammatory secretion and artefactual neural stimulation, but also destroy both cell bodies and axons.

C. Neural Isolation

Specially designed knives have been used to completely isolate different regions of the brain from all neural inputs. This technique has largely overcome the limitations of the electrolytic lesioning method and indicate that there is more than one level of hypothalamic control of pituitary function.

D. Electrical Stimulation

This has proved an informative technique for localizing those brain regions involved in pituitary control. Thus ovulation may be triggered by stimulation of specific regions in the hypothalamus and also of the pre-optic area.

E. Hormone Implantation

Steroid implants have been used to give a great deal of information regarding steroid feedback loci (see Figure 5.6). Thus implants of estrogens or androgens in the arcuate nucleus of male or female rats decreased gonadal weight as did estrogen implants in the mammillary body of female rats. Implants directly into the pituitary or anterior hypothalamus were ineffective. Implants of progesterone into the median eminence inhibited LH secretion but appeared not to affect FSH secretion. Testosterone implanted into the median eminence (but not into the pituitary) resulted in atrophy of the testes and its accessory glands. Moreover, implants of cyproterone (a synthetic anti-androgen that blocks androgen retention by androgen target cells) in the median eminence of immature male rats caused hypertrophy of testes and its accessory glands, and enhanced secretion of LH was indicated. In other experiments (Brodish and Redgate, 1973) local implants of corticosteroids in the median eminence of rats were found to be effective in inhibiting adrenocortical responses to stressful stimuli, whereas such implants in other brain regions were ineffectual.

Although it is currently believed that the primary site of the feedback effect of these steroid hormones is the hypothalamus, nevertheless, it is possible that the glucocorticoids and sex steroids may also have a direct feedback action on the anterior pituitary itself and perhaps other brain regions as indicated in Figures 5.6 and 5.7. There is convincing evidence that steroidal oral contraceptives interfere with FSH and LH secretion, and it is believed that they exert their effect primarily at the hypothalamus or another brain region, thereby suppressing the output of hypothalamic releasing hormones (Diczfalusy, 1971; Klopper, 1973). However, other sites of action, such as interference with gonadotrophin secretion by the pituitary, cannot as yet be excluded.

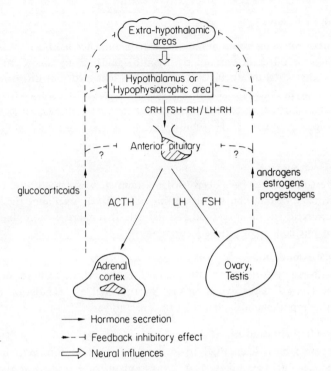

Figure 5.7   Feedback inhibitory action of steroid hormones at
the level of the hypothalamus and anterior pituitary.

In many respects the topographical biochemistry of the brain shows a
remarkable degree of homogeneity from region to region. However, in the
distribution of binding proteins for steroid hormones such as estrogens, androgens
and corticosteroids, various brain regions exhibit considerable dissimilarities. The
regional distribution and biochemical characteristics of such steroid-binding systems
derived largely from studies on the rat brain has been reviewed by McEwen *et al.*
(1972), and there is ample evidence that the adrenal and gonadal steroid hormones
have direct effects on specific regions of the brain. Estradiol and testosterone are
most effective in the pre-optic area and the hypothalamus. The amygdala has not
been studied so extensively, but is also another site of estradiol action. The
corticosteroids are effective in a considerably greater number of neural structures
than sex steroids, and the brain regions sensitive to glucocorticoids include not only
the hypothalamus but also the septum, hippocampus, amygdala, thalamus and
other areas of the brain. There is an impressive parallel relationship between those
brain areas in which steroids are effective following implantation, and those regions
which bind any particular steroid hormone (McEwen *et al.*, 1972).

The role of steroid receptors in the brain is an exciting topic, and although at the
moment not a great deal is known about the mechanism of action of steroids in the
brain, this is a rapidly expanding field. The next few years should witness
considerable advances in this area and help in understanding such aspects as

contraception, immunosuppression and the effects of steroids on sexual differentiation in the central nervous system. The role of steroid hormone receptors and the intracellular mechanism of action of the steroid hormones in various tissues such as uterus, prostate and liver is discussed at length in Chapters 14, 15 and 16. The interactions between the steroid hormones and specific brain regions appear to follow the general receptor mechanisms described in these chapters. Further aspects of the binding of steroid hormones to specific brain receptors have been reviewed by Thomas (1973) and King and Mainwaring (1974).

In this field of steroid–brain interactions, one particular area of investigation that is becoming of increasing interest, involves the striking and permanent changes brought about by transient modulations in the steroid hormone environment at a critical stage of neonatal development. These changes affect the subsequent functional capacity of the brain and are the subject of a review by Brown-Grant (1972). It is likely that steroid sex hormones influence the brain at an important stage of neonatal development and that their presence or absence at this particular time can affect the subsequent sexual attitudes and behavioural patterns of the adult. Although the ovaries and testes are controlled by the same pituitary hormones, when ovaries are transplanted into castrated males they no longer exhibit the characteristic cyclic features of follicular growth and ovulation. That this sex difference in pituitary function does not reside in the pituitary itself, has been shown by transplanting pituitaries from male rats into hypophysectomized females – since these animals then had normal, regular estrous cycles. Current concepts suggest that it is the hypothalamus that is imprinted at an early stage in neonatal development, with either a male or female pattern of activity, and that it is the male pattern that is superimposed on the neutral, or female pattern (see also Chapter 8.III).

In the neonatal male, the testosterone secreted by the testes within a day or two of birth, masculinizes the animal both behaviourally and neuroendocrinologically. The adult will thus exhibit predominantly the male sexual behaviour pattern: mounting, intromission and ejaculation, and a masculine (steady or non-cyclical) release of gonadotrophins. Female rodents given an injection of androgen within a few days of birth will develop into sterile adults that remain in a state of persistent estrous, and it has been suggested that this is due to the development of a non-cyclical pattern of gonadotrophin release. Surprisingly, estrogen injections into the intact neonatal female also result in masculinization of her development (see below). In the castrated neonatal male animal (and the neonatal female), the absence of adequate levels of sex-steroid hormones leads to feminization, with development of lordosis (hollowing of the back) and a cyclical pattern of gonadotrophin release. Moreover, the observation that normal female development ensues following neonatal ovariectomy, demonstrates the irrelevance of the ovarian products to this developmental process.

The interesting observation that injected estrogens also affect sexual differentiation of the rodent brain, has prompted the suggestion that androgens affect brain differentiation, following conversion to estrogens that are formed by aromatization at the site of action with the brain. This idea is supported by the demonstration of the aromatizing enzyme system in neural tissues of rats during the critical period of sexual differentiation – with the activity in male tissue exceeding that in female tissue (Reddy *et al.*, 1974). Furthermore, it has been suggested by these workers that it is the high circulating levels of estrogen binding proteins that, in the perinatal rat, effectively remove the high circulating levels of estrogens, making them unavailable to sensitive brain regions during development. Since they are not bound by this binding protein, androgens (and neonatally administered synthetic estrogens such as diethylstilbestrol) would remain free in the circulation for action at specific loci in the brain. However, although these are very interesting ideas, much further work is necessary before we have a clear understanding of the mechanism of steroid hormone action in sexual differentiation and mating behaviour.

VII. REFERENCES (* indicates review or book)

*Brodish, A., and E. S. Redgate (Eds.) (1973). *Brain-pituitary-adrenal-interrelationships.* S. Karger (Pub.), Basel.

*Brown-Grant, K. (1972). Recent studies on the sexual differentiation of the brain. In R. S. Comline and P. W. Nathanielz (Eds.) 'Foetal and neo-natal physiology'. Cambridge Univ. Press. pp. 527–545.

*Burgus, R., and R. Guillemin (1970). Hypothalamic releasing factors. *Ann. Rev. Biochem.*, 39, 499–525.

Chance, R. E., R. M. Ellis and W. W. Bromer (1968). Porcine proinsulin; characterisation and amino acid sequence. *Science*, 161, 165.

*Costoff, A. (1973). *Ultrastructure of the rat adenohypophysis: correlation with function.* Academic Press, N.Y.

*Diczfalusy, E. (1971). Contraceptive steroids and their mechanism of action. In E. Diczfalusy and U. Borell (Eds), *Control of Human Fertility. Nobel Symp. 15.* Wiley, New York and London. pp. 17–38.

Dierschke, D. J., A. N. Bhattacharya, L. E. Atkinson and E. Knobil (1970). Circhoral (*about an hour*) oscillations of plasma LH levels in the ovariectomized rhesus monkey. *Endocrinology*, 87, 850–853.

Dolais, J., A. J. Valleron, A. M. Grapin and G. Rosselin (1970). Etude de l'hormone lutéinisante humaine (hLH) au cours du nyethémère *Compte rendu hebdomadaire des seances d l'Acad. des sciences,* 270, 3123–3126.

*Flerko, B. (1973). The hypophysiotrophic area and its regulation. In R. O. Scow (Ed), Endocrinology, Proc. IVth Int. Congr. Endocr., Washington. *Excerpta Medica,* Amsterdam. Int. Congr. Series No. 273, pp. 63–66.

*Greenwood, F. C. (1972). Evidence for the separate existence of human pituitary prolactin – a review and results. In A. Pecile and E. E. Müller (Eds), Growth and Growth Hormone; Proc. 2nd Int. Symp. on Growth Hormone, Milan 1972. *Excerpta Medica,* Amsterdam. pp. 91–97.

Greer, M. A., C. F. Allen, P. Panton and J. P. Allen, (1975). Evidence that the *Pars Intermedia* and *Pars Nervosa* of the pituitary do not secrete functionally significant quantities of ACTH. *Endocrinology*, 96, 718–724.

*Harris, G. W., and B. T. Donovan (1966). *The Pituitary Gland*, Vols. 1, 2 and 3. Butterworths, London. 600 pages each.

Hofmann, K., W. Wingender and F. M. Finn (1970). Correlation of adreno-corticotrophic activity of ACTH analogues with degree of binding to an adrenal cortical particulate preparation. *Proc. Nat. Acad. Sci.*, **67**, 829–836.

*King, R. J. B., and W. I. P. Mainwaring (1974). *Steroid-cell interactions*. Butterworths, London, 440 pages.

*Klopper, A. (1973). Endocrinological effects of oral contraceptives. *Clin. Endocrinol. Metab.*, **2**, 489–502.

*Knobil, E., and W. H. Sawyer (Eds) 1974. The pituitary gland and its neuroendocrine control. In *Handbook of Physiology*. Section 7: Endocrinology. Vol. IV. Part 1. Morphology, the neurohypophysis. 584 pages. Part 2. Adenohypophysis. 607 pages. Williams & Wilkins, Co., Baltimore, Maryland.

*McEwen, B. S., R. E. Zigmond and J. L. Gerlach (1972). Sites of steroid binding and action in the brain. In G. H. Bourne (Ed.) *The structure and function of nervous tissue* Vol. V. Structure III and Physiology III. Academic Press, New York. pp. 205–291.

*Porter, J. C., R. S. Mical, N. Ben-Jonathan and J. G. Ondo (1973). Neurovascular regulation of the anterior hypophysis. *Recent Progress Hormone Research*, **29**, 161–198.

*Purves, H. D. (1966) Cytology of the adenohypophysis. In Harris, G. W., and B. T. Donovan (Eds) *The Pituitary Gland*. Vol. 1. Butterworths, London. p. 147–232.

Reddy, V. V. R., F. Naftolin and K. J. Ryan (1974). Conversion of androstene-dione to estrone by neural tissues from fetal and neonatal rats. *Endocrinology*, **94**, 117–121. [See also *Recent Progress Hormone Research* (1975) **31**, 295–319.]

*Reichlin, S. (1973). Hypothalamic-pituitary function. In R. O. Scow (Ed.) *Endocrinology* Proc. IVth. Int. Congr. Endocr., Washington. *Excerpta medica*, Amsterdam. Int. Congr. Series No. 273, pp. 1–16.

Sayers, G. and R. Portanova (1974). Secretion of ACTH by isolated anterior pituitary cells: kinetics of stimulation by CRF and of inhibition by corti-costerone. *Endocrinology*, **94**, 1723–1730.

*Schally, A. V., A. Arimura and A. J. Kastin (1973). Hypothalamic regulatory hormones. *Science*, **179**, 341–350; The LH- and FSH-releasing hormone. In R. O. Scow (Ed.) *Endocrinology*. Proc. IVth Int. Congr. Washington. *Excerpta Medica*, Amsterdam. Int. Congr. Series No. 273, pp. 93–97.

Schwyzer, R., P. Schiller, S. Seelig and G. Sayers (1971). Isolated adrenal cells: Log dose response curves for steroidogenesis induced by $ACTH_{1-24}$, $ACTH_{1-10}$, $ACTH_{4-10}$ and $ACTH_{5-10}$. *FEBS Letters*, **19**, 229–231.

Seelig, S., G. Sayers, R. Schwyzer and P. Schiller (1971). Isolated adrenal cells: $ACTH_{11-24}$, a competitive antagonist of $ACTH_{1-39}$ and $ACTH_{1-10}$. *FEBS Letters*, **19**, 232–234.

*Thomas, P. J. (1973). Review: Steroid hormones and their receptors. *J. Endocrinol.*, **57**, 333–359.

*Ward, D. N., L. E. Reichert, W. K. Liu, H. S. Nahm, J. Hsia, W. M. Lamkin and N. S. Jones (1973). Chemical studies of LH from human and ovine pituitaries. *Recent Progress Hormone Research*, **29**, 533–561.

Wilson, S. C. and P. J. Sharp (1975). Episodic release of luteinizing hormone in the domestic fowl. *J. Endocrinol.*, **64**, 77–86.

Yalow, R. S. and S. A. Berson (1973). Characteristics of 'Big ACTH' in human plasma and pituitary extracts. *J. Clin. Endocrinol. Metab.*, **36**, 415–423.

CHAPTER 6

Adrenal cortex

I. INTRODUCTION

Higher vertebrates possess two ovoid or bean-shaped adrenal glands which sit embedded in fat above each kidney. A cross-section of the gland reveals two clearly separated regions — an inner yellowish coloured core, the *medulla*, surrounded by a red, darker-coloured cortex. The two regions are two distinct glands with separate functions and of different embryological origin, despite their anatomical relationship. The medulla, intrinsically a part of the nervous system, arises in the embryo from the neural crest of the ectoderm and produces the catecholamine hormones — adrenalin (epinephrine) and noradrenalin (norepinephrine). The cortex emanates from the mesoderm at an early stage in the development of the embryo, and in the human, cells originating from this layer are invaded by the medullary cells. In some species of lower vertebrates, the medulla and cortex exist separately. Useful books on the adrenal cortex and its functions include those by Eisenstein (1967), Jenkins (1968), McKerns (1968), Symington (1969), Griffiths and Cameron (1969) and Christy (1971). An informative symposium on the adrenal cortex has also been published (Thorn, 1972).

II. STRUCTURE OF THE ADRENAL CORTEX

In mammals three zones are usually discernible in the adrenal cortex (Figure 6.1):

i) directly beneath the capsule surrounding the gland, is an outer *zona glomerulosa*: these cells are arranged in whorls and appear grouped in clusters,

ii) generally constituting the majority of the adrenal cortex is the *zona*

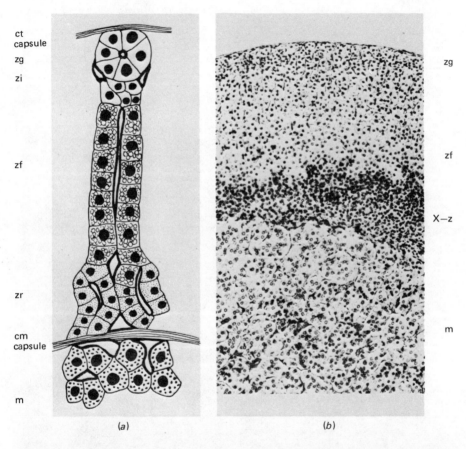

Figure 6.1 Histology of the mammalian adrenal gland. (*a*) Diagram to show zonation of adrenal cortex. Sinusoids are outlined by heavy black lines. (*b*) Section through adrenal cortex of male mouse, 1 month after castration at 3 months of age (x 120). X-zone of densely staining small cells has reappeared between zona fasciculata and medulla, in the region of the zona reticularis. *Abbreviations:* ct capsule, connective tissue capsule of adrenal gland; cm capsule, circum-medullary connective tissue capsule separating cortex from medulla, penetrated by cortical sinusoids which drain into medullary venous sinuses; m medulla of chromaffin cells arranged in lobules; X-z, X-zone characteristic of mouse adrenal cortex in absence of androgen; zf, zona fasciculata consisting of more or less vacuolated cells; zg, zona glomerulosa, poorly defined in mouse; zi, zona intermedia, prominent in rat and other mammals, but not in normal mouse; zr, zona reticularis (replaced by X-zone in castrated mouse). [Reproduced with permission from Gorbman, A., and H. A. Bern (1962). *A textbook of comparative endocrinology.* Wiley, New York, London.]

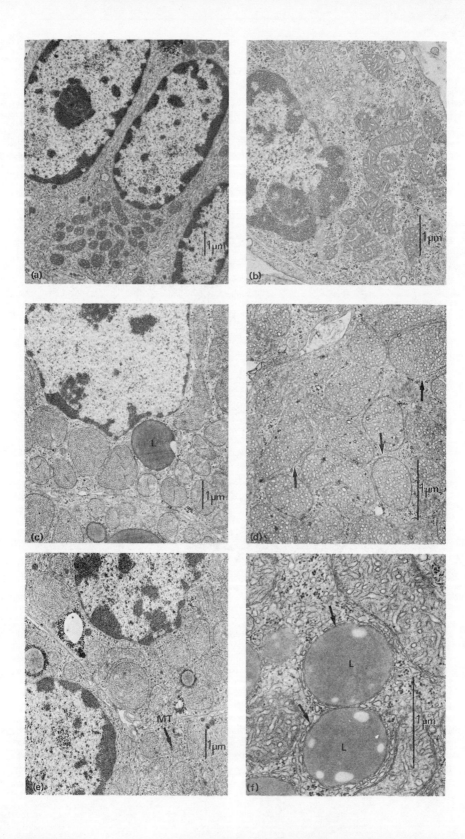

fasciculata arranged in columns of cholesterol-laden cells radiating towards the centre of the gland, and

iii) an inner *zona reticularis* of cells containing little cytoplasmic lipid, arranged in a network system.

These three zones are readily distinguished in man, rat, guinea-pig and rabbit, although in some other species and at particular ages, a clear-cut zonation of this nature is not found. In some mammals, notably the rat and the rabbit, a *zona intermedia* (Figure 6.1a) is evident, lying between the zona glomerulosa and the zona fasciculata.

In the foetal mammal other zones have been observed. In the human there is a considerable region in the inner cortex, designated the *foetal* or *juvenile cortex*, which comprises most of the adrenal gland in the new-born child. This region gradually degenerates and the adult cortex differentiates outside the broad band of the foetal cortex cells that surround the medulla. For further details and photomicrographs depicting the fine structure of adrenocortical tissues the reader is recommended to see Luse (1967) and Symington (1969).

A distinct inner region is discernible in the male mouse up to a month after birth. This zone, located where the zona reticularis is usually found, is called the X-zone (Figure 6.1b) and disappears after the male mouse reaches sexual maturity, or during the first pregnancy in the female. A similar zone is found in the rabbit.

The cells of cortical tissue or *interrenal cells* of non-mammalian vertebrates generally do not present any organized structural arrangement, apart from appearing as cords of cells in a network or irregular pattern. No distinct zonal arrangement is found in any lower vertebrates.

The electron micrographs in Figure 6.2 show the typical cell types found in the rat adrenal cortex. Of especial interest are the differences between mitochondrial shapes in the different zones. The mitochondria in the zona fasciculata appear

---

Figure 6.2   Electron micrographs of perfused-fixed rat adrenal glands. The rat strain was Sprague-Dawley where the zones are not as clearly differentiated as in some other strains. Reproduced by kind permission of Dr G. Bullock, Ciba Labs, Horsham.

(a) *Zona glomerulosa* cells at low magnification showing the close-packed, often very regular cells of this region. The rather dense mitochondria with tubular cristae are very characteristic of this zone. (x 9,400)

(b) *Zona glomerulosa* cell at higher magnification to show the mitchondrial structure. (x 17,000)

(c) *Zona fasciculata.* Many mitochondria fill the cytoplasm of this cell-type and the mitochondria show mainly the vesicular cristae typical of this zone. Lipid droplets (L) are in close proximity to the mitochondria. (x 11,250)

(d) *Zona fasciculata* at a higher magnification showing the detailed structure of the mitochondria. Many are surrounded by smooth endoplasmic reticulum (arrows). (x 25,000)

(e) *Zona reticularis.* Cells from this region contain a large number of smaller distinct mitochondria, which in this strain of rat nearly always contain bundles of microtubules (MT, arrows). (x 11,250)

(f) *Zona reticularis.* Mitochondria and lipid droplets (L) from this region seen at higher magnification. The close relationship between smooth endoplasmic reticulum (arrows) and lipid is clearly visible and very similar to that between smooth endoplasmic reticulum and the mitochondria seen in electron micrograph (d). (x 37,500)

round or ovoid with characteristic vesicular cristae, and their great abundance in this zone deserves particular emphasis, as too does the presence of large numbers of cholesterol-rich lipid droplets. The zona fasciculata is most responsive to ACTH and these cells are primarily responsible for the secretion of cortisol and corticosterone. The regulatory role of ACTH is believed to involve an intimate relationship between the mitochondrial enzymes and cytoplasmic steroid precursors and regulatory agents (see Chapter 11). The zona glomerulosa is unique in being the site of production of aldosterone and the zona reticularis is suggested as the site of adrenal androgen and estrogen biosynthesis although these cells also have the capacity to produce cortisol and corticosterone (Mikail, 1973).

III. ADRENAL BLOOD SUPPLY

The mammalian adrenal has an exceptionally high blood flow-rate and the large volume of blood continuously flowing through the gland arises from three main groups of arteries. These branch into multiple tiny vessels as they approach the gland and as many as fifty different vessels may penetrate the connective tissue capsule. The vascular system of the human adrenal gland has been elucidated by Dobbie, *et al.*, (1968). Two patterns of vascular architecture have been observed in different regions of the human gland (Figure 6.3). One part of the human gland (the 'tail' region) comprises only cortical tissue, whilst other parts (the 'head' and 'body' regions) contain combined cortex and medulla. In the purely cortical 'tail' regions of the gland, the blood flows through the narrow, subcapsular plexus into parallel capillaries between the columns of cells on the zona fasciculata, and thence to the plexus reticularis. This plexus ends abruptly in what resembles a complex

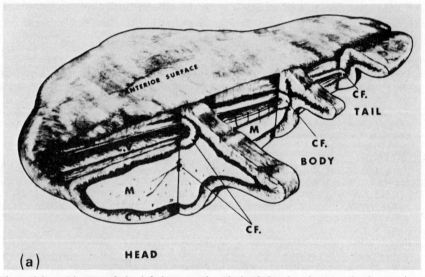

Figure 6.3a Diagram of the left human adrenal gland showing the central vein entering the gland, surrounded by a cuff (CF) of cortical tissue. Note small cuff of cortical tissue which surrounds the branches of the vein in the medulla (M).

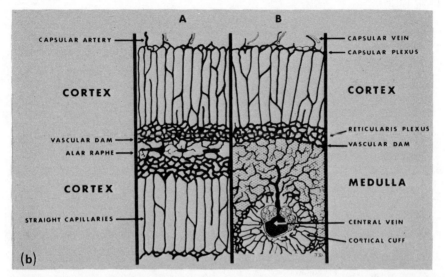

Figure 6.3b This diagram illustrates the two types of circulation present in the human adrenal gland. In the purely cortical regions of the gland, in the tail and in the alae (A), the plexus reticularis is drained by vessels lying in the alar raphe. Where the cortex and medulla are in juxtaposition (B), a type of portal system is found in which the blood is eventually collected in venous sinuses which may then pass through between the muscle pillars of the veins as shown here. [Reproduced with permission of Churchill—Livingstone, Edinburgh, from Symington (1969).]

vascular dam and the blood then passes by relatively few channels, into the sinusoids of the *alar raphae.* In the 'head' and 'body' regions of the gland, blood from the plexus reticularis passes into the branching sinusoids in the medulla. The overriding impression from these structural features is that the adrenal gland is specifically designed to ensure an extremely rich arterial supply and blood drainage system, for all cortical cells.

IV. STEROIDS SECRETED BY THE ADRENAL CORTEX

The adrenal cortex is responsible for the production of a very large number of different steroids and well over 40 different steroids have now been isolated from adrenocortical tissue. However, many are only intermediates or precursors, others are detectable in only minute quantities and some are likely to be extraction artifacts. Of especial interest are those steroids found in adrenal venous blood draining from the gland, and in particular those estimated to be present in higher concentration than in the arterial blood delivered to the cortex. Such steroids may be assumed to be secreted by the adrenal cortex and are shown in Table 6.1.

A. Corticosteroids

The biologically active or important members of this group are depicted in Figure 6.4. The active corticosteroids are all C_{21} steroids having a ketol side-chain

Table 6.1.

Principal steroids secreted by the adrenal cortex

Cortisol
Corticosterone
11-Deoxycortisol
11-Deoxycorticosterone
4-Androstene-3,17-dione
Dehydroepiandrosterone
Dehydroepiandrosterone sulphate
17-Hydroxyprogesterone
17-Hydroxypregnenolone
11β-Hydroxy-4-androstene-3,17-dione
18-Hydroxy-11-deoxycorticosterone
11-Oxoprogesterone
11β-Hydroxyprogesterone
Cortisone
11-Dehydrocorticosterone
Progesterone
Aldosterone
20α-Hydroxy-4-pregnen-3-one
Pregnenolone
Estrone

For further details see: Samuels, L. T. and T. Uchikawa (1967). In Eisenstein (Ed.) *The Adrenal Cortex* Little, Brown & Co., Boston, p. 62, and Baird *et al.* (1969).

($-CO \cdot CH_2OH$, with a characteristic 21-hydroxy group) and the 4-en-3-one conjugated double bond system ($_{O}\overset{\sim}{\sim}$). They differ from one another only in the nature of the functions at C-11, C-17 and C-18.

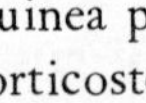

Different species secrete different corticosteroid products. In the rat, rabbit, mouse and in many birds, corticosterone is the predominant product of the adrenal cortex. Although this corticosteroid is secreted by the human adrenal, the most important products here are cortisol and aldosterone and this is also true for various other species including monkey, guinea pig, sheep, cattle, pig and many fish. Such comparative aspects of adrenal corticosteroidogenesis have been comprehensively reviewed (Vinson and Whitehouse, 1970).

The secretion of corticosteroids is subject to a circadian rhythm, being maximal at about 6 a.m. (80—300 ng/ml plasma), and minimal during the evening (about 50 ng/ml plasma). Moreover, it alters considerably in accordance with variations in other hormones which regulate the hormonal status of the animal. Thus there is a wide variation in ACTH secretion throughout the day. Pulses of ACTH are released from the pituitary as shown in Figure 6.5, with consequent stimulatory effects on adrenal corticosteroidogenesis which follow the episodic spurts in ACTH secretion. Features of the circadian rhythm found for the hypothalamo—pituitary—adrenal axis (and other steroidogenic systems) have been reviewed in detail, with particular regard to their relationship to sleep (Daly and Evans, 1974). In man the normal total daily secretion of cortisol is about 15—30 mg, compared with 2—5 mg of corticosterone and 0.1—0.2 mg of aldosterone. The average concentrations of these

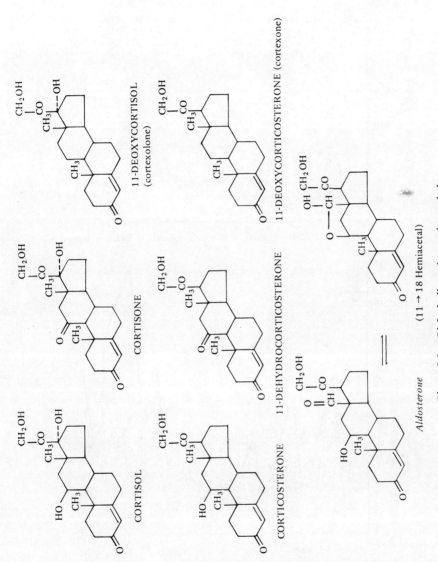

Figure 6.4 Biologically active corticosteriods.

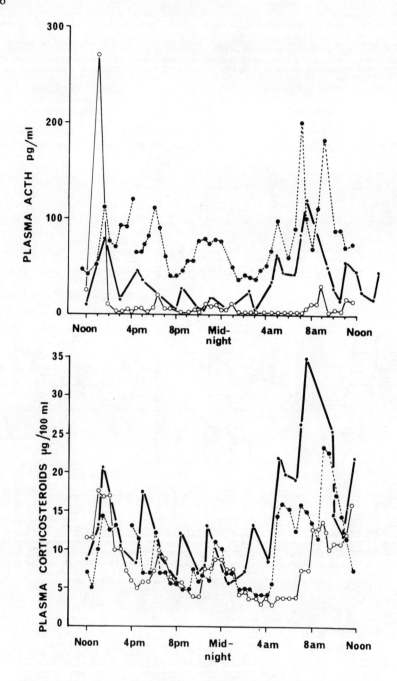

Figure 6.5 Circadian periodicity in concentration of plasma ACTH (by radioimmunoassay) and plasma corticosteroids (by fluorescence assay) in three normal humans. For further details see: Kreiger, Allen, Rizzo and Kreiger (1971), *J. Clin. Endocrinol.*, 32, 266–284; and Berson and Yalow (1968), *J. Clin. Invest.*, 47, 2725–2751.

Table 6.2.

Relative biological potencies of some adrenal corticosteroids and synthetic steroids

Corticosteroid	Life maintaining ability	Liver glycogen deposition	Anti-inflammatory effect	Salt retaining (mineralo-corticoid) effect
Cortisol	1	1	1	1
Corticosterone	0.8	0.3	0.3	1.6
*Prednisolone (1,2-Dehydrocortisol)	2	4	3	1
*Dexamethasone (9α-Fluoro-16 α-methyl-prednisolone)	–	17	28	0.1
Aldosterone	80	0.3	0	300
DOC (11-Deoxycorticosterone)	4	0	0	10

*For structures see Figure 16.1

Data obtained using the adrenalectomized rat for which a life-maintaining dose of cortisol is 2 mg/100 gm body wt/day. The amounts of liver glycogen deposited 1 hr after steroid injections were compared with that obtained after administering $100\,\mu g$ cortisol/100 gm. Anti-inflammatory potency was estimated by the 'granuloma pouch test' which measures the effect of different steroids on the weight of a fibrous deposit (a granuloma) induced by an implanted irritant. Mineralocorticoid activity was evaluated from the Na^+ and K^+ appearing in the urine of adrenalectomized rats on controlled salt and water allowance.

hormones as unconjugated steroids in the peripheral blood system are respectively about 100 ng, 10 ng and 0.1 ng per ml of plasma, although of course these values all vary widely with the hormonal status (e.g. the actual ACTH secretion at any particular time; see Figure 6.5). 11-Deoxycortisol has also been found in human plasma in concentrations of about 10 ng per ml, and this compares with the occurrence of 11-deoxycorticosterone in the plasma of those species in which corticosterone is the predominant corticosteroid. A considerable amount of the steroid hormone content of blood is in the form of *conjugates* as steroid glucuronides and sulphates (Chapter 10). Estimates of total conjugated corticosteroids in normal plasma vary between 50–200 ng per ml.

The corticosteroids may be subdivided into the *glucocorticoids* such as corticosterone and cortisol (which affect carbohydrate metabolism and have anti-inflammatory activity) and the *mineralocorticoids* such as aldosterone and 11-deoxycorticosterone, noted for their Na^+-retaining activity. The biological activities of these adrenocorticoids are shown in Table 6.2 and further details are given in Chapters 15 and 16.

The corticosteroids are rapidly removed from the blood and the half-life of cortisol has been estimated at about 110 min in normal men. This is the time required for the blood concentration of the hormone to be halved. In patients with liver disease the biological half-life is longer (200–800 min). These data compare with estimates of the biological half-life of ACTH in plasma of about 25 min (Berson and Yalow, 1968). Aldosterone is very rapidly eliminated from the blood — within half an hour in normal humans.

B. Adrenal Androgens and Estrogens

Androgenic and other C_{19} steroids secreted by the normal adrenal cortex include androstenedione, 11-hydroxyandrostenedione and dehydroepiandrosterone (DHA) and its sulphate (DHA sulphate). These compounds are the main precursors of the 17-oxosteroids excreted in the urine. However, the total urinary 17-oxosteroids (for many years the only clinical test for assessing androgen production; see Chapter 2.IV) are also derived from ovarian and testicular products, and consequently do not reflect the production of androgens from any one androgen-producing gland.

The production rate of DHA in man exceeds that of cortisol and has been estimated at 25—30 mg/day, while the other adrenal androgens excreted amount to 5—15 mg/day. The blood production rate of androstenedione in normal men and women is about 2 mg/day. Estrogens (mainly estrone) have also been shown to be secreted by the human adrenal, but compared with corticosteroids, in minute amounts — about 10 μg/day (Baird *et al.*, 1969). In normal human peripheral plasma, the most abundant C_{19} steroids present are DHA sulphate and androsterone sulphate (a metabolic product of androstenedione; see Figure 10.8). The levels of these conjugates are similar in men and women at about 1.2 μg/ml and 0.4 μg/ml, respectively, and are compared with other conjugated and unconjugated C_{19} steroids found in human plasma in Table 6.3. (See also Table 8.1.)

The adrenal C_{19} steroids exhibit only relatively weak androgenic activity — androstenedione, DHA and 11-hydroxyandrostenedione having respectively only one fifth, one tenth and one hundredth of the biological activity of testosterone.

C_{19} steroids from the foetal adrenal cortex play an important role in the overall

Table 6.3.
Androgens in human plasma (mean values; μg/100 ml)

Androgen	Men	Women
Sulphate conjugates		
Dehydroepiandrosterone	126	113
Androsterone	43	36
Aetiocholanolone*	1.5	1.7
Testosterone	.11	.02
Glucuronide conjugates		
Androsterone	2.2	1.5
Aetiocholanolone*	1.8	1.5
Unconjugated androgens		
Testosterone	.56	.05
Androstenedione	.11	.18
Dehydroepiandrosterone	.55	.53
Dihydrotestosterone	.05	.02
11β-Hydroxyandrostenedione	.20	.18
Androsterone	.16	.07
Aetiocholanolone*	.07	.18

From: Migeon (1972). See also Table 8.1, page 131.
*3α-Hydroxy-5β-androstan-17-one

production of steroids by the foeto-placental unit and these aspects, together with the pathological conditions (congenital adrenal hyperplasia and virilizing adrenal tumours) leading to hypersecretion of adrenal androgens, have been reviewed (Migeon, 1972) — see subsection VI.

Adrenal androgens all bind to albumin with a low affinity (Forest *et al.*, 1968) compared with the high affinity exhibited by testosterone for its specific testosterone-binding globulin (see Chapter 14.VI).

V. CORTICOSTEROID-BINDING TO BLOOD PROTEINS

It is now recognised that many hormones are transported in the blood, closely associated with, or directly bound to plasma proteins (Daughaday, 1967). Corticosteroids bind to two plasma proteins: albumin and an α-globulin known as transcortin (also referred to as corticosteroid-binding globulin, CBG). Serum albumin has a low affinity but high capacity for cortisol — i.e. this protein can loosely bind a great deal of steroid. Transcortin on the other hand has a high affinity but low capacity for cortisol. The albumin-bound steroid is readily metabolized by the liver, whereas the globulin-steroid complex is not (Baird *et al.*, 1969). About 94% of blood-borne cortisol is protein-bound and of this about 15% is bound to albumin (Dixon *et al.*, 1967). It is thought that only the minor unbound fraction of the steroid hormone is biologically active. The concentration of transcortin in blood has been estimated at about 30 μg/ml and the transcortin in one ml of plasma can bind 200—300 ng of cortisol. Corticosterone can also bind to transcortin, but its affinity for this steroid is less than that for cortisol. In blood aldosterone associates mainly with albumin, although the binding of aldosterone to plasma proteins is much less than that of either cortisol or corticosterone. About 60% of the aldosterone in plasma is albumin-bound.

During pregnancy and estrogen therapy, the concentration of transcortin in plasma increases and abnormally high values are found in women taking steroidal oral contraceptives. Although in the later stages of pregnancy the total blood cortisol levels greatly increase and may even exceed those observed in Cushing's syndrome (see Subsection VI), there are no accompanying symptoms usually associated with a hyper-adrenal condition. This is attributed to the accompanying rise in transcortin concentration which results in a greater proportion of transcortin-bound cortisol and thus about normal levels of the unbound, active steroid. During pregnancy there is a marked increase in unbound aldosterone levels. In the new-born child decreased transcortin levels are observed, with the unbound cortisol representing a greater fraction of the total cortisol than is found in the adult. It is thus important to ascertain free (or unbound) plasma corticosteroid levels, rather than simply the total steroid hormone plasma levels.

The isolation and characterization of transcortin has shown it to be a protein of molecular weight 51,700 containing one binding site per molecule for cortisol (Muldoon and Westphal, 1967).

VI. DISORDERS OF ADRENOCORTICAL FUNCTION

Over the last decade there has been an enormous improvement in the laboratory techniques available for diagnosis of the diseases of the adrenal cortex. These techniques, which allow the determination of picograms (10^{-12} gm) of hormone in blood and urine (Chapter 2) now permit accurate assessments of abnormalities in adrenocortical function. Although relatively rare in occurrence, these disorders may now be very largely alleviated after correct diagnosis and treatment. For detailed descriptions of these disorders and their management see appropriate articles in Eisenstein (1967), Mason (1972), Christy (1971) and Thorn (1972). Recently a text particularly related to the use of ACTH and corticosteroids in medicine has been published (Myles and Daly, 1974) that describes more fully those aspects detailed below.

A. Hypofunction of the Adrenal Cortex

Two major syndromes of adrenocortical hypofunction are known and are accompanied by subnormal production of corticosteroids. In addition to those abnormalities described below, glucocorticoid and mineralocorticoid deficiencies may result from inborn errors of metabolism, e.g. isolated hypoaldosteronism and congenital adrenal hyperplasia (see later).

1. Addison's Disease (Primary Adrenal Insufficiency)

This disorder results from partial or complete destruction of all three zones of the cortex. All functions of the adrenal cortex are usually affected and the clinical features of this condition reflect the lack of glucocorticoids and mineralocorticoids. In the majority of patients it is due to autoimmune adrenal atrophy or tuberculosis although occasionally other causes such as secondary tumours, adrenal haemorrhage, amyloidosis and haemochromatosis have been implicated.

The number of pituitary corticotrophs are increased during the disease, reflecting the hypersecretion of ACTH (> 400 pg/ml plasma) in an attempt to overcome the cortisol deficiency. Although the secretions of all the corticosteroids by the adrenal are decreased during the progress of the disease, the clinical features (arterial hypotension, hypoglycaemia, anaemia, decreased metabolic rate and subnormal serum levels of Na^+ and Cl^-) may be entirely attributed to inadequate levels of cortisol and aldosterone. Pigmentation may occur, due to the high circulating ACTH and MSH levels, the secretions of which both become increased via operation of the negative feedback control system. More severe symptoms may not be apparent until less than 10% of the adrenal cortex remains functional. In Addison's disease, both plasma and urine steroid levels are below normal.

The metabolites of corticosteroids excreted in the urine may fall to 10−20% of normal values and cortisol production rates can vary from 0.5 up to about 10 mg/day (compared with the normal production of 15−30 mg/day). However, since patients with this condition may have basal corticosteroid levels within the accepted normal range, reliance on these determinations alone for diagnosis of Addison's disease is not sufficient. Definitive diagnosis depends upon the demonstration of low corticosteroid production in the presence of high plasma ACTH concentrations. In Addison's disease, because the adrenal is incapacitated and already stimulated fully by high circulating levels of ACTH, additional amounts of ACTH will have no effect. Thus the injection of exogenous ACTH does not change plasma or urinary steroid levels and this forms the basis of the 'ACTH stimulation test'.

2. Secondary Adrenal Insufficiency (Pituitary Insufficiency)

This is a disorder due to the deficient pituitary secretion of ACTH for any reason. Under such circumstances the adrenal cortex atrophies and there is a decrease in the secretion of both glucocorticoids and C_{19} steroids. Aldosterone production, however, remains largely unaffected since it is not substantially under the control of ACTH. Impaired ACTH secretion may be due to interference with either pituitary or hypothalamic function. Thus pituitary tumours may destroy normal pituitary tissue and lead to a decline in ACTH secretion. Pituitary failure can also be a consequence of chronic corticosteroid administration for therapeutic purposes (e.g. for the treatment of rheumatoid arthritis). In this instance, continued corticoid treatment suppresses ACTH secretion by feedback inhibition (see Chapter 5) and sudden cessation of the steroid therapy can leave an incompetent pituitary and result in adrenal insufficiency. Alternatively there may be some malfunction in the production or action of CRH (see Chapter 5) or some other interruption of the hypothalamic-hypophyseal system which leads to impaired ACTH secretion.

The clinical features of adrenal insufficiency are the same as those of Addison's disease, except that pigmentation is absent because of the very low levels of circulating ACTH ($<$ 10 pg/ml plasma), and that even in severe cases the salt balance is less disturbed because the aldosterone secretion is largely independent of ACTH. Moreover, the pituitary defect responsible for ACTH deficiency is often associated with deficiencies in other pituitary hormones which lead to yet further disorders. The diagnostic procedures undertaken are the same as those used for Addison's disease, but in this instance show abnormally *low* plasma ACTH concentrations and the injection of exogenous ACTH should increase plasma or urinary steroid concentrations.

B. Hyperfunction of the Adrenal Cortex

Three types of *lesions* may result in adrenal hyperfunction:

a) *'Adrenal hyperplasia'*. Abnormally increased adrenal function may not always be associated with adrenal growth, however, for simplicity this term is used whether actual enlargement is observable or not.

b) *Benign adenomas*. Such tumours may or may not be responsive to ACTH and thus may be either under pituitary control or not.

c) *Carcinomas*. These are often large tumours and again vary in their degree of pituitary independence (autonomy).

Four *syndromes* of adrenal hyperfunction are known:

1. Cushing's Syndrome

Cushing's syndrome is essentially caused by excessive cortisol production by the adrenal cortex. This term describes the clinical condition deriving from either

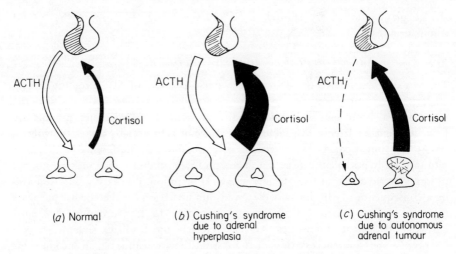

(a) Normal   (b) Cushing's syndrome due to adrenal hyperplasia   (c) Cushing's syndrome due to autonomous adrenal tumour

Figure 6.6   Pituitary–adrenal function in Cushing's syndrome.

adrenal hyperplasia or tumour irrespective of a concomitant pituitary tumour. 'Cushing's disease' usually describes the condition of adrenal hyperactivity in the presence of an ACTH-secreting pituitary adenoma. The pituitary-adrenal relationship that pertains to Cushing's syndrome in hyperplasia and autonomous adrenal tumour is depicted in Figure 6.6. In this diagram (a) represents the normal feedback relationship whereby ACTH stimulates cortisol production which in turn inhibits excessive ACTH production; (b) shows how in adrenal hyperplasia there is excessive ACTH production by the pituitary, the function of which is not inhibited by normal cortisol levels, and the consequence is then overproduction of cortisol; and (c) in autonomous adrenal tumours, the cortisol synthesized in the tumour by an ACTH-independent process, suppresses the pituitary ACTH production and thereby results in atrophy of the normal ACTH-dependent cells of the adrenal cortex.

Determination of the elevated levels of 17-hydroxycorticosteroids in urine or plasma are valuable aids in establishing diagnosis of Cushing's syndrome. Moreover, the various causes of the syndrome may be distinguished by suppression tests with either dexamethasone (see Figure 16.1) — a synthetic steroid which inhibits ACTH output thereby blocking adrenal cortisol production, or with metopirone (metyrapone) — which specifically inhibits 11β-hydroxylation, leading to decreased cortisol production and consequent increased pituitary ACTH output in an effort to restore normal cortisol levels. Stimulation tests employing ACTH injection are also used but are often not very helpful, except when there is no resulting increase in plasma or urinary 17-hydroxycorticoids, since this is almost invariably associated with an autonomous adrenal carcinoma or adenoma. However, the most useful and direct means of differentiating between the various forms of this syndrome is to measure plasma ACTH concentrations, which are high in 'Cushing's disease' but low in autonomous adrenal lesions.

2. Adrenogenital Syndromes (Congenital Adrenal Hyperplasia)

Congenital syndromes exist — rather rarely — in which there is an absence or a limitation of enzymes involved in cortisol biosynthesis. Four of these enzyme deficiencies are known. The syndrome is associated with sexual effects in which the excessive production of androgens by the adrenal cortex results in masculinization of the female and precocious puberty in the male. The enzyme deficiencies result in

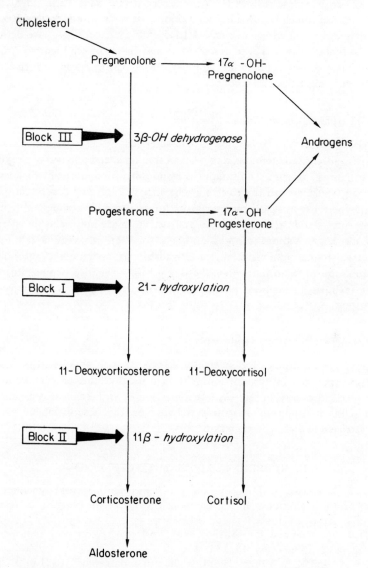

Figure 6.7 Deficiencies in adrenal enzymes found in the different adrenogenital syndromes.

inadequate cortisol production giving rise to excessive ACTH output from the pituitary in an attempt to correct the cortisol levels, but resulting instead in an increased production of androgens.

The biosynthetic pathways for adrenal steroid synthesis and the sites of deficiencies in the enzymes involved in adrenogenital syndromes are outlined in Figure 6.7. The most common form of the syndrome involves a deficiency of adrenal 21-hydroxylase (block I). Another relatively rare form involves the 11β-hydroxylase (block II). A third condition, even rarer, results from a deficiency of the 3β-hydroxy-dehydrogenase (block III), while an exceedingly rare deficiency of the 17α-hydroxylase has been described. It may be seen from Figure 6.7 that the blocks at these different points in the biosynthetic pathway lead to high levels of androgen and progestogen metabolites.

3. Primary Aldosteronism (Conn's Syndrome)

In its classic form this syndrome is characterized by an autonomous adrenal hyperplasia, adrenal adenoma or rarely by a carcinoma, and removal of the tumour effects an immediate cure. The tumour is responsible for abnormally high levels of aldosterone which disturb the electrolyte balance (K^+ loss and Na^+ retention) and produce hypertension. Radioimmunoassays for plasma aldosterone and renin and measurements of aldosterone secretion and excretion are now valuable laboratory aids to diagnosis. Various suppression tests (oral or intravenous salt loading, deoxycorticosterone administration) are available to examine the autonomy or semi-autonomy of aldosterone synthesis by, for example, demonstrating the patient's inability to suppress plasma aldosterone levels after being subjected to such tests.

4. Feminizing and Virilizing syndromes

These very rare syndromes are invariably associated with an adrenal tumour and estrogen or androgen overproduction. Although usually other adrenal steroids are also produced in excess, in rare cases feminization or virilization may be the most apparent clinical condition. Diagnosis is based on the observation of excessive urinary estrogen or androgen excretion.

VII. REFERENCES (*indicates review or book)

Baird, D. T., R. Horton, C. Longcope and J. F. Tait (1969). Steroid dynamics under steady state conditions. In E. Astwood (Ed.) *Recent Progress in Hormone Research*. Academic Press, N.Y. pp. 611–664.

Baird, D. T., A. Uno and J. C. Melby (1969). Adrenal secretion of androgens and oestrogens. *J. Endocrinol.*, 45, 135–136.

Berson, S. A. and R. S. Yalow (1968). Radioimmunoassay of ACTH in plasma. *J. Clin. Invest.*, 47, 2725–2751.

*Christy, N. P. (Ed.) (1971). *The human adrenal cortex*. Harper & Row, New York. 538 pages.

*Daly, J. R. and J. I. Evans (1974). Daily rhythms of steroid and associated pituitary hormones in man and their relationship to sleep. In M. H. Briggs and G. A. Christie (Eds) *Advances in Steroid Biochemistry & Pharmacology*. Vol. 4, Academic Press, London. pp. 61—110.

*Daughaday, W. H. (1967). The binding of corticosteroids by plasma protein. In A. B. Eisenstein (Ed.) *The Adrenal Cortex*. Little, Brown & Co., Boston. pp. 385—403.

*Dixon, P. F., M. Booth and J. Butler (1967). The corticosteroids. In C. H. Gray and A. L. Bacharach (Eds) *Hormones in Blood*. Vol. 2, Academic Press, London. pp. 305—389.

Dobbie, J. W., A. M. Mackay and T. Symington (1968). In V. H. T. James and J. Landon (Eds). *Memoirs of the Soc. for Endocrinology*, No. 1. Cambridge Univ. Press. p. 103.

*Eisenstein, A. B. (Ed.) (1967). *The Adrenal Cortex*. Little, Brown & Co., Boston. 685 pages.

Forest, M. G., M. A. Rivarola and C. J. Migeon (1968). Percentage binding of testosterone, androstenedione and DHA in human plasma. *Steroids*, 12, 323—343.

*Griffiths, K., and E. H. D. Cameron (Eds) (1969). *The Human Adrenal Gland and its Relation to Breast Cancer: 1st Tenovus Workshop*. Alpha, Omega, Alpha Publishing, Cardiff. 111 pages.

*Jenkins, J. S. (1968). *Biochemical Aspects of the Adrenal Cortex*. Edward Arnold Ltd., London, 120 pages.

*Luse, S. (1967). Fine Structure of Adrenal Cortex. In A. B. Eisenstein (Ed.). *The Adrenal Cortex*. Little, Brown & Co., Boston. pp. 1—59.

*Mason, S. (Ed.) (1972). *Clinics in Endocrinology and Metabolism*. Vol. 1, No. 2. Diseases of the adrenal cortex. W. B. Saunders Co. Ltd., London. 598 pages.

*McKerns, K. W. (Ed.) (1968). *Functions of the Adrenal Cortex*, Vols 1 and 2. Appleton-Century-Crofts, New York. 1176 pages.

*Migeon, C. J. (1972). Adrenal androgens in man. *Amer. J. Med.*, 53, 606—626.

Mikail, Y. (1973). A study of some of the histological and histochemical features of the zona reticularis. *Acta Anat. (Basel)*, 84, 498—508.

Muldoon, T. G. and U. Westphal (1967). Steroid—protein interactions: isolation and characterization of corticosteroid-binding globulin from human plasma. *J. Biol. Chem.*, 242, 5636—5643.

*Myles, A. B. and J. R. Daly (1974). *Corticosteroid and ACTH treatment*. Edward Arnold, London. 230 pages.

*Symington, T. (1969). *Functional Pathology of the human adrenal gland*. Churchill—Livingstone Ltd, Edinburgh & London.

*Thorn, G. W. (Ed.) (1972). Symposium on the Adrenal Cortex. *Amer. J. Med.*, 53, 529—684.

*Vinson, G. P., and B. J. Whitehouse (1970). Comparative aspects of adrenocortical function. In M. H. Briggs (Ed.) *Advances in Steroid Biochemistry and Pharmacology*, Vol. 1. Academic Press, London. p. 163—342.

CHAPTER 7

Ovary

I. INTRODUCTION

The paired ovaries in all known mammalian species perform two functions: gametogenic, in the production of ova, and endocrine, in the production of steroid hormones. The ripening and release of the ova proceeds through a regular cycle of events controlled by the trophic hormones follicle stimulating hormone (FSH), luteinizing hormone (LH) and prolactin. The release of the trophic hormones from the pituitary is under the local control of releasing hormones from the hypothalamus, which in turn are controlled by the steroid hormones. The mechanism by which the ovarian periodicity is regulated is perhaps the most complicated inter-relationship of hypothalamus, pituitary and an endocrine organ. Although considerable variation exists for accomplishing this precise control throughout the mammalian kingdom, there are many relationships which are common, whether one considers the estrous cycle of the lower mammals or the menstrual cycle of the primate.

Detailed reviews on the ovary have been published by Donovan and van der Werff ten Bosch (1965), Schwartz and Hoffman (1972), Short (1972), Kragt and Dahlgren (1972) and Eskes *et al.* (1974).

II. OVULATION

At birth the human female ovary contains approximately 2 million germ cells or oocytes. By the time the age of puberty has been reached, the number of

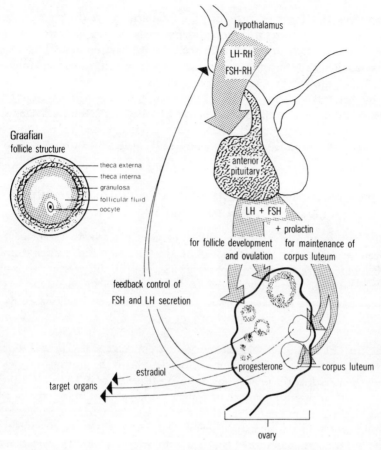

Figure 7.1   Interrelationships between hypothalamus, pituitary ovary and uterus.

primordial follicles, each of which is potentially able to ovulate and be fertilized, has dropped to 200,000–300,000. It is probable that no new ones are formed during post-natal development. The primordial follicles ripen into Graafian follicles (Figure 7.1) and burst to release the ova.

 In primates, including women, generally only one follicle ripens at a time. The mechanism by which a single follicle matures each month is unknown. Many other animals of course produce and release many ova at one time. After ovulation the ovum or ova pass down the Fallopian tube where fertilization by the spermatozoa from the male can take place. The fertilized ova are implanted in the uterine wall and then begin to divide to form the blastocysts. If fertilization does not take place the ova pass out of the uterus and the cycle begins again. In women, ovulation takes place approximately every 28 days from puberty until menopause.

 In the follicle the cell layer surrounding the germ cell is referred to as the *granulosa* layer, while the stroma cells immediately adjacent to this are the *theca interna* (Figure 7.1). As proliferation takes place, fluid accumulates between the granulosa cells and forms a small cavity containing the *follicular fluid*. During maturation of the follicle the theca interna cells enlarge and are extensively vascularized, in contrast to the granulosa cells, which have no direct blood supply before ovulation. The mature follicle is known as the Graafian follicle in recognition of the Dutch scientist Reinier de Graaf, who first described it (see review by Setchell in Eskes *et al.*, 1974). When it reaches maturity, the follicle ruptures on the surface of the ovary. Following ovulation the follicle collapses, and the granulosa and theca interna cells rapidly proliferate and at the same time become intensely vascularized. This ruptured follicle is transformed into the *corpus luteum*.

III. GONADOTROPHIN AND OVARIAN STEROID SECRETION BEFORE PUBERTY

With the introduction of sensitive radioimmunoassay methods, recent advances have been made in our understanding of the pituitary and ovarian hormone secretions which take place before puberty. FSH and LH are present for example both in the rat pituitary and blood very soon after birth. FSH especially, is secreted in increasing amounts to reach a peak at day 10 thereafter decreasing to day 25 (Figure 7.2). This FSH peak is paralleled by secretion of estradiol-17β from the ovary.

In the first 10 days of life the rat ovary differentiates and degenerates. Primary follicles develop from the attachment of follicle cells to the growing oocytes and the primary interstitial tissue develops. In the next period (day 10 to day 20) there is rapid growth of a great number of follicles although the larger type of antral (Graafian) follicles do not yet appear. It is at this time that ovarian steroid synthesis begins presumably in the interstitial tissue. The third period (day 20—puberty) is characterized by the appearance of large antral follicles (Figure 7.2). Ovulation does not normally take place in the rat until day 35—40, but in the last period of development before puberty precocious ovulation can be induced by exogenous gonadotrophin.

The exact relationship between ovary, hypothalamus and pituitary in terms of control of their secretions during these periods is not yet understood. In view of the parallel levels of estradiol and FSH it is difficult to postulate a feedback mechanism. However, it is known that exogenous estradiol lowers the high blood levels of FSH caused by ovariectomy in the prepubertal rat.

IV. GONADOTROPHIN AND STEROID SECRETION DURING THE MENSTRUAL CYCLE

Follicles are capable of maturing in the initial stages without stimulation by gonadotrophins. That the continued growth of the follicle requires gonadotrophins has been known for a long time, but the exact nature of these hormones has only recently been investigated. Originally it was thought that FSH caused follicle growth and stimulated estrogen secretion, whereas LH was essential for the rupture

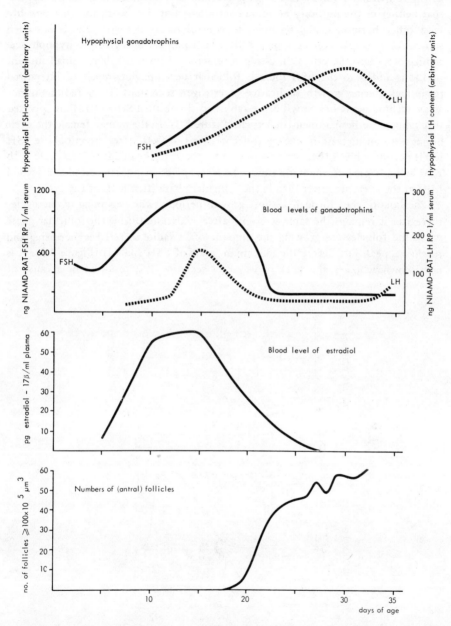

Figure 7.2 Pituitary gonadotrophin content, hormone levels in the blood and follicular development in the immature rat. [Data from Meijs-Roelofs, *Ph.D. thesis*, Erasmus University, Rotterdam; Ojeda and Ramirez (1972); Kragt and Dahlgren (1972); and Meijs-Roelofs *et al*. (1973).]

of the follicles and stimulation of progesterone secretion. Recent evidence suggests that neither of the pituitary hormones act alone, but they work together possibly with other hormones, e.g. prolactin to control the ovulatory cycle. It has been shown for example that very pure FSH or LH preparations given to hypophysectomized rats have no effect on estrogen secretion. However, when a small amount of LH is added to the FSH there is follicular development, repair of interstitial tissue and uterine growth (indicative of estrogen secretion). Using radioimmunoassay techniques it has now been established that both FSH and LH are secreted throughout the human menstrual cycle (Figure 7.3). In the human female the cycle begins with an increase in plasma concentrations of FSH. After the initial rise FSH levels decline while LH levels continue to increase. In the middle of the cycle both FSH and LH peak at the same time. The levels of FSH in the luteal phase (second half) of the cycle are lower than in the follicular phase (first half) of the cycle.

The oocyte goes through a short growth period at the beginning of the cycle, thereafter it remains the same size until after ovulation. During the follicular phase while the follicles are growing the amount of estradiol secreted is increasing and reaches a peak just before the maximum levels of FSH and LH (Figure 7.3). It is not known whether the peak of estradiol secretion is a result of or a cause of

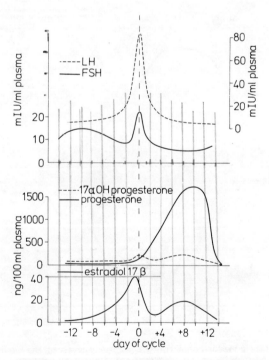

Figure 7.3 Levels of LH, FSH, progesterone, 17α-hydroxyprogesterone and estradiol-17β in the normal human menstrual cycle. Day 0 is the day of maximum LH levels in plasma. [Data taken from D. T. Baird (1971) and G. T. Ross *et al.* (1970).]

follicular development. Again it is not known what the function is, if any, of the 17-hydroxyprogesterone which progressively increases during the first half of the cycle and peaks at the same time as LH and FSH. It may be just a reflection of increased steroid biosynthesis. The initial increase in the level of progesterone occurs at the peak of FSH and LH secretion and reaches a maximum in the middle of the luteal phase (Figure 7.3).

V. THE ROLE OF GONADOTROPHINS IN OVULATION

It has been clearly shown that under the right conditions LH administration will cause ovulation. It is also apparent that an acute surge of LH is necessary. However, the apparent lack of activity of pure LH in the rat, already referred to, taken together with the coincident high levels of FSH and prolactin, in addition to LH, might indicate that LH alone is not responsible for causing ovulation.

VI. FUNCTION OF STEROIDS SECRETED DURING FOLLICULAR PHASE

The actual mechanism by which LH is released probably entails an increase in LH-releasing hormone. The secretion of the releasing hormone must be triggered off by a mechanism operating at exactly the right time when the follicle is mature. This mechanism is thought to be mediated by increased steroid secretion, most probably estradiol, which peaks just before the LH surge (Figure 7.3). It has been clearly shown in a number of species that estradiol will induce ovulation. However, there appear to be additional factors which operate with the estradiol. In the rat this is a time of day signal while in the rabbit it is the stimulus of mating.

VII. THE CORPUS LUTEUM

The life of the corpus luteum in the human female is about 14 days, but it can be as short as 7 days. Although it has been known for a long time that this temporary gland is maintained by LH it may be that other hormones, e.g. prolactin, are also involved.

If pregnancy has not been established, the corpus luteum regresses (luteolysis) and the levels of all ovarian steroids decline. This decline in steroid levels may be the signal for the commencement of the next cycle. However, as yet the sequence of events necessary to initiate the cycle remains unknown. In the event that fertilization and implantation have occurred, then 8 days after ovulation human chorionic gonadotrophin (hCG) can be detected in the mother and the corpus luteum is preserved by the placental trophic support. Progesterone levels remain elevated. Of especial interest is the fact that human placentae do not secrete *17α-hydroxy-progesterone*, its presence therefore in the maternal peripheral plasma represents corpus luteum function exclusively. The duration of secretion of this steroid is equivalent to the functional life span of the corpus luteum during pregnancy. With this convenient tag, workers have been able to estimate that the steroidogenic activity of the luteal tissue persists for only 9—10 weeks of pregnancy at which time progesterone levels increase as a result of placental steroidogenesis while 17α-hydroxyprogesterone falls to undetectable levels.

In the sheep, it has been established that the uterus secretes prostaglandin $F_{2\alpha}$ (see p. 145) which causes destruction of the corpus luteum. Removal of the uterus causes prolongation of the life of the corpus luteum. Moreover this action of the uterus is very local, because removal of the uterine horn on the opposite side to the corpus luteum does not affect its life. There appears then to be a corpus luteal—uterine cycle; the corpus luteum stimulates the uterus to secrete prostaglandin $F_{2\alpha}$ which in the end destroys the corpus luteum. In the human female the present evidence indicates that the life of the corpus luteum is not controlled by the lytic action of the uterus. It has been shown that although prostaglandins are present in the uterus, hysterectomy has no effect on the life of the human corpus luteum and hysterectomized women continue to have normal ovulatory cycles.

VIII. STEROIDS SECRETED BY THE OVARY

In general, the secretion of a particular steroid by an organ such as the ovary can be demonstrated if its concentration is higher in the venous effluent than in peripheral plasma. By this method it has now been shown that practically every steroid in the pathway from pregnenolone to estradiol is secreted by the ovary. For example, it has been established that progesterone, 17α-hydroxyprogesterone, dehydroepiandrosterone, androstenedione, testosterone, estrone and estradiol-17β are all secreted by this organ. The levels of some of these steroids in peripheral plasma throughout the human menstrual cycle are given in Figure 7.3. The concentrations of estradiol-17β in ovarian vein plasma are about 10 times higher than estrone. The difference in the concentrations of DHA and testosterone in ovarian venous blood compared to peripheral blood is not great (about 2/1), this is in contrast to androstenedione which is about 20/1 indicating that in woman the ovary is an important source of this androgen. Furthermore there is a mid-cycle peak of androstenedione but not of testosterone or DHA secretion.

IX. CELLULAR SOURCE OF OVARIAN STEROIDS

It is generally accepted that the theca interna cells during the follicular phase secrete estrogens and that the corpus luteum secretes progesterone in the luteal phase. Estrogen is also secreted during the second half of the cycle and it is thought that this is derived from the corpus luteum. The synthesis of steroids in the ovary is controlled mainly by LH. FSH on the other hand is thought to be concerned mainly with stimulating cellular development, although Moon *et al.* (1975) have now shown that FSH stimulates estradiol-17β synthesis from testosterone in cultured rat ovarian tissue.

In vitro studies with the different ovarian tissues incubated with ^{14}C-acetate have shown that the isolated follicle will convert acetate mainly to estrogens. The corpus luteum on the other hand forms mainly progesterone. In the human follicle, but not in the bovine, estrogens are also formed in the corpus luteum. Both hCG

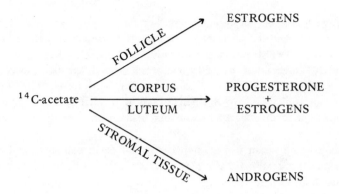

Figure 7.4 Summary of *in vitro* studies with different tissues isolated from the ovary showing main steroids formed from ^{14}C-acetate.

and LH stimulate the incorporation of ^{14}C-acetate into steroids in the follicle *in vitro*. The stroma or interstitial tissue has been shown to form predominantly androstenedione, dehydroepiandrosterone and testosterone plus small amounts of estrogens from acetate. Recent work suggests that estrogen formation may be associated with the *outer* or *cortical* portion of the ovarian stroma. The exact role of this tissue is unknown. Steroidogenesis in the stromal tissue is also stimulated by LH and hCG *in vitro*. A summary of the steroids formed from ^{14}C-acetate by the different ovarian tissues is given in Figure 7.4 (Besch and Buttram, 1972).

X. DISORDERS OF OVARIAN FUNCTION AND ORAL CONTRACEPTIVES

As discussed in Section IV of this chapter the normal human ovary goes through cyclic changes in hormone levels accompanied by ovulation and followed by breakdown of the endometrium (menstruation) if pregnancy does not take place. Abnormalities in ovarian function have many causes and will only be dealt with briefly here. For more extensive reviews, especially with respect to clinical assessment, the reader is referred to Schwarz and Hoffman (1972), Erzin *et al.* (1973), Hafez and Evans (1973), Eskes *et al.* (1974) and Hall *et al.* (1974).

The disorders of ovarian function can be divided into

(i) Failure of sexual maturation (primary amenorrhea), or

(ii) Failure of established sexual function (secondary amenorrhea).

Both of these may be due to dysfunction of the ovary itself or indirectly due to dysfunction of the hypothalamic—pituitary axis. In addition diseases of the ovary may be associated with other endocrine and metabolic disturbances (e.g. congenital adrenal hyperplasia, Cushing's syndrome, obesity, hyper- and hypothyroidism).

Primary amenorrhea may be due to congenital hypoplasia, absent or damaged ovaries and, rarely, to ovarian tumours. In these cases when the age of puberty is reached, gonadotrophins are released but they have little or no effect on the ovaries. Estrogen and progesterone levels will remain low and plasma gonadotrophin levels will be abnormally high. In patients with gonadotrophin deficiency there may be distinctive lesions in the hypothalamus or pituitary (e.g. caused by tumours). However, in the majority of cases it is generally assumed that there is simply a failure to secrete LH/FSH releasing hormone(s).

In primary amenorrhea the first menstrual period has never occurred. The complete failure of established sexual function is referred to as *secondary amenorrhea*, or as *oligomenorrhea* when periods occur infrequently. The reasons for these abnormalities may be endocrine but also metabolic, systemic or psychological.

An example of ovarian dysfunction caused by other endocrine and metabolic diseases is *congenital adrenal hyperplasia* (see Chapter 6.VI). In these cases there is an increased androgen secretion by the adrenal gland resulting in an inhibition of the secretion of gonadotrophins by the pituitary.

High androgen levels are also found in another ovarian dysfunction, the *polycystic ovary syndrome* (Stein Leventhal Syndrome). In this disease there is a hypothalamic-pituitary dysfunction characterized by excess ovarian or adrenal androgens. It can be divided into a number of classes depending on the cause; the common feature is the presence of polycystic ovaries. The present evidence suggests that the basic disturbance is the hypothalamic cyclic centre which controls the production and release of gonadotrophins. The latter are still formed, but not in a cyclic manner or in the right amounts to stimulate the ovaries to form estrogens. Instead of which, androgens are formed and ovulation does not take place. In some cases, the normal functions of the ovary may be restored by treatment with clomiphene. This anti-estrogen acts on the hypothalamus causing gonadotrophin release from the pituitary, in addition it may also act directly on the ovaries. In general clomiphene is used in cases of ovulatory failure where levels of gonadotrophins are low.

Ovarian tumours are formed by the different hormone-secreting cell types in the ovary (granulosa, theca, and hilus cells, etc.) with the consequence that excess androgens and/or estrogens are secreted. Much more common though are the non-functional tumours such as the various types of cystadenomas. The clinical syndromes produced by the functional tumours are virilization and precocious puberty. The frequency of occurrence of ovarian tumours is greatly increased in patients with dysgenetic gonads.

Oral contraceptives. Analogues of progesterone and estradiol are extensively used as oral contraceptives. There are two main types. One contains both progestogen and estrogen and acts by inhibiting ovulation. The other contains a low amount of progestogen ('the minipill') and probably acts mainly by increasing the viscosity of the cervical mucus and thus inhibiting the penetration of the spermatozoa. The ovulation inhibitory action probably occurs via inhibition of the LH−RH/FSH−RH release from the hypothalamus preventing the mid-cycle surge of gonadotrophins. The analogues of progesterone used contain extra substituents (e.g. 6-methyl, 17-acetoxy) which slow down the normal rapid metabolism of progesterone (Cooke and Vallance, 1965, Fotherby and James, 1972). 19-Nor compounds (e.g. norethisterone acetate) are also extensively used. 17-Ethinyl substituted and various other derivatives of estradiol are used as the estrogen component.

XI. REFERENCES (* indicates review or article)

Baird, D. T. (1971). Steroids in blood reflecting ovarian function. In David T. Baird and J. A. Strong (Eds), *Control of Gonadal Steroid Secretion*, University Press Edinburgh Pfizer Medical Monograph, 6, 175—189.

*Besch, P. K., and V. C. B. Buttram (1972). Steroidogenesis in the human ovary. In H. Balin and S. Glasser (Eds), *Reproductive Biology. Excerpta Medica*, Amsterdam, 552—571.

Cooke, B. A., and D. K. Vallance (1965). Metabolism of megestrol acetate and related progesterone analogues by liver preperations *in vitro. Biochem. J.*, 97, 672—677.

*Donovan, B. T., and J. J. van der Werff ten Bosch (1965). In H. Barcroft, H. Davson and W. D. M. Paton (Eds), *Physiology of puberty*. Monographs of the physiological Society, No. 15. London, 1—216.

*Eskes, T. K. A. B., H. L. Houtzager and E. V. van Hall (Eds) (1974). Ovarian function. Proceedings of the Reinier de Graaff Tercentenary Symposium, 8—11 August, 1973. *Excerpta Medica*, Amsterdam.

*Ezrin, C., J. O. Godden, R. Volpé and R. Wilson (Eds) (1973) *Systematic Endocrinology*. Harper & Row.

*Fotherby, K., and F. James (1972). Metabolism of synthetic steroids. In M. H. Briggs and G. A. Christie (Eds), *Advances in Steroid Biochemistry and Pharmacology*, 3, 67—165. Academic Press, London and New York.

*Hafez, E. S. E., and T. N. Evans (Eds) (1973). *Human reproduction, conception and contraception*. Harper & Row.

*Hall, R., J. Anderson, G. A. Smart and M. Besser (1974). *Fundamentals of Clinical Endocrinology*. Pitman Medical, London.

Kragt, C. L., and J. Dahlgren, (1972). Development of neural regulation of follicle stimulating hormone (FSH) secretion. *Neuroendocrinology*, 9, 30—40.

Meijs-Roelofs, H. M. A., J. Th. J. Uilenbroek, F. H. de Jong and R. Welschen (1973). Plasma oestradiol-17β and its relation to serum follicle stimulating hormone in immature female rats. *J. Endocr.*, 59, 295—304.

Moon, Y. S., J. H. Dorrington and D. T. Armstrong (1975). Stimulatory effect of FSH on estradiol-17β by hypophysectomized rat ovaries in organ culture. *Endocrinology*, 97, 244—247.

Ojeda, S. R., and V. D. Ramirez (1972). Plasma levels of LH and FSH in maturing rats: response to hemigonadectomy. *Endocrinology*, 90, 466—472.

*Ross, G. T., C. M. Cargille, M. B. Lipsett, P. L. Rayford, J. R. Marshall, C. A. Strott and D. Rodbard (1970). Pituitary and gonadal hormones in women during spontaneous and induced ovulatory cycles. *Recent Progress in Horm. Res.*, 26, 1—48.

*Schwarz, N. B., and J. C. Hoffman (1972). Ovulation: basic aspects. In H. Balin and S. Glasser (Eds), Reproductive Biology. *Excerpta Medica*, Amsterdam, 552—571.

*Short, R. V. (1972). Role of hormones in sex cycles. In C. S. Austin and R. V. Short (Eds), *Hormones in Reproduction*, Book 3. Cambridge University Press, 42—72.

CHAPTER 8

Testis

I. INTRODUCTION

The testes fulfil a dual role analogous to that of the ovaries, i.e. an endocrine function in the formation of steroid hormones and a germinal one in the production of spermatozoa. The seminiferous tubules are the site of spermatozoa production and they occupy approximately 85 per cent of the gland volume. They are highly coiled (in the rat there are about 6 separate tubules) and are embedded in connective tissue containing the Leydig (interstitial) cells, the site of steroidogenesis (Figure 8.1). In contrast to the seminiferous tubules, the Leydig cells have an excellent blood and lymphatic supply. The whole testis is surrounded by a dense white capsule, the tunica albuginea.

The testes are different from the ovaries in that there are no marked cyclic changes in the production of the steroid hormones (however, seasonal changes in the function of the testes in some species are well known). Apparently the same two hormones controlling the ovary, FSH and LH, also control the testis. They are secreted by the male pituitary gland under the control of releasing hormones from the hypothalamus (Figure 8.1) (the male 'LH' is also referred to as ICSH, interstitial cell stimulating hormone, and is thought to be biologically identical with LH of the female which affects luteal cells, however they do appear to differ immunologically). The effect of FSH in the male (together with testosterone) is to promote spermatogenesis and the growth of the seminiferous tubules, while LH stimulates the growth and steroid hormone production of the Leydig cells. One of the main products of the Leydig cells is testosterone. In addition to its role in sperma-

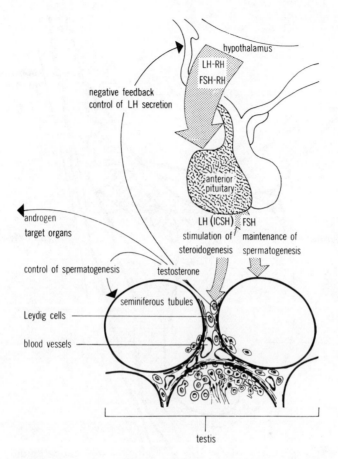

Figure 8.1 Interrelationships between hypothalamus, pituitary, the testis and testosterone dependent tissues.

togenesis, this steroid (probably after conversion to 5α-dihydrotestosterone in its target tissues, see Chapter 14) has important anabolic and androgenic effects òn bone, muscle and hair growth and maintains the prostate, seminal vesicles and other accessory organs. It also plays an important role in the mating behaviour of the male.

Detailed reviews on the testis have been published by Johnson *et al.* (1970), Rosenberg and Paulsen (1970), Eik-Nes (1970), James *et al.* (1973) and Brandes (1974).

II. MORPHOLOGICAL RELATIONSHIP OF THE EPIDIDYMIS TO THE TESTIS

The epididymis is closely associated with the posterior surface of the testis overlapping its posterolateral aspect (Figure 8.2). The head of the epididymis

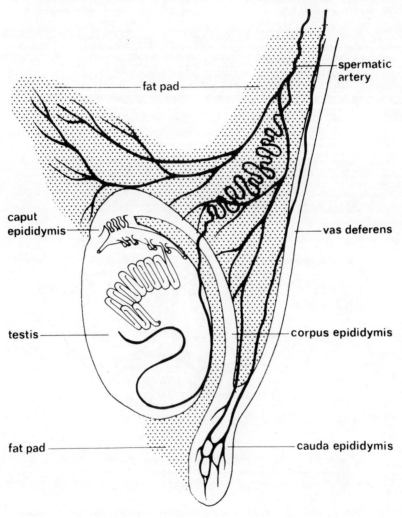

Figure 8.2   Morphological relationship of the epididymis to the testis. (From Cooke *et al.* 1973; reproduced by permission of IPPF.)

(caput) is connected to the testis by the *ductuli efferentes*, a group of six or more tubules. The attenuated body of the epididymis (corpus) extends from the head to the tail of the epididymis (cauda). The *vas deferens* is a continuation of the tail of the epididymis and passes into the spermatic cord. The spermatic artery arises from the aorta and before reaching the testis it supplies branches to the head of the epididymis and the epididymal fat pad. Veins emerge from the posterior aspect of the testis and pass up the spermatic cord in an extremely tortuous course through the pampiniform plexus.

Both ends of the seminiferous tubules open into the rete testis through the short tubuli recti. The lumina of the tubules and the rete testis are filled with spermatozoa suspended in fluid; this fluid is probably a mixture of a secretion from the seminiferous tubules themselves and a second secretion probably formed in the rete or tubuli recti.

III. DEVELOPMENT OF THE TESTES AND STEROIDOGENESIS

In the embryo, the testes grow from a ridge of mesodermal cells in the neighbourhood of the primitive kidney. During the first 8 weeks of human embryonic life the development of the testes is identical to that of the ovaries and no distinction is visible. Then the characteristics of each gonad become apparent. Tubular structures (seminiferous tubules) develop surrounded by connective tissue containing fibroblasts, blood vessels and interstitial (Leydig) cells. During this time the testes gradually descend from the abdominal cavity towards the lower region of the abdomen. The testes in the human foetus usually drop into their suspending bag or scrotum during the 8th month of pregnancy. From this time on during childhood there is little change in testis structure and the gland is apparently functionless.

The classic work of Jost (see review 1970) into the development of the rat and rabbit foetus has led to the surprising conclusion that the foetal testes play an important role in determining the phenotypic sex of the developing foetus. Castration of 19-day old rabbit foetuses *in utero* showed that in the absence of the testes all the body sexual characteristics became feminine. It was concluded from these and other experiments that the *basic developmental trend of the gonadless body is essentially feminine*, and that the *testes impose masculinity and repress femininity*. The foetal testes cause retrogression of the Mullerian ducts (presumptive uteri) and tubes which persist in the absence of the testicular influence, and stimulate the development of the epididymis, vas deferentia and seminal vesicles from the Wolffian ducts (these ducts regress in the absence of the testes). Androgens such as testosterone can replace foetal testes in their masculinizing effects, but fail to inhibit the development of the Mullerian ducts. This suggests that the *foetal testis produces two kinds of morphogenetic substances*; a Mullerian duct inhibitor, which has still to be isolated and identified, and a masculinizing factor similar to testosterone (see also p. 95).

These observations lead to the conclusion that at about the time Leydig cells first appear and the testis becomes recognizable as such, this organ acquires certain of the enzymes for steroidogenesis. Evidence is now accumulating that the foetal testis is capable of steroidogenesis at this stage of development. Direct demonstration of the secretion of testosterone by the foetal testis has not yet been possible for technical reasons. On the other hand, androgens have been isolated from plasma of neonatal animals. For example in the rat, the levels of testosterone decline from day 1 to day 25. From day 25 plasma levels rise gradually to adult levels (Miyachi *et al.*, 1973). This postnatal decline in plasma levels of testosterone is reflected by histochemical changes in Leydig cells which provide evidence of regression of enzymic activity after the first week of life. It has been suggested that two distinct generations of Leydig cells exist in the rat and that the appearance of the second

130

generation coincides with the secretion of gonadotrophins shortly before puberty (see Odell and Swerdloff, 1975).

IV. CONTROL OF STEROIDOGENESIS

A. LH and FSH

The stimulation of the biosynthesis and secretion of androgens by the testis is mainly a result of the action of LH, this has been shown both *in vivo* and *in vitro*.

Present evidence indicates that there may be more than one hormone or factor controlling the secretion of testosterone in the testis. This is not an uncommon feature of the control of the secretion of tissues. For example, prolactin, LH and FSH are needed to maintain functional corpora lutea. It has been shown in the perfused rabbit testis that FSH acts synergistically with LH to increase testosterone secretion (Johnson and Ewing, 1971). This is illustrated in Figure 8.3. In the absence of exogenous gonadotrophic hormone, during the first 2 h of perfusion with an artificial medium, secretion of testosterone declined to a basal amount. When administered alone, FSH did not significantly alter secretion from this basal amount. Secretion was increased in the presence of LH and when combined with FSH further increases in the testosterone production occurred. It was also found that FSH increased the maximum increase obtained with large doses of LH. Thus suggesting that FSH may act at different sites or by different mechanisms. The synergistic effect of FSH and LH on the secretion of testosterone *in vivo* (but not

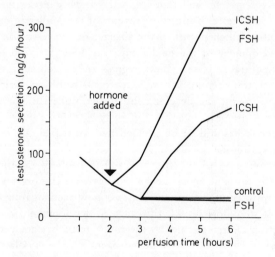

Figure 8.3 Testosterone secretion by rabbit testis perfused *in situ* with medium only (control) or medium containing ICSH (30 ng/ml) and/or FSH (15 ng/ml). (B. H. Johnson and L. L. Ewing, *Science,* 173, pp. 635–637 (1971). Copyright © 1971 by the American Association for the Advancement of Science.)

in vitro) has also been shown in the rat (Swerdloff, Jacobs and Odell, 1972; Safoury and Bartke, 1974; Odell and Swerdloff, 1975).

B. Other Hormones

It is well established that *prolactin*, in addition to its effects on the mammary gland, influences ovarian steroidogenesis and regulates lipid metabolism in the ovary. Prolactin is also present in the pituitaries of male mammals. Recent evidence (Hafiez *et al.*, 1972) suggests that it may also act synergistically with LH to stimulate steroidogenesis in the rat testis. There is at present little evidence to suggest the *prostaglandins* have a function in regulating testosterone production in the testis. This is in contrast to their important role in luteolysis in some species and their effect on ovarian and adrenal steroidogenesis. Evidence presented mainly by Eik-Nes for the dog testis indicates that the rate of *blood flow* in the spermatic artery (and consequently factors which regulate blood flow) will determine the rate of secretion of testosterone from the testes.

V. STEROIDS SECRETED BY THE TESTES

The action of androgens in the body is very clearly demonstrated by the characteristic changes in the male at puberty. As androgen production begins, the testes enlarge followed by growth of the penis and axillary and pubic hair. The beard develops and the voice deepens. Increased muscle protein is laid down and there may be a dramatic increase in weight and height.

The main steroids secreted by the testis with androgenic properties are testosterone, androstenedione and dehydroepiandrosterone. 5α-Dihydrotestosterone is secreted in small amounts but is mainly formed by peripheral conversion of testosterone (see Chapter 14). Estrogens are also secreted by the testes; estradiol-17β is synthesized and secreted by the testes of several species. The horse testes are unusual in producing and secreting large amounts of the estrogens equilin and equilenin. Plasma levels and secretion rates for testicular steroids in man and the rat are given in Table 8.1.

Table 8.1.

	Plasma levels (μg/100 ml)		Testicular secretion rate (mg/24 h)		Androgenic Potency capon comb	seminal vesicle weight
	man	rat	man	rat		
testosterone	0.7	0.2	6.2	0.075	100	100
androstenedione	0.1	0.03	— — —	0.010	25	10
dehydroepiandrosterone	0.5	0.125	0.15	— — —	10	3
5α-dihydrotestosterone	0.05	— — —	n.d.	— — —	100	— — —
estradiol-17β	0.003	0.0002	0.030	0.0001	— — —	— — —

(From *The Testis*, Cooke *et al.*, 1973)

VI. CELLULAR SOURCE OF TESTICULAR STEROIDS

It is generally accepted that the Leydig cells are the main site of testicular androgen biosynthesis. It has been suggested that cells in the seminiferous tubules may also be a source of steroid hormones that influence the differentiation of the germinal cells (Lacy and Pettitt, 1970). There are steroid converting enzymes in the seminiferous tubules although they are generally of much lower activity than those in the Leydig cells. With the exception of cholesterol, steroids from the interstitial tissue pass freely into the seminiferous tubules and thus precursors of active androgens formed in the interstitial tissue may be further converted in the tubular compartment. The enzymes that are present in the seminiferous tubules include 17- and 20-hydroxysteroid dehydrogenase and 5α-reductase. The quantitative importance of seminiferous tubular steroid metabolism with respect to spermatogenesis remains to be determined.

The cellular site of testicular estrogen biosynthesis is still not clear, although Dorrington and Armstrong (1975) have now demonstrated that FSH stimulates estradiol-17β synthesis in cultured rat Sertoli cells.

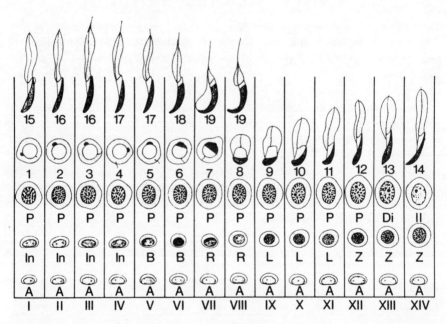

Figure 8.4 Composition of the fourteen cellular associations observed in the seminiferous epithelium in the rat. Each column consists of the various cell types composing a cellular association or stage of the cycle (identified by Roman numerals at the base of the figure). The various cellular associations succeed one another from stage 1 to stage 14. The succession of the 14 cellular associations constitutes the cycle of the seminiferous epithelium. Abbreviations: A, In, B: Type A, Intermediate and type B spermatogonia; R, L, Z, P, Di: primary spermatocytes at pre-leptotene, leptotene, zygotene, pachytene and diakinesis, respectively; II: secondary spermatocytes; 1—19: successive stages of spermiogenesis (From B. Perey, Y. Clermont and C. P. Leblond, 1961). Reproduced by permission of Y. Clermont.

VII. SPERMATOGENESIS

The male has no cycle comparable to the estrous cycle of the female, but what has to be coordinated is the equivalent of maturation of the ovum, i.e. the process of spermatogenesis and subsequent transport of the spermatozoa from the seminiferous tubules. The successive stages in the development of the spermatozoa are given in Figure 8.4.

One feature of the seminiferous tubules is that the different cells in any cross-section always form one of a number of constant associations. For example just after the spermatozoa have been shed (Clermont Stage IX, Figure 8.4) there are A_1 spermatogonia in the basal compartment, leptotene and pachytene spermatocytes in the adluminal compartment between pairs of Sertoli cells and new spermatids embedded in the luminal margin of the Sertoli cells. The cell associations are quite invariable: certain cells are never found associated with certain other cells. Moreover, the rate of development from one cellular association to another can be judged by noting the most advanced cell types containing radioactivity in their nuclei at various times after an injection of ^{3}H-thymidine. This substance is incorporated into DNA during spermatogonial mitoses and during the preleptotene stage of the meiotic prophase, but not thereafter. The time taken for the same cellular association to reappear is very constant for each species and ranges from 8 to 16 days. More detailed reviews of spermatogenesis have been published by Perey *et al.* (1961), Monesi (1972) and Steinberger (1971).

VIII. HORMONAL CONTROL OF SPERMATOGENESIS

The role of gonadotrophins in the maintenance of spermatogenesis is demonstrated by the effects of hypophysectomy which causes spermatogenesis to cease at the level of primary spermatocytes and there is a quantitative decrease of type A spermatogonia. Replacement of LH in hypophysectomized animals will qualitatively restore spermatogenesis, but quantitatively germ cell numbers remain below normal. The possible role of FSH in spermatogenesis is less clear, although it is thought that it maintains the Sertoli cells and is required for the last stages of spermatid maturation.

Large doses of testosterone maintain spermatogenesis in hypophysectomized rats and it is generally assumed therefore that the effect of LH on spermatogenesis is not direct but is mediated through stimulation of testosterone production. However, there remains a quantitative decrease in type A spermatogonia in hypophysectomized rats which is not restored, by either testosterone or LH. If pregnenolone, dehydroepiandrosterone or androstenedione are given instead of testosterone similar effects are found in hypophysectomized rats.

Administration of estrogens or small doses of testosterone to intact animals suppress spermatogenesis through suppression of gonadotrophins. Large doses of testosterone result in a 20–40% decrease in spermatogenesis.

A working *hypothesis* for the hormonal control of spermatogenesis proposed by Steinberger (1971) is as follows: 'Formation of type A spermatogonia is probably controlled by testosterone. The further development of spermatogonia up to primary pachytene spermatocytes does not require either gonadotrophins or steroid hormones. The second reduction division for the formation of spermatids requires testosterone. The early steps of spermatid formation may be under no hormonal control or require testosterone, whereas the last stages of spermatid maturation require the presence of FSH'.

IX. DISORDERS OF TESTIS FUNCTION

Disorders of the testis can be divided into the following groups. Several of the primary hypogonadic syndromes can be classified into more than one group depending on the severity of the disease.

HYPOGONADISM

A. *Primary*

    1) Deficiency of Leydig cell and seminiferous tubule function, e.g. cryptorchism

    2) Deficiency of seminiferous tubules alone, e.g. Kleinfelter's syndrome

    3) Deficiency of Leydig cell function, e.g. disorders of testosterone biosynthesis

B. *Secondary*

Hypogonadotrophic hypogonadism

MALE SEXUAL PRECOCITY

Precocious puberty

Testis tumours

TESTICULAR FEMINIZATION

These disorders of the testis are assessed by use of the following:

    i)   trophic and steroid hormone measurements in plasma

    ii) histologic and biochemical studies on testis biopsies

    iii) chromosomal studies

    iv) sperm counts

Previously androgen secretion was determined by '17-keto steroid' measurements in urine. However these assays are unreliable because they reflect both adrenal gland and testis steroid production, and furthermore small changes in testosterone production are not detectable. Reliable radioimmunoassays are now extensively used for plasma testosterone measurements as well as for assay of LH and FSH in plasma.

The following is a brief description of some of the testis disorders. For more extensive reviews especially with respect to clinical assessment the reader is referred to Steinberger and Steinberger (1972), Ezrin *et al.* (1973), Hafez and Evans (1973), James *et al.* (1973), Hall *et al.* (1974).

HYPOGONADISM

In primary hypogonadism one or both specific functions of the testis (i.e. germinal and endocrine) are lost. In secondary hypogonadism there is a lack of gonadotrophin secretion and a consequent dysfunction of the testis.

Cryptorchism (undescended testis). This is a failure of the testis to descend into the scrotum which in normal males usually occurs at about 8 months of gestation. Unilateral cryptorchism is about five times commoner than bilateral cryptorchism. The incidence of cryptorchism in children at birth is 3.4%, falling to 1.7% after one month and 0.4% after one year. There is about 40 times greater incidence of neoplasia in cryptorchid testes compared with normal testes.

Present evidence suggests that if the human testes remain outside the scrotum after the age of 5 years, irreversible changes take place; the testes then become incapable of spermatogenesis thereafter. The reason is that the intra-abdominal temperature is $2-3°C$ higher than scrotal temperature and this is sufficiently high to prevent normal spermatogenic development. Leydig cell function is not so sensitive to these higher temperatures and therefore the cryptorchid testes form testosterone. However gradually total testicular degeneration may occur due to complete testicular fibrosis resulting in loss of Leydig cell function. If the undescended testes are moved to the scrotum (either by surgery — orchidopexy — or by chorionic gonadotrophin treatment) before the age of five years, then normal testicular maturation occurs, but after this time the chances of normal development are very much reduced.

Kleinfelter's syndrome is the commonest form of male primary hypogonadism and is due to a cytogenetic abnormality resulting in a deficient seminiferous tubule function. In the true Kleinfelter's syndrome at least two X chromosomes and a Y chromosome are present, giving a total of 47 or more chromosomes. Before puberty, development is normal, but at puberty development of the male characteristics is generally diminished. Frequently gynaecomastia (breast development) occurs. Usually the levels of plasma FSH are high, the LH levels are normal but the testosterone plasma levels are low. The testes are small and firm, there is a lack of spermatogenesis and a variable degree of Leydig cell hyperplasia. hCG administration produces no or subnormal activation of Leydig cell testosterone secretion. This lack of response of the testis to trophic hormone stimulation implies that there is a deficiency in one or more of the biosynthetic pathways leading to testosterone biosynthesis.

Deficiency of Leydig cell function. The development of secondary sex characteristics which normally occurs at puberty will not be seen in this deficiency because of the low or absent testosterone formation in the Leydig cells. No increase in testosterone is detectable after LH administration. Spermatogenesis can be 'restored' in some of these patients by administration of testosterone.

Secondary male hypogonadism. The normal rise in pituitary gonadotrophin secretion which occurs at puberty and stimulates testosterone secretion in the testis Leydig cells does not occur in secondary male hypogonadism. The secondary sex characteristics do not develop and the testes remain very small and contain immature seminiferous tubules and poorly differentiated Leydig cells. Gonadotrophin therapy in these patients stimulates Leydig cell function, increases testosterone production and secondary sex characteristics develop.

MALE SEXUAL PRECOCITY
Premature development of the testis resulting in spermatogenesis and appearance of secondary sex characteristics can take place in boys before the age of 9. This is due to early activation of the hypothalamic – pituitary mechanism for the formation of gonadotrophins. Excessive testosterone production can also occur in patients with congenital adrenal hyperplasia (Chapter 6.VI).

Testicular tumours
There are 3 main groups of testicular tumours.

1) Germinal cell tumours (seminoma, teratoma, combined seminoma and teratoma)
2) Sertoli cell tumours
3) Leydig cell tumours

The incidence of testicular tumours is 2–3/100,000 men/year, accounting for 1–2% of all malignant tumours in men. Both Sertoli and Leydig cell tumours (which only account for about 1–2% of testis tumours) have been reported to secrete estrogens. Leydig cell tumours sometimes but not always secrete androgens.

TESTICULAR FEMINIZATION
Patients with testicular feminization usually have external genitalia and breast characteristics of phenotypic females, but genetically they are normal males and they have normal plasma testosterone levels (46, XY). Internal genitalia other than the testis are absent. This syndrome not only occurs in man but also in the mouse, rat, dog and cow. It is assumed that the lack of masculinization of these genetically male subjects is due to a defect in testosterone action during foetal life and puberty. It has been demonstrated that in androgen target organs in normal animals, testosterone is converted to 5α-dihydrotestosterone which is then transferred to the nucleus, bound to a protein receptor (see Chapter 14). It has been postulated that in testicular feminization one or more steps of this mechanism are defective.

X. REFERENCES (*indicates review or article)

*Brandes, D. (Ed.) (1974). *Male accessory sex organs. Structure and function in mammals.* Academic Press, New York, San Francisco, London.
*Cooke, B. A., H. J. van der Molen and B. P. Setchell (1973). In R. G. Edwards

(Ed.), *The Testis. Research in Reproduction*, Vol. 5, no. 6. International Planned Parenthood Federation.

Dorrington, J. H. and D. T. Armstrong (1975). Follicle Stimulating Hormone stimulates estradiol-17β synthesis in cultured Sertoli cells. Proc. Nat. Acad. Sci., 72, 2677–2681.

*Eik-Nes, K. B. (Ed.) (1970). *The Androgens of the Testis*. Marcel Dekker Inc., New York.

*Ezrin, C., J. O. Godden, R. Volpé and R. Wilson (Eds) (1973). *Systematic Endocrinology*. Harper & Row.

*Hafez, E. S. E. and T. N. Evans (Eds) (1973). *Human reproduction, conception and contraception*. Harper & Row.

*Hall, R., J. Anderson, G. A. Smart and M. Besser (1974). *Fundamentals of Clinical Endocrinology*. Pitman Medical, London.

Haviez, A. A., A. Bartke and C. W. Lloyd (1972). The role of prolactin in the regulation of testis function: the synergistic effects of prolactin and luteinizing hormone on the incorporation of $1\text{-}^{14}C$ acetate into testosterone and cholesterol by testes from hypophysectomized rats *in vitro*. *J. Endocr.*, 53, 223–230.

*James, V. H. T., M. Serio and L. Martini (Eds) (1973). *The Endocrine Function of the Human Testis*, Vol. I and II. Academic Press, New York and London.

*Johnson, A. D., W. R. Gomes and N. L. VanDemark, (Eds) (1970). *The Testis*, Vol. I, II and III. Academic Press, New York and London.

Johnson, B. S. and L. L. Ewing (1971). *Follicle-stimulating hormone in the regulation of testosterone secretion in rabbit testes. Science*, 173, 635–637.

*Jost, A. (1970). Hormonal factors in the sex differentiation of the mammalian fetus. *Phil. Trans. Roy. Soc. Lond. B*, 259, 119–130.

Lacy, D. and A. J. Pettitt (1970). Sites of hormone production in the mammalian testis and their significance in their control of male fertility. *British Medical Bull.*, 26, 87–91.

Miyachi, Y., E. Nieschlag and M. B. Lipsett (1973). The secretion of gonadotrophins and testosterone by the neonatal male rat. *Endocrinology*, 92, 1–5.

*Monesi, V. (1972). Spermatogenesis and the spermatozoa in reproduction in mammals, Book I. In C. R. Austin and R. V. Short (Eds), *Germ cells and fertilization*. Cambridge University Press. pp. 46–84.

Odell, W. D. and R. S. Swerdloff (1975). The role of testicular sensitivity to gonadotropins in sexual maturation of the male rat. *J. Steroid Biochemistry*, 6, 853–857.

Perey, B., Y. Clermont and C. P. Leblond (1961). The wave of the seminiferous epithelium in the rat. *Amer. J. Anat.*, 108, 49–77.

*Rosenberg, E. and C. A. Paulsen (Eds) (1970). *The Human Testis*. Plenum Press, New York and London.

Safoury, S. E. and A. Bartke (1974). Effect of FSH and LH on plasma testosterone levels in hypophysectomized and in intact immature and adult male rats. *J. Endocr.*, 61, 193–198.

*Steinberger, E. (1971). Hormonal control of mammalian spermatogenesis. *Physiol. Rev.*, 51, 1–22.

*Steinberger, E. and A. Steinberger (1972). Testis: basic and clinical aspects in reproductive biology. In H. Balin and S. Glasser (Eds). *Reproductive Biology Excerpta Medica*, Amsterdam, 144–267.

138

*Swerdloff, R. S., H. S. Jacobs and W. J. Odell (1972). Hypothalamic-pituitary-
gonadal interrelationships in the rat during sexual maturation. In B. B. Saxena,
C. G. Beling, H. M. Gandy (Eds), *Gonadotrophins*. Wiley-Interscience, New
York, 546—561.

CHAPTER 9

Foeto-placental unit

I. INTRODUCTION

The foetus and placenta complement each other in their ability to form the huge amounts of steroids which are produced during human pregnancy. This discovery led to the concept of the foeto-placental unit as a steroidogenic system. According to this concept 'the foetus and placenta' form a functional unit to carry out steroid biosynthetic reactions together, which the placenta *per se* or the foetus *per se* are incapable of completing (see review, Diczfalusy, 1969). This has led to the elucidation of the individual pathways of steroid metabolism in the placenta and different organs of the foetus.

An important clinical aspect of steroid secretion during human pregnancy is that the amounts produced may give an index of foetal—maternal well-being. Progesterone for example is mainly formed as a result of maternal-placental synthesis and therefore reflects placental function. Estriol formation, on the other hand, relies on precursors from the foetus and therefore reflects foetal well-being. The biosynthetic pathways leading to these steroids were discussed in Chapter 4. The secretion of the pregnancy hormones and their biological and clinical significance will now be discussed as follows:

II. Chorionic gonadotrophin secretion.

III. Secretion of steroid hormones and the control of parturition.

IV. Clinical assessment of the endocrine function of the foetus and placenta.

II. CHORIONIC GONADOTROPHIN SECRETION

The placenta is remarkable in being able to synthesize trophic hormones independently of the hypothalamus or pituitary gland. There are two main hormones that are secreted, namely human placental lactogen (hPL) and human chorionic gonadotrophin (hCG). They are secreted in abundance in the first few weeks of pregnancy and during this time may well play an important luteotrophic role, because in the absence of the maternal pituitary, pregnancy is not terminated. Their roles after this time however are still unclear. hPL was so named because of its lactogenic properties, but it also has somatotrophic, mammotrophic, luteotrophic and various metabolic actions. However, it is difficult to ascribe all these properties

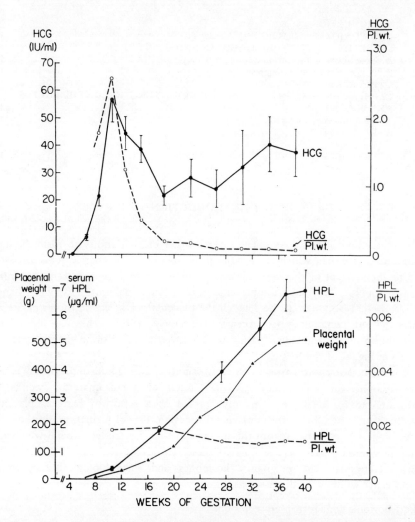

Figure 9.1 Secretion patterns of hCG and hPL during normal pregnancy (from Selenkow *et al.*, 1969). Reproduced by permission of Excerpta Medica Foundation.

to hPL in view of the fact that many of the studies have been carried out with impure preparations. The biological properties of hCG are very similar to those of LH but they differ in chemical structure, immunologically and in their metabolic half-life (hCG has a much longer half-life than LH).

Secretion of hCG during normal human pregnancy differs markedly from hPL (Figure 9.1) (Selenkow *et al.*, 1969). Serum hCG is detectable during the first 6 weeks of pregnancy, rises to a peak around the 10th week, falls to low levels around week 18 and thereafter rises steadily. The rise in hCG in the first 10 weeks is even more striking when considered in relation to placental weight. hPL rises steadily and in parallel with placental weight throughout pregnancy.

III. SECRETION OF STEROID HORMONES AND CONTROL OF PARTURITION

Excellent reviews on these subjects have been published by Ryan (1969), Findlay (1972), Heap (1972), Liggins (1972), and Liggins *et al.*, (1973).

A. Role of ovarian secretion during pregnancy

Some animal species require ovarian steroids for maintenance of pregnancy, whereas others do not. The latter category depends on the synthesis of the steroids in the foetus and placenta. Further classification can also be applied with regard to gestational length (Figure 9.2) and species requirement for total or partial ovarian secretion. In general animals with short gestation periods of 60 days or less require the ovary for pregnancy maintenance.

B. Progesterone and estrogen secretion

In the human, during pregnancy, progesterone is synthesized via maternal cholesterol in the placenta except during the early stages of pregnancy when it is derived from the corpus luteum. Some idea of the life of the corpus luteum and its progesterone secretion can be gauged by the secretion of 17α-hydroxyprogesterone which is formed exclusively by the corpus luteum and not by the placenta (Chapter 7, Figure 7.3). This may have some useful clinical applications in investigations of early foetal death due to poor corpus luteum function. The dependence of pregnancy on progesterone can easily be demonstrated in experimental animals by removal of the ovaries, which initiates abortion.

In the first trimester of human pregnancy, the levels of progesterone in plasma are about the same or slightly above those of the luteal phase of the menstrual cycle. Thereafter there is a progressive increase which sharply declines after removal of the placenta (Figure 10.4). In the sheep, comparatively low levels of progesterone are found during the first half of pregnancy which increase markedly around day 80 (Figure 9.3b) and then during the last few days of pregnancy there is a rapid decline. In the rat and skunk there is also a sharp drop in progesterone levels

Duration of pregnancy

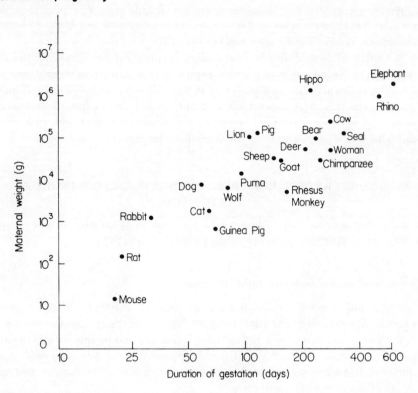

Figure 9.2 The normal duration of gestation in relation to body size in different species (from Findlay, 1972). (Reproduced by permission of IPPF.)

before parturition. The possible fall in progesterone levels immediately before parturition in the human has been a matter of controversy. Csapo *et al.*, have published data collected from different laboratories (Csapo *et al.*, 1971) showing that there is a decrease before parturition. These results were in contradiction to earlier work (Llauro *et al.*, 1968; Yannone *et al.*, 1968). Turnbull *et al.* (1974) showed that although there is no dramatic fall in progesterone levels just before parturition, there is a progressive decrease from 36 weeks to term. Furthermore this decrease in progesterone is accompanied by an increase in estradiol (Figure 9.3a).

In human pregnancy estriol secretion is detectable at about 6–8 weeks and thereafter increases (Chapter 10, Figure 10.4). The precursor of estriol, DHAS, originates in the foetal adrenal gland, most probably in the foetal zone (Cooke, 1970). Subsequent metabolic steps take place in the placenta and the foetal liver as described in Chapter 4. In the sheep the secretion of estrogen is very low during pregnancy except just before parturition when there is a sudden peak of secretion of total unconjugated estrogens (Figure 9.3b).

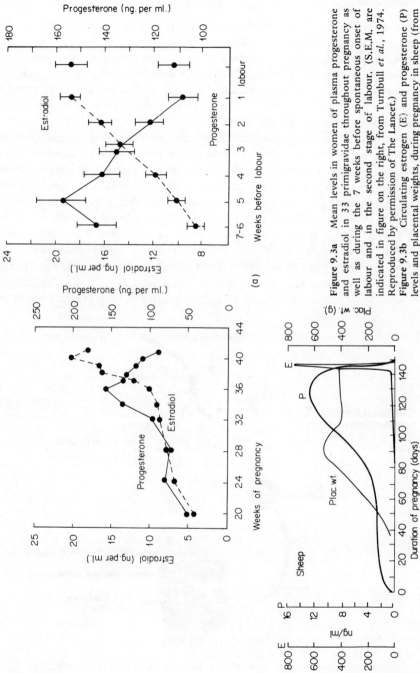

Figure 9.3a Mean levels in women of plasma progesterone and estradiol in 33 primigravidae throughout pregnancy as well as during the 7 weeks before spontaneous onset of labour and in the second stage of labour. (S.E.M. are indicated in figure on the right, from Turnbull *et al*, 1974. Reproduced by permission of The Lancet.)

Figure 9.3b Circulating estrogen (E) and progesterone (P) levels and placental weights, during pregnancy in sheep (from Findlay, 1972). Reproduced by permission of IPPF.

C. Parturition

One of the functions of progesterone is thought to be to block myometrial activity during pregnancy. This has clearly been shown in the rabbit by Csapo and coworkers, but there is some doubt whether or not it applies to all species. If progesterone does block myometrial activity, a withdrawal of progesterone might be expected to occur just before parturition subsequently causing the myometrium to contract and expel the foetus. Decreases in progesterone have been observed to occur in some species as discussed above.

In recent years, much progress has been made in determining the factors which control parturition in the sheep. This animal may well serve as a model for further investigation of the control of parturition in other species. It would appear that the foetal lamb plays an important role in initiating parturition. Initial evidence for this important conclusion came from the observation that sheep grazing in the mountains of Idaho often had prolonged pregnancies ending with death due to the large size of the foetuses. The cause of this was eventually traced to a weed *Veratrum californicum* which the sheep ate during early pregnancy. This alkaloid-containing weed caused severe brain damage to the foetus, but not to the mother. This suggested that the foetal brain was playing some part in determining the initiation of labour. It was also found that the foetal lamb pituitary was often

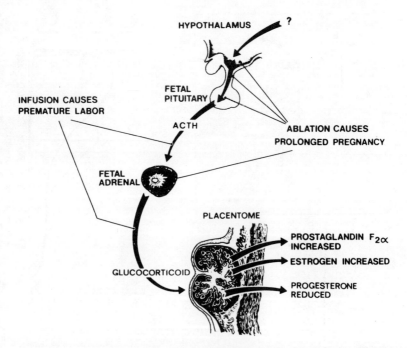

Figure 9.4 Schematic diagram of the pathway by which the foetal lamb influences endocrine events in the ewe. Also shown are the experimental procedures that have been used to modify the activity of the pathway (from Liggins, *et al.*, 1973). Reproduced by permission of Academic Press.

missing and the foetal adrenals were atrophic. Further work showed that disruption of the hypothalamic/pituitary/adrenal axis in normal lambs prolonged pregnancy by many weeks. Administration of ACTH or adrenal corticosteroids was found to induce premature labour in sheep within 4–5 days after day 133 of pregnancy (normal gestation period in the sheep is 147 days). Withdrawal of progesterone does occur before parturition in the sheep, which might lead to the conclusion that the foetal adrenal corticosteroids cause the decrease in progesterone synthesis which consequently leads to the initiation of parturition. However it was found that administration of large quantities of progesterone at the time of parturition or induced labour did not prevent birth of the foetal lambs. This suggested that there was another factor involved. This factor has now been found to be a prostaglandin. A large increase in $PGF_{2\alpha}$ has been found to occur in the maternal cotyledons (but not in the foetus) 24 hours before the onset of labour and increases up to labour. The prostaglandins are well known for their muscle contractile properties. Figure 9.4 summarizes the known factors involved in parturition in the sheep.

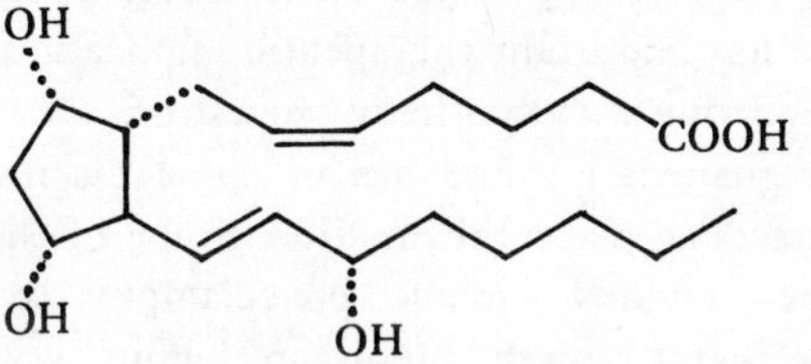

Prostaglandin $F_{2\alpha}$

IV. CLINICAL ASSESSMENT OF THE ENDOCRINE FUNCTION OF THE FOETUS AND PLACENTA

The assays of progesterone, estrogens and chorionic gonadotrophins are now widely used to assess foetal maternal well-being and provide much useful information to the clinician. However it is still a matter of discussion as to whether they are of significant prognostic value. In many cases, by the time an abnormal change in hormone secretion has occurred irreversible metabolic changes have already taken place. The following is a brief description to indicate the possible use of hormone assays during pregnancy. For a more detailed description the reader is referred to an excellent review by Klopper (1969).

A. Chorionic gonadotrophin

A lot of the early work on hCG measurements was carried out using biological assays which has led in some cases to erroneous conclusions. Radioimmunoassays have now superseded the biological assay and much more reliable data are being assembled. It is probable that hCG assays in pregnancy may be more useful than previously thought, especially in early pregnancy. For example in one study it was found that patients with threatened abortion in early pregnancy with normal hCG levels went successfully to term whereas patients with low hCG levels aborted. Clinically there was no difference in these two groups of patients. In late pregnancy hCG hormone assays have given a less reliable index of placental function. Large fluctuations in hCG levels occur in late pregnancy and little is known about the factors controlling hCG production and secretion. When more is known about normal values and these controlling factors it may be that hCG assays will prove to be more useful in the future.

B. Progesterone

Most of the studies on progesterone secretion have been carried out by measuring the amount of its main metabolite, pregnanediol, excreted in maternal urine and the progesterone levels in maternal plasma. It is apparent from the numerous studies carried out that abortion tends to occur when the excretion of pregnanediol is low. However it would seem that pregnanediol measurements have little prognostic value in recurrent abortion; pregnanediol output shows little change until the foeto-placental unit is irretrievably damaged. It has also been found that progesterone deficiency is not a major cause of recurrent abortion, but rather a consequence of it. This of course has important therapeutic implications and rules out the treatment of threatened abortion with synthetic progestins.

In spite of these findings pregnanediol values are of some diagnostic value, especially in late pregnancy in assessing placental function. Some of the obstetric complications where it has been studied include pre-eclamptic toxaemia of pregnancy, retarded intra-uterine foetal growth, premature labour, postmaturity, diabetes and rhesus incompatibility. As with any of the hormonal assessments of endocrine function it is highly desirable to carry out serial measurements of pregnanediol from the same patient over a long period. This is especially true with pregnanediol where large fluctuations occur in day-to-day excretion.

C. Estrogens

Estriol is quantitatively the most important estrogen excreted during pregnancy. It is usually measured in maternal urine, although recently plasma methods have become available. Again serial measurements of estriol are highly desirable. Estriol is a product of the foetus and placenta (see Chapter 4) and therefore reflects the well-being of the foetus more than pregnanediol measurements. Measurements of this steroid are very simple to perform and have been automated (see review, Grant and Hall, 1970). Estriol measurements have been found to be useful in the following clinical conditions: prolonged pregnancy, retarded foetal growth, pre-eclamptic toxaemia, intra-uterine foetal death, diabetes and rhesus incompatibility. Most of these conditions lead to a lowering of estriol excretion and consequently in these circumstances determination of estriol has a diagnostic value. These measurements are especially useful in retarded foetal growth and help the clinician to decide when delivery should take place. However until it can be determined what the controlling factors are which determine estriol synthesis and secretion, the potential of this type of assay will not be fully realized.

V. REFERENCES (*denotes review or book)

*Cooke, B. A. (1970). Biosynthesis of dehydroepiandrosterone sulphate in human foetal adrenal glands: Pathways, localization and development of enzymes. Symposium on Reproductive Endocrinology, held in Edinburgh, 1969. *Proc. Royal Soc. Med.,* Livingstone, Edinburgh, 84—94.

Csapo, A. I., E. Knobil, H. J. van der Molen and W. G. Wiest (1971). Peripheral plasma progesterone levels during human pregnancy and labour. *Am. J. Obstet. Gynec.,* 110, 630—632.

*Diczfalusy, E. (1969). Steroid metabolism in the foetoplacental unit. In A. Pecile and C. Finzi, (Eds) The Foeto-Placental Unit. Proceedings of an international symposium held in Milan, Italy, September 4—6, 1968. *Excerpta Medica Foundation,* Amsterdam. pp. 65—109.

*Findlay, A. L. R. (1972). The control of parturition. In *Research in Reproduction,* Vol. 4, No. 5. The International Planned Parenthood Federation.

*Grant, J. K., and P. F. Hall (1970). The automation of steroid analyses. In M. H. Briggs, (Ed.) *Steroid Biochemistry and Pharmacology.* Vol. I. Academic Press, London and New York. pp. 419—452.

*Heap, R. B. (1972). Role of hormones in pregnancy. In C. R. Austin and R. V. Short, (Eds). *Hormones in Reproduction,* Book 3. Cambridge University Press. pp. 73—105.

*Klopper, A. (1969). The assessment of placental function in clinical practice. In A. Klopper and E. Diczfalusy, (Eds) *Foetus and Placenta.* Blackwell Scientific Publications, Oxford and Edinburgh. pp. 471—555.

*Liggins, G. C. (1972). The foetus and birth. In C. R. Austin and R. V. Short, (Eds) *Hormones in Reproduction,* Book 2. Cambridge University Press. pp. 72—109.

*Liggins, G. C., R. J. Fairclough, S. A. Grieves, J. Z. Kendall and B. S. Knox (1973). The mechanism of initiation of parturition in the ewe. *Recent Progress in Horm. Res.,* 29, 111—150.

Llauro, J. L., B. Runnebaum and J. Zander (1968). Progesterone in human peripheral blood before, during and after labour. *Am. J. Obstet. Gynec.,* 101, 867—873.

*Ryan, K. J. (1969). Theoretical basis for endocrine control of gestation — a comparative approach. In A. Pecile and C. Finzi, (Eds) The Foeto-Placental Unit. Proceedings of an international symposium held in Milan, Italy, September 4—6, 1968. *Excerpta Medica Foundation,* Amsterdam. pp. 120—131.

*Selenkow, H. A., B. N. Saxena, C. L. Dana and K. Emerson (1969). Measurement and pathophysiologic significance of human placental lactogen. In A. Pecile and C. Finzi, (Eds) The Foeto-Placental Unit. Proceedings of an international symposium held in Milan, Italy, September 4—6, 1968. *Excerpta Medica Foundation,,* Amsterdam. pp. 340—362.

Turnbull, A. C., A. P. F. Flint, J. Y. Jeremy, P. T. Patten, M. J. N. C. Keirse and A. B. M. Anderson (1974). Significant fall in progesterone and rise in estradiol levels in human peripheral plasma before onset of labour. *The Lancet,* January 26th, 101—104.

Yannone, M. E., J. R. McCurdy and A. Goldfien (1968). Plasma progesterone levels in normal pregnancy, labour and the puerperium. *Am. J. Obstet. Gynec.,* 101, 1058—1061.

CHAPTER 10

Liver and kidney

I. INTRODUCTION

In the intact organism steroid hormones are normally secreted into the blood-stream from the adrenal cortex, gonads and other steroid producing tissues. At the same time both the liver and kidney are metabolizing these active hormones to inactive products which are excreted in the urine. The circulating blood levels of active steroid hormones are, therefore, dependent upon both the rate of steroid secretion into the blood and the rate of removal of the hormone from the blood (Figure 10.1). Clearly the metabolic processes for the inactivation and removal of steroid hormones are important in regulating the hormonal status of the body. When these metabolic processes are disrupted, as for example in liver disease, steroids will disappear from the blood system more slowly. Thus the normal half-life of cortisol is about 100 min, whereas for patients with liver disease this half-life may be greatly extended (up to 7 hr; Dixon *et al.*, 1967).

II. CONJUGATED STEROIDS

Essentially the effect of the liver and kidney enzymes is to reduce double bonds in the steroid nucleus and introduce hydroxyl functions that serve as loci for the further introduction of hydrophilic groups. The process involves the conversion of the lipophilic steroids (that are sparingly soluble in water) into metabolites that are readily water soluble and can therefore be easily eliminated in the urine. The final excretion products are usually steroids conjugated as β-glucosiduronates (glucuron-

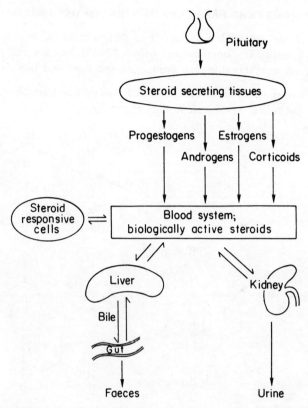

Figure 10.1 Simplified scheme for the overall metabolism of steroid hormones.

ides) or sulphate esters (Figure 10.2). Glucuronides are formed from uridine diphosphoglucuronic acid using the enzyme glucuronosyl transferase (found in liver microsomes) with the liberation of uridine diphosphate. The sulphate ester formation is catalysed by sulphokinases requiring ATP and Mg^{2+} and using 3′-phosphoadenosine-5′-phosphosulphate as substrate.

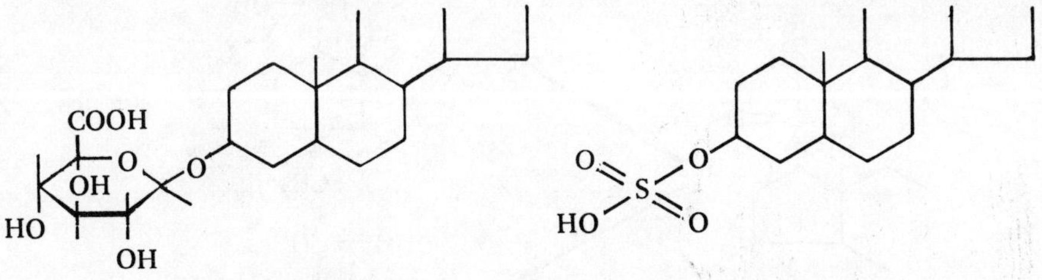

(a) steroid β-glucosiduronate
(also termed glucuronide)

(b) steroid sulphate

Figure 10.2 Conjugated steroids.

III. GENERAL FEATURES OF STEROID METABOLISM

Although there are a bewildering number of different steroid metabolites (for a comprehensive survey see Dorfman and Ungar, 1965), there are really only a few enzymic conversions involved in their production and these may be simplified as:

i) Reduction of the 4-en-3-one conjugated double bond system to produce a 3-hydroxyl function; this can produce the following:

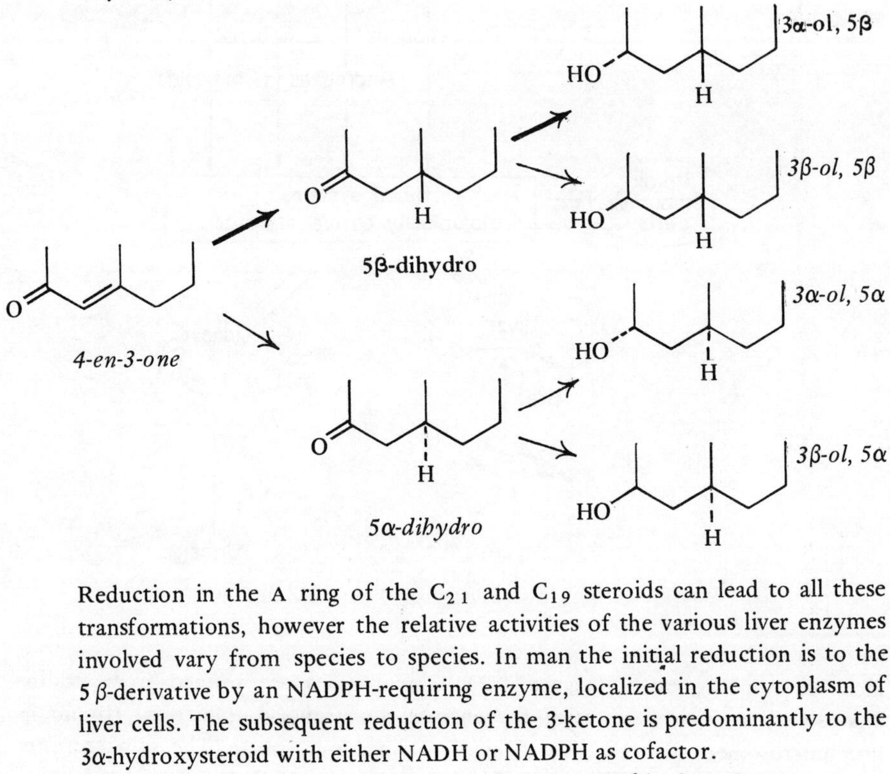

Reduction in the A ring of the C_{21} and C_{19} steroids can lead to all these transformations, however the relative activities of the various liver enzymes involved vary from species to species. In man the initial reduction is to the 5 β-derivative by an NADPH-requiring enzyme, localized in the cytoplasm of liver cells. The subsequent reduction of the 3-ketone is predominantly to the 3α-hydroxysteroid with either NADH or NADPH as cofactor.

ii) Reduction of the 20-ketone function to a 20α- or 20β-hydroxyl group:

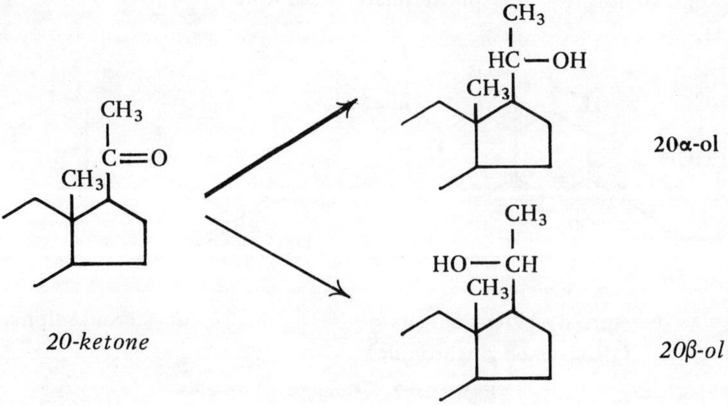

The 20α-ol predominates and this reduction usually occurs after that of the 3-ketone.

iii) Generation of a ketone function at the C-17 position either by oxidation of the 17-hydroxyl group in C_{19} steroids, or by cleaving off the C-21,20 side-chain of C_{21} steroids containing a 17α-hydroxyl group:

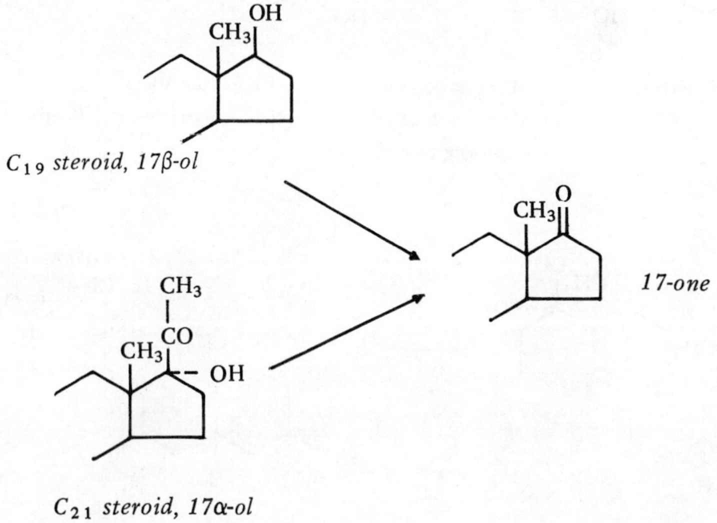

C_{19} steroid, 17β-ol

17-one

C_{21} steroid, 17α-ol

IV. PROGESTERONE AND 17α-HYDROXYPROGESTERONE

The catabolites of progesterone and 17α-hydroxyprogesterone produced by the liver are mainly the 5β-pregnanes and the 3α- and 20α-hydroxy-derivatives as shown in Figure 10.3. The circulating progesterone, emanating largely from the ovary during the luteal phase of the menstrual cycle and from the placenta during pregnancy, is largely metabolized in the liver to pregnanediol. The principal urinary products of 17α-hydroxyprogesterone are pregnanetriol and some aetiocholanolone. Large amounts of pregnanediol (20—70 mg/day) and pregnanetriol (up to 7 mg/day) are found in the urine of women during late pregnancy (see Figure 10.4) arising from high production of progesterones by the placenta. In the luteal phase of the cycle 3—7 mg/day of pregnanediol are found. During the follicular phase of the menstrual cycle and during the menopause the level of urinary pregnanediol in the female (Table 10.1) falls to about 0.5 mg/day similar to that found in the male, and is largely of adrenal origin. Similarly, low levels of pregnanediol (about 0.7 mg/day) and pregnanetriol (about 0.3 mg/day) are found in children of both sexes.

The catabolism of progesterones in non-endocrine glands other than liver appears to differ; thus the predominant products in the uterus are the 5α-pregnanes and the 3α- and 20α-hydroxy-derivatives.

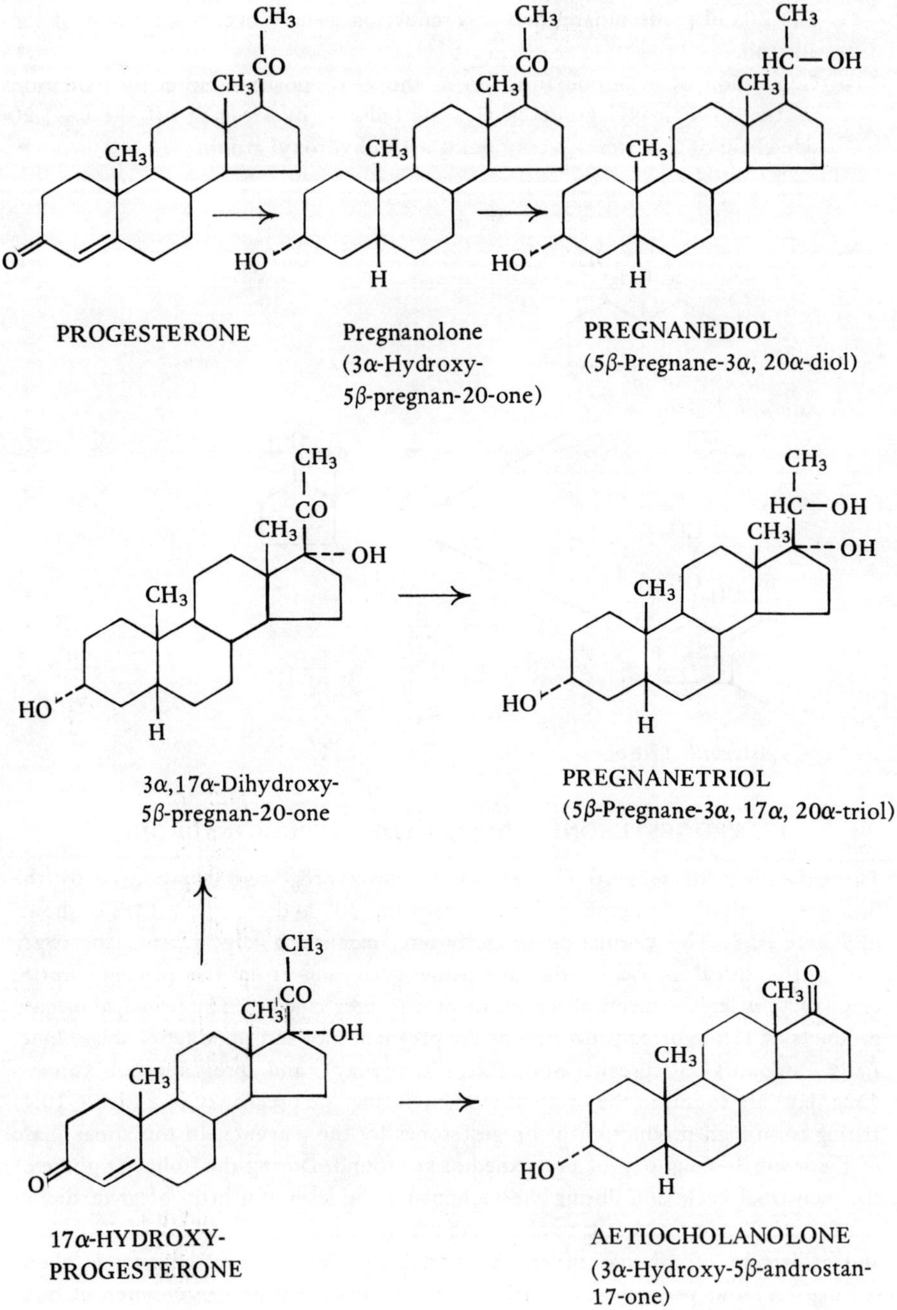

Figure 10.3 Principal catabolic pathways for the conversion of progesterone and 17α-hydroxyprogesterone (human). Other hepatic catabolites such as the 5α-dihydro steroids and the 3β-hydroxy derivatives are also produced, but in small amounts.

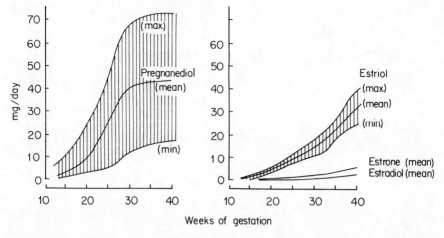

Figure 10.4 Urinary pregnanediol and C_{18} steroids during human pregnancy. During pregnancy increasing amounts of progesterone are produced by the placenta and this is reflected in a consistent rise in the daily excretion of pregnanediol in the urine. Pregnanediol output rate increases rapidly during the first three months and reaches a maximum after about eight months when it remains constant until parturition. Following delivery and elimination of the placenta, there is a dramatic fall in its output, and urinary pregnanediol has proved a useful assessment of placental function. Measurements of urinary estriol may be of greater value however, since this also provides information on the status of the foetal circulation.

V. CORTICOSTEROIDS

A. Aldosterone

Because of the relatively low levels of aldosterone secreted under normal circumstances ($100-150\ \mu g$/day in the human; plasma concentration about 8 ng/100 ml) the accumulation of sufficient material to identify the structures of catabolites has been a particular problem. Despite these difficulties, however, more than a dozen metabolites have been identified. Following injection of tracer amounts of radioactive aldosterone (Flood *et al.*, 1961), 90% of the injected

Table 10.1.
Urinary concentrations of C_{21} and C_{18} steroids during the menstrual cycle in normal women.

	μg steroid/24 hours*			
	Follicular Phase	Ovulatory Phase	Luteal Phase	Menstruation
Pregnanediol	1000	1000	4000	500
Pregnanetriol	1000	1400	1600	700
Estrone	7	20	16	4
Estradiol	3	8	5	1
Estriol	7	25	20	8

*Confer: *Recent Progress Hormone Res.* (1970) **26**, 49 and Loraine and Bell, 1968.

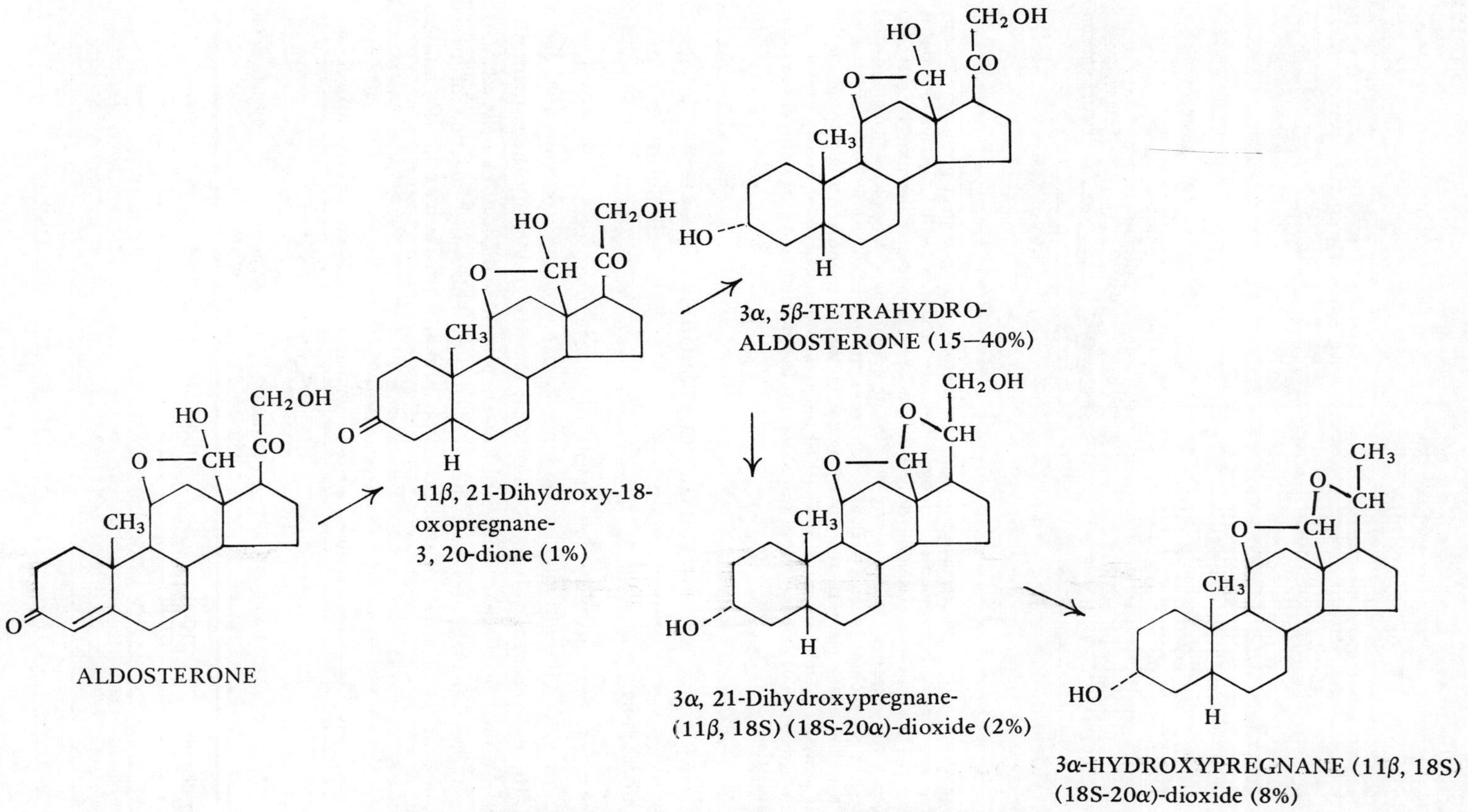

Figure 10.5 Some of the main urinary metabolites of aldosterone.

radioactivity was recovered in the urine within 2 days, of which only 0.1% was unchanged aldosterone. Rather more than half of the urinary metabolites of aldosterone appear as glucuronide conjugates – the 18-glucuronide of aldosterone itself accounting for less than 10% of the administered activity. Conjugation occurs mainly in the liver although some conjugates may be produced in the kidney (Leutscher *et al.*, 1965). Many laboratories have demonstrated that 3α, 5β-tetrahydroaldosterone is the main metabolite accounting for 15–40% of the secreted products (Figure 10.5). The catabolites of aldosterone are, in general, reduction products and bicyclic acetal metabolites as illustrated in Figure 10.5. Procedures that have been used for identification of the urinary metabolites of aldosterone have been discussed by Kelly and Lieberman (1964) and Rosenfeld *et al.* (1967).

B. Glucocorticosteroids

The principal glucocorticoids are cortisol and corticosterone. In man the former steroid predominates, but in some species (rat, rabbit, mouse) corticosterone is the major secretory steroid product of the adrenal cortex. Minor quantities of 11-deoxycortisol and 11-deoxycorticosterone are also secreted.

The liver contains reductases capable of reducing the 4–5 double bond of unsaturated 3-ketosteroids to either the 5α- or 5β-reduced product, usually with loss of the biological activity with which the steroid is normally associated. It appears that there are two specific reductases in the liver for each steroid – a microsomal enzyme which results in the 5α-product and a soluble enzyme which produces the 5β-product. All these reductases operate irreversibly and require NADPH. Cortisol, like aldosterone, is converted mainly to the 5β-isomers, whereas corticosterone and testosterone (see later) are converted to relatively equal mixtures of the 5α- and 5β-isomers.

Further metabolism of these 5α- and 5β-isomers in the liver occurs by reduction of the 3-ketone, 11β-hydroxyl, and 20-ketone as outlined in Figures 10.6 and 10.7. The kidney also contains several of these reducing enzymes. The properties of the hydroxy-steroid dehydrogenases (reversible enzymes) and oxo-reductases (irreversible enzymes) responsible for these reductions have been reviewed by Dorfman and Ungar (1965, Chapter VI). Most of the urinary metabolites of the glucocorticoids are found in the urine as the glucuronide conjugates.

Any malfunctioning of the thyroid hormone production system affects the blood levels of corticosteroids, and this is believed to be due to an effect at the level of the liver enzyme (11β-dehydrogenase) responsible for converting cortisol to cortisone. Whereas both cortisol and corticosterone exert a feedback inhibitory effect on the pituitary production of ACTH, cortisone has little or no such feedback inhibitory effect. For this reason the 11β-dehydrogenase plays an important role in regulating the blood circulating level of cortisol. This 11β-dehydrogenase is stimulated by thyroid hormones, and elevated levels of thyroid hormones have been shown both to increase the oxidation of cortisol to

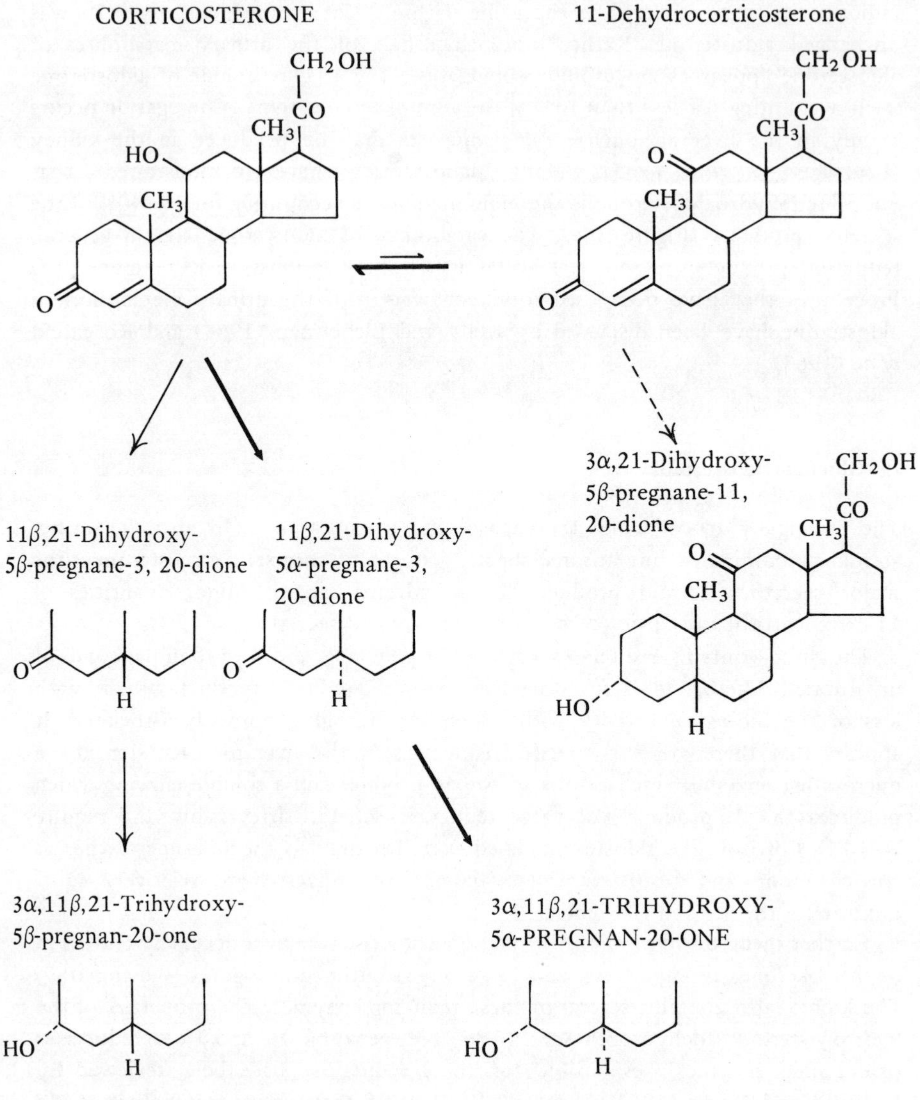

CORTICOSTERONE   11-Dehydrocorticosterone

Figure 10.6   Principal metabolites of corticosterone.

cortisone and also to stimulate the endogenous production of cortisol. Moreover, decreased levels of thyroid hormone are associated with a decreased production of cortisol and a decreased rate of metabolism of the 11β-hydroxy steroids.

VI. C_{19} STEROIDS

The main precursors of testosterone are androstenedione and dehydro-epiandrosterone with androstenediol and 17α-hydroxyprogesterone acting as

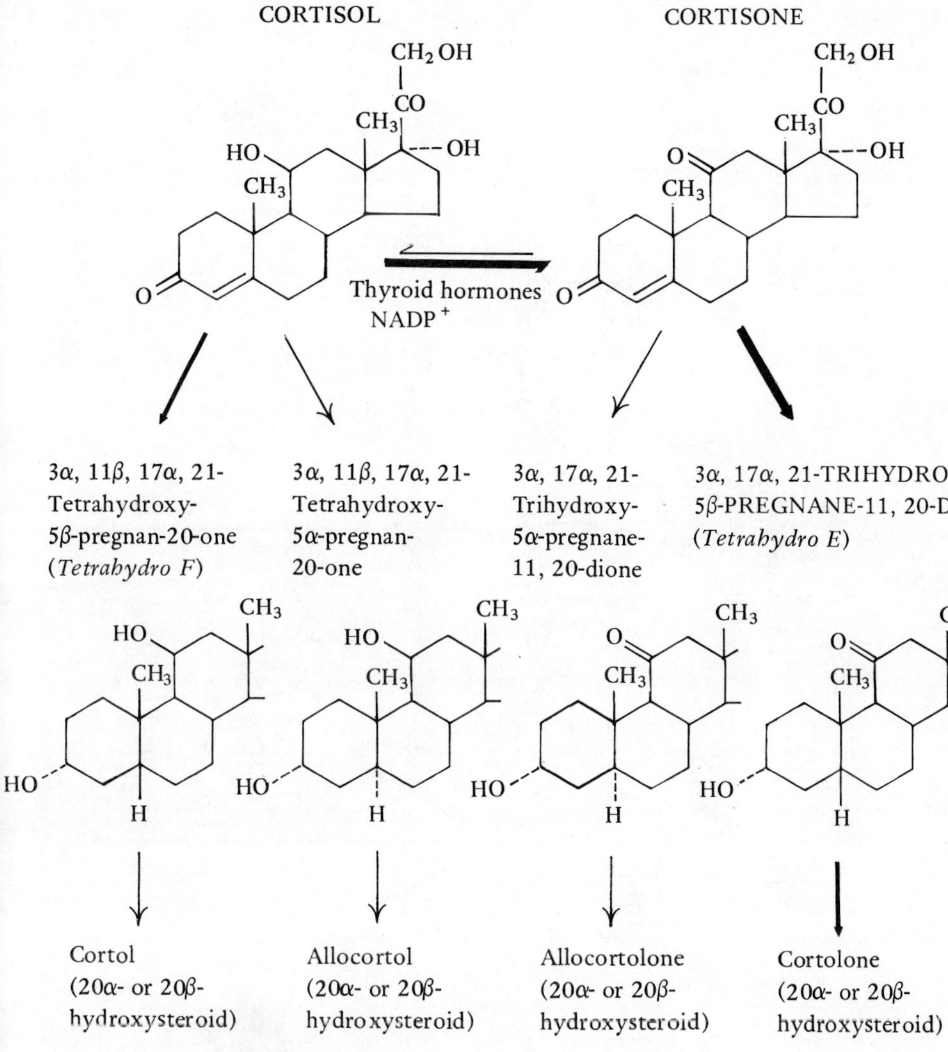

Figure 10.7 Principal metabolites of cortisol. In man the principal urinary metabolites of cortisol and cortisone are Tetrahydro E and, to a lesser extent, Tetrahydro F.

additional sources (see Figure 4.5). The adrenal cortex, as well as the testis, is an important source of androgens. In addition to androstenedione and 11β-hydroxy-androstenedione, the adrenal gland produces large quantities of dehydro-epiandrosterone sulphate. This latter conjugated steroid is also produced by the foetus, and particularly during the later stages of pregnancy functions as an important precursor for the estrogens produced by the placenta (see Chapter 4.VIc and Chapter 9).

The main pathways for metabolism of the important C_{19} steroids are shown in

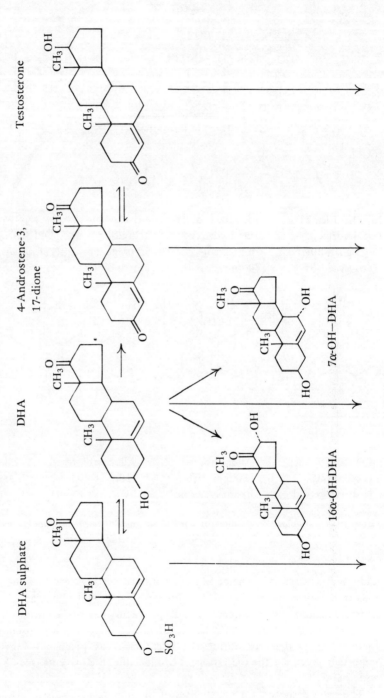

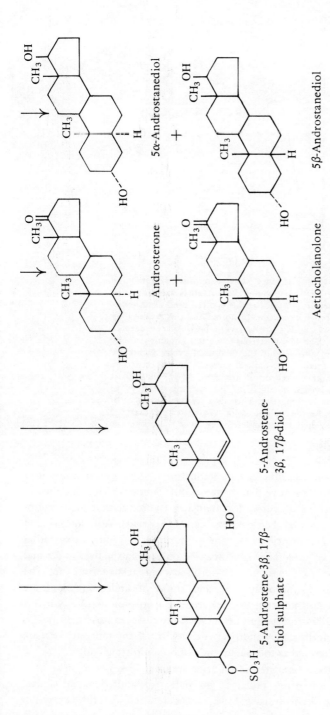

Figure 10.8 Metabolism of the principal androgens. The sulphated steroids are excreted as such, the other metabolites are conjugated with glucuronic acid before excretion in the urine.

5α-Androstanediol

+

5β-Androstanediol

Androsterone

+

Aetiocholanolone

5-Androstene-3β, 17β-diol

5-Androstene-3β, 17β-diol sulphate

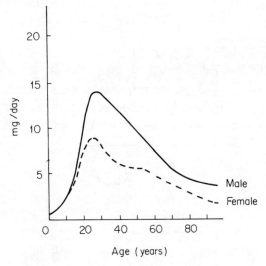

Figure 10.9 Urinary 17-oxosteroids excreted by normal men and women. Mean values are shown for total urinary 17-oxosteroids — often used as an index of androgen excretion. In normal females, peak values of 7–12 mg/day are observed between the ages of 20–30. The 17-oxosteroid excretion remains virtually constant throughout the menstrual cycle. In normal males there is a marked increase at puberty to a maximum excretion of between 12–17 mg/day at 20–30 years of age. In old age this declines to between 2–8 mg/day. There is a reasonable degree of overlap between amounts of 17-oxosteroids excreted by individual males and females, over the entire age range.

Figure 10.8. Dehydroepiandrosterone and its sulphate may be reduced in the liver to the 17β-hydroxysteroid derivative 5-androstene-3β,17β-diol, which is excreted in the urine as the sulphate or glucuronide conjugate. Hydroxylation of dehydro-epiandrosterone at the 7α- and 16α-position can also occur. Testosterone and androstenedione are interconvertible via the action of a 17β-hydroxysteroid dehydrogenase and both of these androgens may be reduced in the liver to 5α- and 5β-hydroxysteroids. The principal urinary products of testosterone are the glucuronides of 5α- and 5β-androstanediol, and those of androstenedione are androsterone (3-hydroxy-5α-androstan-17-one) and aetiocholanolone (3α-hydroxy-5β-androstan-17-one). Dihydrotestosterone (17β-hydroxy-5α-androstan-3-one) is believed to be the biologically active androgen, derived from, and more active than, testosterone. It, too, is excreted as the glucuronide of 5α-androstanediol.

Most (but not all) of the 17-oxosteroids in urine are of androgenic origin and the urinary 17-oxosteroids are often taken as an index of androgens in clinical investigations. Following hydrolysis of the conjugates and careful extraction procedures, some of the non-androgenic 17-oxosteroids can be removed (e.g.

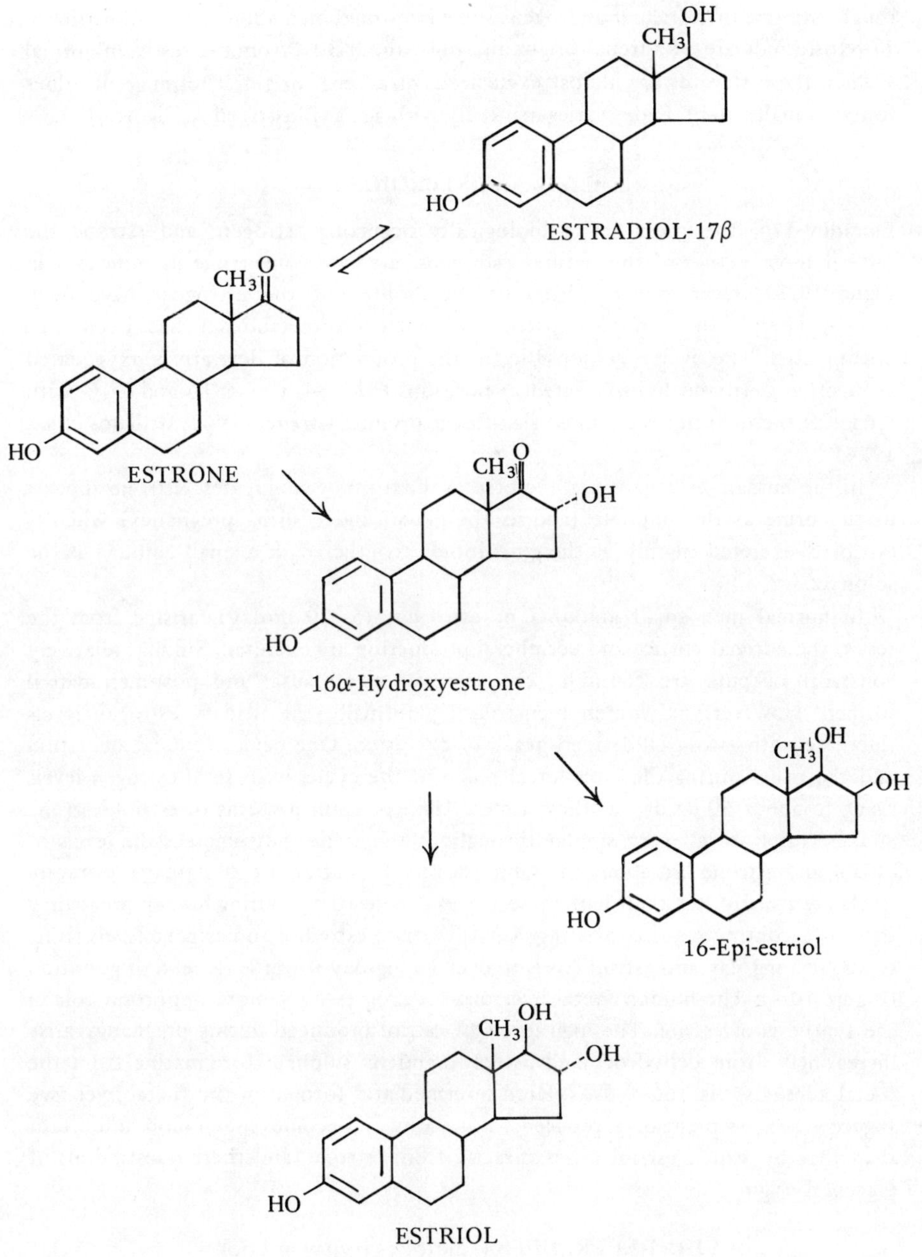

Figure 10.10 Principal metabolites of the estrogens.

estrone, by alkali washing) to yield an extract which is reasonably representative of the urinary metabolites of androgens. However, these metabolites afford only a rough estimate of testicular androgens since in normal men about 70% of the urinary 17-oxosteroids are of adrenal origin and only about 30% from the testis; in normal women these steroids are almost exclusively of adrenal origin. The range of values found in males and females varies markedly with age as illustrated in Figure 10.9.

VII. C_{18} STEROIDS

Estradiol-17β, the most active biologically occurring estrogen, and estrone the second most active of the natural estrogens, are interconvertible as indicated in Figure 10.10. Over twenty different metabolites of the estrogens have been identified and the complex pattern of estrogen metabolism has been well documented. The liver is responsible for the production of derivatives oxygenated at position C-16 and hydroxylated at positions C-2, C-4, C-6, C-16 and C-18, with estriol as the quantitatively most significant product (Breuer, 1962; Williams *et al.*, 1974).

In the human, estrogens are excreted in the form of conjugates. Estrone appears in the urine as the sulphate (and as the glucuronide during pregnancy) whereas estriol is excreted mainly as the glucuronide together with a small amount as the sulphate.

In normal men small amounts of estrogens (5–20 μg/day), arising from the testis, the adrenal cortex and peripheral production are excreted. Similar, relatively constant, outputs are found in the urine of menopausal and post-menopausal women. However, in women menstruating normally the urinary estrogen levels fluctuate with two well-defined peaks of excretion. One peak occurs at ovulation and the other during the later luteal phase of the cycle, with total estrogen levels rising to about 50 μg/day at these times. The excretion patterns of estriol, estrone and estradiol are all very similar throughout the cycle, but whereas the levels of estriol and estrone are about the same (peak values at about 20 μg/day), estradiol levels are usually less than half these values (Table 10.1). During human pregnancy there is a continuous rise in estrogen output, with estradiol and estrone levels rising to about 2 mg/day and estriol levels to over 10 mg/day towards the end of gestation (Figure 10.4). The human foetal liver plays a progressively more important role in the synthesis of estriol. The high levels of estriol produced during pregnancy arise increasingly from dehydroepiandrosterone and its sulphate (originating from the foetal adrenals) via 16α-hydroxylated intermediates formed in the foetal liver (see Figure 4.14). As pregnancy proceeds, this pathway becomes much more important than that by which estriol arises directly from estrone (and thereby estradiol) of placental origin.

VIII. REFERENCES (*indicates review or book)

*Breuer, H. (1962). The metabolism of the natural estrogens. *Vitamins and Hormones*, 20, 285–335.
*Dixon, P. F., M. Booth and J. Butler (1967). The corticosteroids. In C. H. Gray &

A. L. Bacharach, (Eds), *Hormones in blood*. Academic Press, London and New York. Vol. 2, 305—389.

*Dorfman, R. I. and F. Ungar (1965). *Metabolism of Steroid hormones*. Academic Press, New York and London.

Kelly, W. G. and S. Lieberman (1964). Isolation and characterization of human urinary metabolites of aldosterone. In E. E. Baulieu and P. Robel (Eds), *Aldosterone, a symposium*. Blackwell, Oxford, pp. 103—129.

Flood, C., D. S. Layne, S. Ramcharach, E. Rossipal, J. F. Tait and S. A. S. Tait (1961). An investigation of the urinary metabolites and secretion rates of aldosterone and cortisol in man and a description of methods for their measurement. *Acta Endocrinol.*, 36, 237—264.

Loraine, J. A. and E. T. Bell (1968). *Fertility and contraception in the human female*. Livingstone, Edinburgh.

Leutscher, J. A., E. W. Hancock, C. A. Camargo, A. J. Dowdy and G. W. Nokes (1965). Conjugation of 1,2-^{3}H-aldosterone in human liver and kidneys and renal extraction of aldosterone and labelled conjugates from blood plasma. *J. Clin. Endocrinol. Metab.* 25, 628—638.

*Rosenfeld, R. S., D. K. Fukushima and T. F. Gallagher (1967). Metabolism of adrenal cortical hormones. In A. B. Eisenstein (Ed.) *The Adrenal Cortex*. Little, Brown & Co., Boston. pp. 103—131.

Williams, J. G., C. Longcope and K. I. H. Williams (1974). 4-Hydroxyestrone: a new metabolite of Estradiol-17β from humans. *Steroids*, 24, 687—701.

Hormonal Mode of Action in Regulating Steroid Hormone Biosynthesis

CHAPTER 11

Control of glucocorticoid synthesis by ACTH

I. INTRODUCTION

The biochemistry of the adrenal cortex and the mode of action of ACTH in controlling its steroidogenic capability is a field that has attracted the interest of many workers over the past few decades. Many aspects of this subject have been comprehensively reviewed (Garren et al., 1971; Gill, 1972, 1975; Kowal, 1970b; Schulster, 1974a; Wicks, 1974).

Earlier chapters in this book have documented relevant features concerning the ACTH molecule and its mode of secretion from the pituitary (Chapter 5. IIIA) as well as the important structural aspects of the adrenal cortex and its pattern of steroid products (Chapter 6). In this chapter, the details of the biochemical system through which ACTH is thought to regulate glucocorticosteroid synthesis in adrenocortical cells are discussed.

ACTH regulates the functioning of adrenal cortex in a very general manner (see Chapter 5.IIIA). Not only does this pituitary hormone control the synthesis of the corticosteroids and adrenal androgens, it also regulates the growth and size of the gland and the replication of adrenocortical cells. These trophic effects of ACTH (for review see Gill, 1975) are most evident in the enlargement of the gland occurring in Cushing's disease and in the adrenocortical atrophy observed following hypophysectomy. The zona fasciculata—reticularis of the adrenal cortex is highly responsive to ACTH and cells in this region are principally concerned with glucocorticoid synthesis; the zona glomulerosa, on the other hand, is relatively unresponsive to ACTH and is more concerned with mineralocorticoid synthesis (see Chapter 12).

A discussion of the ACTH steroidogenic mechanism necessitates examination of several different aspects, including: the role of cell membrane receptors for the protein hormone, adenylate cyclase, and the mediatory function of cyclic AMP, cyclic AMP-dependent protein kinase and protein phosphorylation, and the possible involvement of protein and RNA synthesis. Each of these areas is discussed in turn and some attempt is made to correlate the data obtained from the large number of studies performed in this field to provide some working models for the action of ACTH. It must be emphasized, however, that despite the considerable efforts of large numbers of researchers, the detailed mechanism of this complex process is still far from clear and these models remain at best unproven, at worst speculative. Nevertheless significant advances have been made in recent years and it is clear that there is much to be discovered about the delicate and finely-tuned mechanism by which ACTH can switch on the steroidogenic machinery of adrenal zona fasciculata—reticularis cells with such speed, specificity and precision. Moreover, studies in this field have enhanced our understanding of many other cellular control systems, particularly those concerning the ways in which other protein hormones act on their target endocrine tissues (cf. Chapters 12 and 13), as well as some of the processes affecting cellular growth.

II. ACTH IN BLOOD

Before we can interpret studies in this field it is important to know what levels of ACTH actually occur in the living animal.

The plasma concentrations of ACTH under a variety of different conditions have been measured and the data from numerous laboratories have been summarized (Sayers, 1967). Estimates range from $0.4-6\,\mu$ units ACTH/ml* plasma for normal humans under normal conditions, and in subjects undergoing surgery the concentration increases to $4-12\,\mu$ units ACTH/ml plasma. Comparison of the concentrations in man and rat shows that they are quantitatively very similar under a variety of circumstances. The concentration of ACTH in the normal rat under normal circumstances is less than $5\,\mu$ units/ml blood and rapidly rises to $10\,\mu$ units/ml blood after ether anaesthesia and scalding. Even one week after adrenalectomy the ACTH concentration in the rat (maintained on saline without

---

*ACTH (IIIrd Int. Standard, sub-cut. activity): 1 international unit is approx. 10 μg ($1\,\mu$U = 10 pg). (Bangham, Mussett and Stack-Dunne: *Bull. World Health Org.* 1962, 27, 395—408).

steroid replacement therapy) only increases to 32 μ units/ml blood, and this is elevated to a maximum of 100 μ units/ml blood after extreme stress.

Blood-borne ACTH is inactivated rapidly and in the rat the half-life of endogenous ACTH may be as short as 1 min. About 20% of injected ACTH is taken up by the rat kidney, and the liver is also involved in the rapid degradation of the hormone. Because of the episodic nature of its secretion (see Figure 6.5), its short life-span in the circulation and the ability of adrenal tissue to bind and concentrate the hormone, assays of ACTH concentrations in blood samples unfortunately give little indication as to the actual concentration of ACTH present at its site of action at the adrenocortical cell. For these reasons, it is difficult to ascribe values to what is often, but vaguely, referred to as 'physiological concentrations' – nevertheless it seems reasonable to regard concentrations above the highest recorded blood concentrations (i.e. > 100 μ units/ml or > 1 ng/ml) as 'non-physiological'. This is an important consideration since studies *in vitro* may show effects only at very high hormonal concentrations (e.g. ACTH effects on fat cells), or else may at very high hormonal concentrations show responses which are different in character from those elicited at very low concentrations.

One important effect of ACTH (among many others – see Chapter 5.III) is its action *in vivo* to stimulate blood-flow through the adrenal gland - an effect which results in both an increased supply of blood-borne components such as steroid precursors, cofactors and oxygen, as well as an increased rate of removal of secretion products from the gland. In this context it is important to note that the adrenal gland structure ensures an extremely rich blood supply and an efficient drainage system for all cortical cells (Chapter 6.III). When adrenal tissue or isolated cells are studied using *in vitro* systems, this stimulatory effect of ACTH on blood-flow rate is lacking. This exemplifies one of the difficulties in comparing *in vivo* and *in vitro* data in this field, and this is just one way in which the results obtained from any experiment can be influenced by the particular system employed.

III. ADRENAL SYSTEMS EMPLOYED FOR ACTH STUDIES

Much important and informative work has been done *in vivo*, utilizing intact or surgically treated (e.g. hypophysectomized) animals, by cannulating the adrenal vein and measuring blood-borne products from the adrenal following injection of ACTH and other compounds. However, these studies suffer from the disadvantages of complex effects (such as effects on blood-flow rate) and the inconvenience associated with analysis of blood samples.

Simple *in vitro* techniques have been devised in which glands, fragments or slices are incubated in the presence of added agents, in a simple buffer solution. Again much information has derived from these studies, but such *in vitro* incubations, where medium merely bathes the outer surface of the tissue fragment, are poor substitutes for the *in vivo* situation in which each cell is plentifully supplied with blood. This is evident from the relatively poor steroid output, normally not more than 20% of the *in vivo* secretion rate, obtained from such incubations in response to ACTH and the high concentrations of hormone that are required to elicit these responses.

In recent years various systems have become available for studying the responses of whole adrenal cells. The adaptation of ACTH responsive mouse adrenal cortex tumours to tissue culture has provided an extremely useful system for studies into the biochemistry of ACTH action on these tumour cells. It is also now possible to prepare isolated adrenal zona fasciculata—reticularis cells from normal tissue by a variety of enzymic disaggregation techniques employing collagenase or trypsin and the advantages of such systems have been discussed in Chapter 3.IV. The sensitivity and magnitude of the steroidogenic response to ACTH of the isolated cell system are of particular note. Median effective doses for ACTH of $6-120\ \mu$ units/ml have been reported (i.e. responses are obtained with concentrations of ACTH that are found in blood) and maximal stimulatory effects of ACTH of up to 100-fold have been found.

By the use of sophisticated techniques for the purification of cells isolated by enzymic disaggregation procedures (Tait *et al.*, 1974), it is now possible to study the behaviour of single cell types as opposed to the somewhat complex mixture of cell types that have been studied hitherto. This may moreover allow some understanding of the interplay between the different cells of the adrenal cortex, and the way in which products from one cell-type may be utilized by another.

One advantage provided by the *in vivo* system is the facility for examining the dynamic functioning of the gland. Thus changes in secretion rate may be monitored. The *in vitro* superfusion system of continuous incubation, developed independently by Tait and by Saffran (see Chapter 3.III), allows the study of the dynamic response of adrenal tissue *in vitro* and overcomes the difficulties associated with the complex milieu of the *in vivo* system. Recently a superfusion system for isolated cells has been developed and it is now possible to observe the rapid responses of isolated zona fasciculata—reticularis cells using this technique (Schulster and Jenner, 1975). Important differences between studies employing conventional static incubation procedures and those using dynamic superfusion systems have emerged (see later, Subsection X).

Subcellular fractionation of adrenal tissue has provided much information about the subcellular localization of enzymic systems involved in steroidogenesis. Moreover, much knowledge has derived from the use of mitochondrial preparations and membrane fractions, and cell-free systems have proved useful for adrenal protein synthesis studies.

IV. ACTH MEMBRANE RECEPTORS

The concept of *receptors* originated with pharmacological studies on the action of various drugs and has been developed to account for the specificity of protein hormone target cell interactions. Thus a protein hormone *receptor* is considered as an element of the target cell that specifically recognizes the hormone and acts in initiating the cellular response to the hormone. This bifunctional character — that in response to its interaction with the hormone, a stimulus is generated that in turn triggers a measurable response – is intrinsic to the concept of *receptors*. The *receptor site* itself may be regarded as a pattern of forces forming a part of some structural system of the cell, and with which the hormone can specifically associate in a manner that results in the hormonal response (cf. Steroid Receptors p. 249).

It is important to recognize that specific 'binding' of a hormone to various fractions (plasma membranes or other subcellular organelles) prepared from homogenized cells, may or may not be part of a *receptor* function. The primary criteria for experimental definition of *hormone receptors* must be obtained from studies with intact cells or isolated organs that define the specificity, dose-response characteristics, the parameters of reversibility of action and equilibrium dissociation constants etc. Only then can final criteria be established from cell-free studies. This latter is possible for the hormones acting through the adenylate cyclase system (generating cyclic AMP; see following subsection) because the characteristics of specificity and cyclic AMP production shown by the intact cell *receptor* can survive the homogenization procedure. Thus 'binding', linked to adenylate cyclase activity studies, may be evaluated as a measure of *hormone receptor* activity and correlated with intact cell studies.

A number of ACTH analogues have been synthesized and the effect of these synthetic manipulations on the steroidogenic capabilities of such molecules has been evaluated (Table 5.4). This has been useful in identifying molecular structural features related to particular biological functions. These structure–function studies have demonstrated that only a portion of the total ACTH molecule is essential for steroidogenic activity. Thus although ACTH comprises a single polypeptide chain of 39 amino acid residues, the full complement of amino acids involved in the activation of the ACTH *receptor* resides between positions 4–10 of the ACTH structure (see Chapter 5.III).

The ACTH molecule has been coupled to very large inert polymers such as cellulose, agarose and polyacrylamide and the complex thus produced (comparable in size to the adrenal cell itself) shown to retain the capacity to stimulate adrenal steroidogenesis. Thus using an isolated adrenal cell suspension prepared by collagenase disaggregation, it has been shown that β^{1-24}-ACTH diazotized to beads of polyacrylamide can stimulate steroidogenesis, and that this biological activity is not due to cleavage of active peptides from the complex (Richardson and Schulster, 1972). Such studies show that ACTH can stimulate steroidogenesis without entering the adrenal cell, and support the idea that specific *receptors* for ACTH are located on the outer surface of the cell membrane.

Extracts of adrenal tumour cells have been used (Lefkowitz *et al.* 1970b) to demonstrate the direct binding of iodinated ACTH to its biologically significant site. Purified monoiodo [^{125}I] ACTH, that was biologically active and free of non-radioactive ACTH, was shown to bind to purified extracts of adrenal cells containing ACTH-sensitive adenylate cyclase, and an intimate relationship between [^{125}I] ACTH-binding and the activation of adenylate cyclase was evident. These workers (Lefkowitz *et al.*, 1971) have reported the detection of two orders of receptors – a high affinity site (representing only about 0.1% of the total *receptor* proteins) of apparent dissociation constant (K'_d): 1×10^{-12} M and a lower affinity site of K'_d: 3×10^{-8} M. It is however possible that these observations derive from the presence of only one order of *receptor* and more than one species of [^{125}I] ACTH molecule, or different types of cell. Other workers have reported the presence of '*receptors*' in rat adrenal fractions of K'_d: 1×10^{-13} M and 1×10^{-11} M (Wolfsen *et al.* 1972). A plasma membrane-enriched fraction has been isolated from bovine adrenal cortex and this membrane fraction is believed to contain an ACTH *receptor* (Finn *et al.* 1972); it binds ACTH and ACTH analogues and fragments, and moreover contains an ACTH-sensitive adenylate cyclase. The ready accessibility of this material will aid further studies into *receptor* mechanisms and the character-ization of those regions of the ACTH polypeptide molecule that are involved in binding and those related to biological activity. This *receptor* preparation may moreover prove valuable for use in a '*radio-receptor*' assay for ACTH. *Radio-receptor assays* for a large number of different hormones have now been developed utilizing the different specific *receptors* in their various target tissues, and recent years have shown increased interest in this field. This topic has been reviewed (Schulster 1974b). For details of association and dissociation constants see p. 249.

Using isolated adrenal cells, divergent effects of ACTH and its *o*-nitrophenyl sulphenyl derivative (NPS-ACTH) have been found (Moyle *et al.*, 1973), and these studies implied the presence of two *receptors* for ACTH in the adrenal cell population used – either in the same cell or in different cell types. Again using intact isolated adrenal cells, examination of the binding characteristics of purified, biologically active ^{125}I-labelled ACTH and correlation of this binding with steroidogenesis and cyclic AMP production has also demonstrated the presence of at least two *receptors* for ACTH (McIlhinney and Schulster, 1975). One *receptor* was of low affinity (apparent K'_d: 1×10^{-8} M) and present in some 30,000 sites /cell; another was of much higher (>40-fold) affinity and present in far fewer sites.

Calcium is required at a point somewhere between the binding of ACTH and the activation of adenylate cyclase by the hormone (Lefkowitz *et al.*, 1970a). In the absence of calcium, cell membrane particles derived from adrenal tumour cells were unaffected in their ability to bind ACTH, whereas the activation of adenylate cyclase by ACTH was totally inhibited. Following the exogenous addition of high concentrations of Ca^{2+} (2 mM), both ACTH activation of adenylate cyclase and ACTH binding were inhibited. Although the details of this inhibitory action of exogenous calcium have not been elucidated, it has been suggested that as well as affecting adenylate cyclase and its substrate interaction, calcium is also involved directly in the interaction between ACTH and its receptors (see later, Subsec-tion VII).

Although ACTH binding sites of various affinities have been reported, it must again be emphasized that all substances that bind hormones are not necessarily *receptors*. Before such a binding component derived from homogenized cells may be considered to be a *receptor*, it is necessary to establish its binding characteristics. Thus it must be shown to have a specificity and affinity for the activating hor-mone, analogues, competitive inhibitors and inactive hormones, that is similar to that found in intact cells. Moreover, it must have an association constant greater than or equal to (but not smaller than), that derived from whole cell *receptor* studies. However, it is now clear that for many hormones there are specified binding sites in whole cells (which may be termed *acceptors*) that fulfil the above criteria yet are not *receptors* directly linked to the functional hormone response system. This concept of *acceptors* and *receptors* for protein hormone binding has recently been reviewed and the functional significance of such acceptors discussed (Birnbaumer *et al.* 1974). It is suggested that *acceptors* may represent either a hormone-specific catabolizing system, or a large proportion of *receptor* molecules that are 'uncoupled' from the enzyme or function they regulate. Alternatively they may act as short-term storage devices, sited near to *receptors* and functioning to extend the biological life-span of the hormone and increase the local hormone concentration for the *receptor*.

For ACTH, many of these ideas have yet to be substantiated, and much work remains to be done before we have a clear understanding of this exceedingly complex aspect of the steroidogenic control system.

V. ADENOSINE 3′,5′-CYCLIC MONOPHOSPHATE (CYCLIC AMP)

There is a considerable body of evidence supporting the role of adenosine 3′,5′-cyclic monophosphate (*cyclic AMP*) as an intracellular *secondary messenger* mediating the actions of a variety of different hormones (see Robison *et al.*, 1971). According to this *secondary messenger* concept, a hormone is initially secreted by one type of cell and travels to the cells of its target tissue, where it stimulates the internal formation of a secondary messenger. This change in the information content of the target cells has been proposed as the essential function of hormones. So far the only secondary messenger that has been identified is cyclic AMP — although others (such as cyclic GMP) may exist, their role has yet to be established. Reviews by Jost and Rickenberg (1971) and others to be found in Greengard and Robison (1974) cover further work in this field.

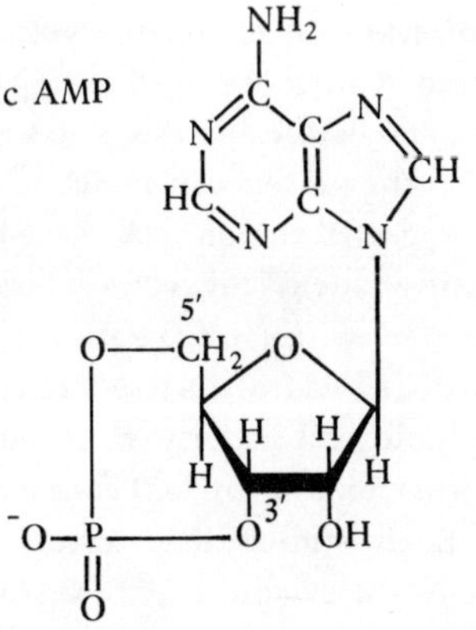

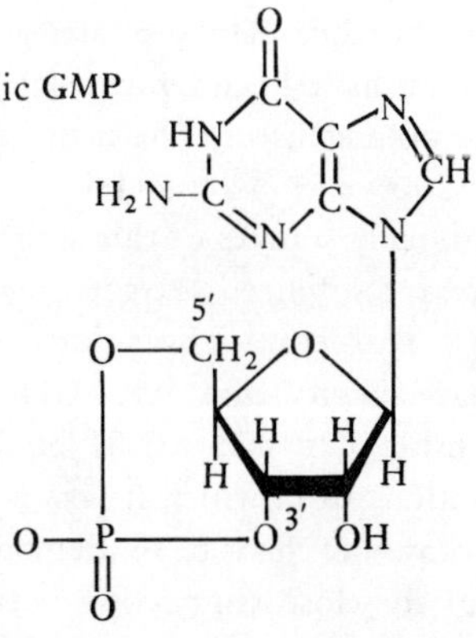

The suggestion for involvement of cyclic AMP in the ACTH stimulation of corticosteroidogenesis was prompted initially by the studies in 1957 of Haynes and Berthet. Their data implied that this effect of ACTH involved phosphorylase activation. Fumarate and NADP$^+$ both stimulated corticosteroidogenesis in homogenates of bovine adrenal cortex. The biosynthesis of corticosteroids requires NADPH at several points in the pathway (Figure 4.8) and Haynes' studies with homogenates suggested that NADPH availability played a key role in steroidogenesis. However, although the concept of an intermediary role for cyclic AMP has been given much corroborative evidence by recent studies, the remainder of the Haynes—Berthet scheme involving stimulation of phosphorylase and provision of NADPH is now seen to be inadequate.

A. Adenylate cyclase

The level of cyclic AMP within a cell at any particular time is regulated by the activities of at least two enzymes: adenylate cyclase and a specific cyclic AMP phosphodiesterase. The formation of cyclic AMP from ATP is catalysed by adenylate cyclase whilst its breakdown to 5'-AMP is regulated by phosphodiesterase.

It has been found that the methods used for the homogenization and fractionation of various tissues (e.g. liver and erythrocytes) influence the sedimentation properties of the adenylate cyclase preparation. Nevertheless, it has been ascertained that adenylate cyclase is located in the cell membrane of many tissues such as rat fat cells, liver and the α and β cells of isolated islets of Langerhans, and dog and pigeon erythrocytes. For the adrenal cortex, however, the membranal location of adenylate cyclase is not yet clearly established and to some extent its occurrence at the level of the cell membrane has been suggested by inference from work on other, more extensively studied tissues. Nevertheless, studies on mouse adrenal tumour cells support this idea, since the ACTH responsive adenylate cyclase of these cells was found associated only with particulate fractions, and the presence of adenylate cyclase has been found in the low speed centrifugate ('membrane-nuclear' fraction) obtained from homogenates of beef adrenal. Further data supporting the localization of adenylate cyclase at the cell membrane have been provided by Kelly and Koritz (1971) working with bovine adrenal homogenates. The majority of the adenylate cyclase was found in the low speed (2000 x g) pellet and it was shown that the presence of intact cells and nuclei were unlikely sources of this activity. Mouse adrenal tumour cells have been used to prepare a 'solubilized extract' of ACTH-sensitive adenylate cyclase (Lefkowitz et al. 1970b). This extract was further fractionated without separation of its ACTH-binding capacity and its ACTH-responsive adenylate cyclase activity. A clear relationship between ACTH binding and biological activity was evident for this preparation, from which it was concluded that binding of ACTH to its biologically significant site had been demonstrated. Such studies have emphasized that a particularly close connection between adenylate cyclase and the ACTH *receptor* site can be demonstrated (see Subsection IV).

From a simple model for the kinetics of adenylate cyclase activation by hormones, and if this system is described as one in equilibrium or in a steady state, it may be permissible to regard it as an allosteric enzyme system with hormones as heterotrophic activators (De Haën, 1974; Rodbard, 1974).

B. Phosphodiesterase

The methylxanthines, such as theophylline and caffeine, are noted for their inhibitory effect on cyclic AMP phosphodiesterase – the enzyme that inactivates cyclic AMP by converting it to 5'-AMP. For many hormones, the enhancement of their effects by theophylline and other methylxanthines has been used as good circumstantial evidence that these hormones exert their effects via adenylate cyclase (cf. Robison *et al.* 1971, p. 41).

The methylxanthines, however, have a wide variety of effects other than the inhibition of phosphodiesterase (which inhibition requires rather high concentrations). Thus methylxanthines stimulate glycogen synthetase, inhibit the adenosine stimulation of cyclic AMP production by guinea-pig brain tissue, as well as inhibit adrenal protein synthesis. It is likely that it is because of its inhibitory effect on adrenal protein synthesis, that earlier studies in this field found that most concentrations of theophylline inhibited, rather than potentiated, the ACTH effect on steroidogenesis.

However, recent studies have demonstrated a potentiating effect of theophylline. Thus after pre-incubation of bisected adrenals with theophylline, cholesterol side-chain cleavage activity (an index of corticosteroidogenesis) was increased, and this stimulation was observed in the absence of added ACTH or cyclic AMP, under incubation conditions during which protein synthesis was not inhibited (Leier and Jungmann, 1971). Moreover, in the hypophysectomized rat, both the basal and the ACTH stimulated corticosterone secretion was increased by acute theophylline administration. The effect of theophylline and other methylxanthine inhibitors of phosphodiesterase, in potentiating both the cyclic AMP levels and the steroidogenic effect of submaximal concentrations of ACTH, has now been demonstrated using both *in vivo* and *in vitro* systems (Peytremann *et al.* 1973a; Mackie and Schulster, 1973). An important aspect of such studies would appear to be the selection of a dose of inhibitor (e.g. 1 mM theophylline) which was without effect on protein synthesis in the adrenal system employed. It is particularly impressive to be able to use an 'inhibitor' to demonstrate an enhancement of the ACTH effect, since the usual criticism of non-specific effects (see Subsection X) cannot apply and the data presented in these studies thus strongly support the idea that the potentiating effect of theophylline on steroidogenesis is due (at least partly) to the endogenous accumulation of cyclic AMP.

As a further facet of this concept, phosphodiesterase activity can be stimulated *in vitro* by imidazole and, since this takes place in whole cells, those hormones which exert their effect via cyclic AMP should be inhibited by imidazole. Such an inhibitory effect has been demonstrated for a variety of hormonally responsive systems (cf. Robison *et al.*, 1971) and the ACTH steroidogenic response of rat adrenal quarters is inhibited by imidazole. However, other processes such as precursor incorporation into protein and RNA are also inhibited by imidazole and it must clearly be regarded as a non-specific inhibitor.

C. Studies on the role of cyclic AMP

Many workers have now shown that cyclic AMP or dibutyryl cyclic AMP (a lipophilic derivative) added to the adrenal tissue of various species is able to enhance corticosteroid synthesis in a manner similar to that of ACTH itself. In particular, the study of Karaboyas and Koritz (1965) is of importance in that it showed that the site in the steroidogenic pathway at which exogenously added cyclic AMP was acting was at a point between cholesterol and pregnenolone, the same as that defined ten years previously as the locus of the ACTH steroidogenic effect.

Substantial evidence for an intermediary role of cyclic AMP in the ACTH response has been provided by Grahame-Smith *et al.* (1967). Using quartered rat adrenal glands, it was found that increasing concentrations of ACTH produced increasing concentrations of cyclic AMP whilst steroidogenesis was proportionately stimulated (Figure 11.1). Similar results were observed *in vivo* after injecting ACTH into hypophysectomized rats (Figure 11.2). Another important observation by these workers was that ACTH increased the cyclic AMP content of adrenal quarters *in vitro* within a minute and before there was any measurable increase in ACTH-induced steroidogenesis. Moreover, the relative potencies of ACTH analogues (e.g. α-melanocyte stimulating hormone and N-α-acetyl-α^{1-24} ACTH) in increasing cyclic AMP levels were reflected in their potencies as steroidogenic agents. It was

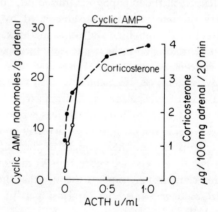

Figure 11.1 The relationship between ACTH dose, adrenal cyclic AMP concentration (o———o; nmoles/g adrenal tissue) and rate of corticosterone synthesis (•− − −•; μg/100 mg adrenal/20 min incubation) by rat adrenal quarters *in vitro*. From Grahame-Smith *et al.* (1967). Reprinted with permission. Copyright by American Society of Biological Chemists.

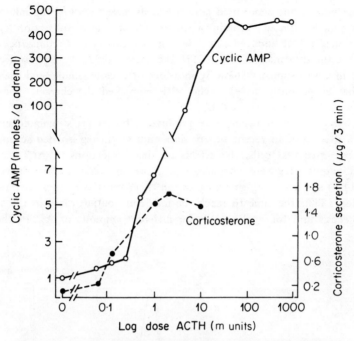

Figure 11.2 The relationship between the increase in adrenal cyclic AMP concentration (○———○; nmoles/g adrenal tissue) and corticosterone secretion (●———●; μg/3 min) in response to various doses of ACTH administered intravenously to the rat. Redrawn from Grahame-Smith *et al.* (1967). Reproduced with permission. Copyright by American Society of Biological Chemists.

not possible to dissociate the ability of polypeptide molecules structurally related to ACTH to stimulate adrenal cyclic AMP from their capacity to increase steroid synthesis. These studies further suggested that ACTH acted by increasing adenylate cyclase activity (rather than acting by some alternative mechanism such as inhibiting the phosphodiesterase).

In dynamic studies using superfused adrenal glands (see Chapter 3.III), the response to continuous infusions of different concentrations of ACTH and cyclic AMP has been observed (Schulster *et al.*, 1970). Decapsulated adrenals were used, consisting of zona fasciculata—reticularis and medulla, from rats hypophysecto-mized 3—4 hours previously, and the characteristics of the steroid output curves obtained by continuous ACTH infusions were reproduced by continuous infusions of cyclic AMP. Similar rates for the decay in steroidogenesis were found after the first hour of infusion of equipotent doses of ACTH and cyclic AMP, and this implies that the factor(s) regulating the declining corticosterone output during later time periods in this superfusion system are similar for both stimulators. Moreover, cyclic AMP, at each dose studied, exerted its maximum steroidogenic effect earlier than an equivalent dose of ACTH, thus showing that the kinetics of the response accord with the concept of an intermediary role for cyclic AMP.

Other studies using superfused adrenal glands have described the inhibition by cycloheximide — a known protein synthesis inhibitor (see Subsection X) of the ACTH or cyclic AMP induced response. Under a variety of circumstances, it was shown that the dynamics of the ACTH and the cyclic AMP response were both inhibited in a very similar fashion by infusions of cycloheximide, and again it was found that exogenously added cyclic AMP mimicked the characteristics of the steroidogenic stimulation by ACTH.

The characteristics of cyclic AMP production by ACTH stimulated cells have also been examined. In recent superfusion studies utilizing isolated adrenal (zona fasciculata—reticularis) cells, the effects of single injections of ACTH on corticosteroid output rates were compared with those on cyclic AMP production rates (Figure 11.3) and a striking similarity in the characteristics of these two responses was evident. Thus the time to reach the maximum output rate was the same for steroidogenesis and for cyclic AMP, for different amounts of ACTH; the initial

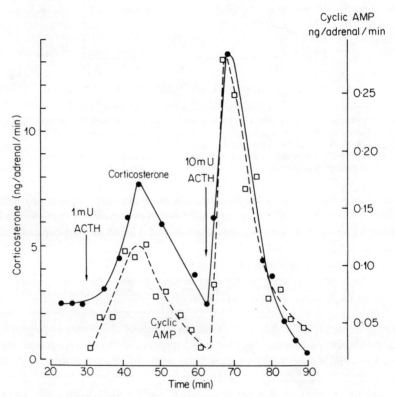

Figure 11.3 Superfused, isolated rat adrenocortical cells: comparison of the cyclic AMP output rate (□– – –□; ng/min from the cells equivalent to one adrenal) and corticosterone output rate (●———●; ng/min from the cells equivalent to one adrenal). ACTH (1 and 10 mU) was administered as a single rapid injection into the flowing stream of incubation medium at the times indicated by the arrows. One min fractions of the superfusate were assayed. Reprinted with permission of *J. Steroid Biochem.* from Schulster and Jenner (1975).

stimulatory rates and the decay rates for the two responses were very similar; the ratios of the peak heights (maximum output rates) produced in response to different amounts of ACTH were the same for cyclic AMP and steroidogenesis — as were also the ratios of areas under the curves (total response).

Thus the results obtained from these studies into the dynamic characteristics of the adrenal response are consistent with the concept of an intermediary role for cyclic AMP in the ACTH effect, and provide additional strong support for this concept.

In accord with earlier observations, superfusion studies by Pearlmutter *et al.* (1971) have shown that it is the total amount of ACTH presented to the adrenal, rather than the concentration of the hormone, that modulates its response. This observation is consistent with the concept of an adrenal cell *receptor* as the initial site of action of ACTH, since effectively all available molecules of the hormone would be bound by a receptor protein of high binding-affinity until saturation of all the available *receptor* sites. The response to dibutyryl cyclic AMP was, like that to ACTH, dependent upon the total dose. In contrast, the overall steroidogenic response of the superfused adrenal to cyclic AMP was concentration dependent. Dibutyryl cyclic AMP is noted for its ability to stimulate adrenal steroidogenesis at 30- to 50-fold lower concentrations than cyclic AMP itself, and Pearlmutter *et al.* (1971) have suggested that the dibutyryl cyclic AMP penetrating into the adrenal cells remains trapped inside, possibly by conversion to a (protein-bound?) form that is unable to leak out of the cell. The consequent intracellular binding of dibutyryl cyclic AMP would account for the similarity of its dose-response characteristics to those of ACTH. It was further suggested that the discrepancy between the effect of exogenous ACTH (response being dependent upon total amount) and cyclic AMP (response dependent upon its concentration) arises from the binding capabilities of the adrenal cell. Thus whereas ACTH is bound with high affinity and the cell is efficiently able to take up all the available hormone, cyclic AMP remains largely unbound. In this case, the rate of penetration of cyclic AMP into the cell and its consequent steroidogenic potency would be proportional to its concentration in the surrounding medium.

It should be emphasized that it is necessary to add remarkably high concentrations of exogenous cyclic AMP in order to stimulate steroidogenesis (e.g. half maximal effective doses of 3 mM cyclic AMP are reported for isolated adrenal cells: see Figure 11.4). There is a large discrepancy between the small increases in cyclic AMP associated with ACTH stimulation of steroidogenesis and the effectiveness of exogenously added cyclic AMP. However, it is reasonable to suppose that ACTH, interacting via membrane *receptors*, and exogenously added cyclic AMP, acting at some subsequent intracellular locus, would show a somewhat different pattern of steroidogenesis.

Using isolated adrenocortical cells and conventional static incubation procedures, the dose-response characteristics and time-course relationships have been examined. Following ACTH addition the consequent cyclic AMP and corticosterone accumulation has been measured (Beall and Sayers, 1972; Mackie *et al.*, 1972). The data from these studies are entirely consistent with the contention that

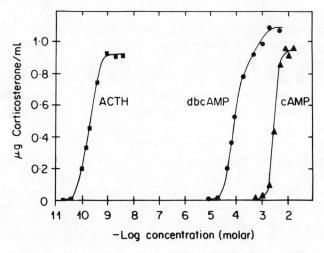

Figure 11.4 Corticosterone secretion by isolated rat adrenal cells in response to ACTH (■), dibutyryl cyclic AMP (●) and cyclic AMP (▲). Reprinted by permission of the copyright owner from Free *et al.* (1971). Copyright by the American Chemical Society.

cyclic AMP is a mediator of ACTH stimulated adrenal steroidogenesis. Thus increased cyclic AMP output was apparent within 1 minute of ACTH addition and before any discernible increase in steroidogenesis. Moreover, as shown in Figure 11.5, those concentrations of ACTH that stimulated steroidogenesis also increased cyclic AMP output in this system. However, these data also demonstrate that increased cyclic AMP outputs are obtainable by increasing the ACTH concentration beyond that necessary to stimulate maximum steroidogenesis. Thus at a concentration of ACTH (10^{-3} units/ml) which was maximal for steroidogenesis, cyclic AMP outputs were only 12% of maximum. This correlates well with the data obtained *in vivo*, (Figure 11.2) and there appears to be an enormous reserve adrenal capacity for cyclic AMP production. Only a small fraction of the cells' potential for cyclic AMP production need be activated in order to trigger maximal steroidogenesis. It is of interest in this context, that examination of the binding of ^{125}I-labelled ACTH to intact cells has demonstrated the existence of 'spare' *receptors* for ACTH, and it has been calculated that maximum steroidogenesis is elicited when about 12% of the total binding sites are filled (McIlhinney and Schulster, 1975). From this it seems clear that the large amounts of cyclic AMP produced at high (more than maximal for steroidogenesis) concentrations of ACTH are associated with the filling of these 'spare' *receptors* (of low affinity; see Subsection IV) that are not directly involved in steroidogenesis. Whether the filling of the high affinity receptor sites for ACTH (that appear to directly relate to steroidogenesis) is also associated with cyclic AMP production is as yet unclear.

Using isolated adrenal cells, divergent effects of ACTH and its *o*-nitrophenyl sulphenyl derivative (NPS–ACTH) have been observed (Moyle *et al.*, 1973) and this data suggests that either very small amounts of cyclic AMP are involved in the

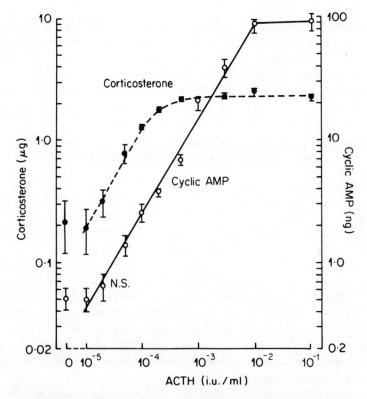

Figure 11.5 Effect of different concentrations of ACTH on isolated rat andrenocortical cells. Cyclic AMP levels (○———○; ng/hr) and corticosterone accumulated (●— — —●; μg/hr) from cells derived from 2 adrenals are shown on a logarithmic plot (Means ± S.E.M.). All steroid and cyclic AMP outputs from ACTH stimulated samples were compared with the respective outputs at 1 x 10^{-5} i.u. ACTH/ml and shown to be significantly different ($p < 0.05$; paired t-test) except where indicated (N.S. = not significant). Reproduced by permission of the copyright owners from Mackie *et al.* (1972). Copyright by North-Holland Pub. Co.

steroidogenic effect of ACTH or that factor(s) other than cyclic AMP mediate this action.

Apart from the data of Moyle *et al.* (1973) other studies have queried the obligatory mediatory role of cyclic AMP. Thus Sharma (1973) has proposed that the ACTH effect on the isolated adrenal cell is via two different mechanisms operating at two different steps in the conversion of cholesterol to pregnenolone: one is cyclic AMP dependent and the other is cyclic AMP independent. Measurements of the dynamics of steroidogenesis by isolated adrenal cells using a column perfusion technique (Lowry and McMartin, 1974) have indicated a sigmoid increase with time in the rate of ACTH stimulated steroidogenesis. The effect of added cyclic AMP appeared to be more rapid (a hyperbolic response), and it was therefore suggested that cyclic AMP might not be the sole intracellular mediator of ACTH action.

In conclusion, although a considerable body of evidence has now accumulated strongly supporting an obligatory role for cyclic AMP mediating the steroidogenic effect of ACTH, nevertheless several aspects remain to be clarified before this idea can be unequivocally accepted. It is now obvious that the role of cyclic AMP is more complex than the straightforward mediatory role that was originally conceived for it.

VI. INTRACELLULAR CYCLIC AMP RECEPTOR PROTEIN AND CYCLIC AMP-DEPENDENT PROTEIN PHOSPHOKINASE

The existence in adrenal cells of a cyclic AMP binding protein has been convincingly demonstrated. Subcellular fractions obtained from bovine adrenal cortex have been examined for binding of [^{3}H]cyclic AMP, using equilibrium dialysis to separate the unbound from the bound material. Although binding activity was observed in all subcellular fractions, it was greatest in the microsomal fraction and soluble cytoplasm. By further fractionation of the microsomes, it has been found that the microsomal cyclic AMP binding activity is associated predominantly with the endoplasmic reticulum rather than with free ribosomes. Trypsin, protease and heating to 50°C all inactivated [^{3}H]cyclic AMP binding substance found in the microsomes and soluble cytoplasm, whereas ribonuclease and deoxyribonuclease were without effect. The protein nature of the cyclic AMP binding material indicated by these studies has been confirmed following its purification (Gill and Garren, 1971).

The binding affinity of the receptor has been examined and a Scatchard plot (cyclic AMP bound against the ratio of bound over unbound cyclic AMP) exhibited a linear relationship, from which a single type of non-interacting binding site was suggested (Garren et al., 1971). The measured binding constant K_d was about 3×10^{-8} M and the molarity of the binding sites was estimated at 1×10^{-7} M. However, additional binding sites were demonstrable at high cyclic AMP concentrations (10^{-4} M). (See p. 250 for discussion of Scatchard plot.)

It has been concluded that cyclic AMP is not metabolized or covalently associated with the receptor protein since, following trichloroacetic acid precipitation or boiling, all the unbound radioactive material released from the receptor behaved chromatographically like cyclic AMP. The specificity of the receptor protein for cyclic AMP has been assessed by determining the ability of several nucleotides to compete with [^{3}H]cyclic AMP for binding sites on the protein. Other cyclic 3'5'-nucleotides (cyclic IMP, cyclic GMP and cyclic CMP) are very much less efficient than cyclic AMP in competing for binding sites on the receptor although they do bind to it.

A protein phosphokinase has been found associated with cyclic AMP receptor protein in the soluble cytoplasmic fraction derived from adrenal cortex tissue. This protein phosphokinase activity was stimulated by cyclic AMP, and the enzyme catalysed the phosphorylation of exogenously added histone, protamine and phosphorylase kinase, as evidenced by the incorporation of [^{32}P] into protein, using [γ-^{32}P]ATP as substrate (Gill and Garren, 1970). Similar cyclic AMP-dependent protein kinases have been found in many other tissues, including ovary, testes, skeletal muscle and liver. With saturating concentrations of histone as the exogenously added substrate, cyclic AMP was found to stimulate adrenal protein kinase activity with a K_m value (half maximal stimulation) of 1.4×10^{-8} M cyclic AMP, and a maximal stimulation of about 4-fold above the basal value was observed.

Both the subcellular distribution and nucleotide specificity of the cyclic AMP receptor protein and the cyclic AMP-dependent protein kinase are very similar. Like the cyclic AMP receptor protein, protein kinase activity is located in adrenal microsomes as well as the soluble cytoplasmic fraction of the cell, and after further fractionation of the microsomes most of the cyclic AMP-dependent protein kinase is found in the endoplasmic reticulum, as opposed to the free ribosomes. As a consequence of the continued association of both receptor and kinase activities in the endoplasmic reticulum, despite extensive washing and protein purification procedures, it has been suggested that they exist together in this structure in a unified regulatory complex.

The existence of such a unified complex has been demonstrated by its sedimentation as a single front in the analytical ultracentrifuge, as well as by its migration as a single band containing both cyclic AMP-receptor and kinase activities after polyacrylamide gel electrophoresis (Gill and Garren, 1971). Moreover, incubation of cyclic AMP with the receptor—kinase complex dissociated the cyclic AMP-bound receptor from the kinase, which was thereby activated. This dissociated cyclic AMP-bound receptor migrated identically with purified receptor (obtained following chromatography on DEAE-cellulose) instead of migrating with the protein kinase as previously. The kinase thus activated had no cyclic AMP-receptor activity and no longer responded to the nucleotide. The protein kinase was similarly activated when the cyclic AMP-receptor protein was differentially denatured by heating. Moreover, addition of increasing amounts of purified receptor protein to protein kinase increasingly suppressed the kinase activity, while cyclic AMP completely restored the activity. From these studies, the model depicted in Figure 11.6 has been proposed to explain the cyclic AMP stimulation of protein kinase activity. The cyclic AMP-receptor protein is envisaged as a repressor of the protein kinase when complexed with it. Cyclic AMP, by binding to the receptor protein, causes the receptor to release the kinase, which is thereby fully activated.

One difficulty with this concept arises from the observation by Butcher that overall cyclic AMP concentrations in non-stimulated adrenal tissue are about 300—600 nM with the K_d of the receptor protein and the K_m of the phosphokinase about 10—50 nM. The endogenous levels of adrenal cyclic AMP are therefore 10—100 times higher than the K_d and K_m values of the cyclic AMP-receptor and the kinase. Consequently this receptor should always be fully saturated with cyclic AMP and the phosphokinase fully active; it is therefore difficult to envisage this acting as a control system. One explanation of the apparent anomaly may be that extensive binding or compartmentalization of cyclic AMP occurs within the cell, with a consequent decrease in its effective free concentration. Alternatively the characteristics of activation of functional protein kinase within the cells may be quite different from those determined for the overall protein kinase activity in a cell-free system, using an exogenously added protein substrate.

The effect of ACTH on the state of activation of cyclic AMP-dependent protein kinase within isolated adrenal cells has been examined (Richardson and Schulster, 1973) and ACTH found to cause its complete activation within 2 minutes. This activation followed a sigmoid log dose—response curve with half-maximal stimulation at about 10^{-3} units (ACTH/ml) and theophylline potentiated the ACTH effect on protein kinase activity. Although some low ACTH concentrations that elicited a clear (submaximal) steroidogenic response failed to cause a clear increase in overall protein kinase activity, nevertheless an important role for protein kinase in the action of ACTH on intact adrenocortical cells was evident from these studies.

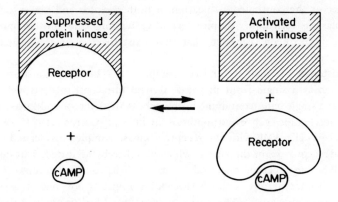

Figure 11.6 Model proposed for the activation of protein kinase by cyclic AMP. Cyclic AMP, in binding to its receptor protein, causes an allosteric change in this protein that results in the dissociation of the receptor protein from the protein kinase. This enzyme can now assume the catalytically active form. For further details see text and Garren *et al.* (1971); Gill (1972).

The exact function of the cyclic AMP-dependent protein kinase and the nature of the intracellular substrate that it phosphorylates are still unknown. A role for protein synthesis in the ACTH effect is clear (see Subsection X). However, although a purified preparation of protein kinase can catalyse the incorporation of $[^{32}P]$ from $[\gamma\text{-}^{32}P]$ ATP into protein tightly associated with ribosomes added to the incubation medium, and this ribosomal phosphorylation has been postulated to modulate the translation of stable messenger RNA (Gill, 1972), there is as yet no evidence that ACTH acting on intact cells can give rise to such a phosphorylation of ribosomes within the cell. Cyclic AMP-dependent protein kinase activity has been demonstrated in a variety of cell membrane preparations including the adrenal, and this raises the possibility that local increases in cyclic AMP concentrations, in the region of the adrenal cell membrane, can activate specific, membrane-bound species of protein kinase.

VII. THE ROLES OF CALCIUM AND PROSTAGLANDINS

As early as 1953 Birmingham and coworkers showed that Ca^{2+} played an important role in steroidogenesis, however it is now clear that Ca^{2+} is involved at several loci in this process and the precise nature of its role is still far from clear. As discussed earlier (Subsection IV) a requirement for calcium ions has been demonstrated for the ACTH stimulation of adenylate cyclase, and several earlier studies implied that Ca^{2+} may be required for ACTH binding to the adrenal cell membrane. However, Lefkowitz et al., (1970a) have shown that Ca^{2+} (2 mM) directly inhibited the binding of ACTH to cell membrane particles prepared from adrenal tumour cells; nevertheless Ca^{2+} was required for the stimulation of adenylate cyclase in these particles (although 1 mM Ca^{2+} was again inhibitory).

On the other hand, the ACTH stimulation of adenylate cyclase in isolated whole adrenal cells from normal rats was not inhibited even by 7 mM Ca^{2+} in the incubation medium (Sayers et al., 1972), and it was suggested as an explanation of this discrepancy that, in the intact cells, adenylate cyclase is confined to a compartment (probably on the inner plasma membrane) which remains unaffected by changes in the Ca^{2+} content of the external medium, and that for activation by ACTH it normally requires only trace amounts of Ca^{2+}. Following the suggestion that Ca^{2+} is in some way involved in the transmission of the signal produced by the ACTH-receptor interaction (i.e. somewhere between binding and adenylate cyclase activation) (Lefkowitz et al., 1971), it may be argued that a high concentration of Ca^{2+} can amplify the signal for the stimulation of adenylate cyclase despite some inhibition of ACTH binding.

Further studies using isolated adrenal cells have shown that in the absence of Ca^{2+}, low concentrations of ACTH do not stimulate steroidogenesis or cyclic AMP production (Haksar and Péron, 1973; Bowyer and Kitabchi, 1974); ACTH concentrations had to be increased 10,000-fold before a response was evident. However, dibutyryl cyclic AMP stimulated steroidogenesis even in the absence of Ca^{2+} (although the response was then reduced). In this way, apart from an involvement at the membrane, Ca^{2+} has also been implicated at various other loci in the steroidogenic stimulation by ACTH. Thus de novo protein synthesis appears to be an integral part of the ACTH mechanism (see Subsection X), and both ACTH and cyclic AMP-stimulated amino acid incorporation into protein require the presence of Ca^{2+}; moreover addition of Ca^{2+} alone will increase the incorporation of amino acid into protein in an in vitro cell-free system (Farese, 1971a, b, c). Direct effects of Ca^{2+} on isolated adrenal mitochondria have also been noted, and Ca^{2+} (in the presence of succinate, isocitrate and $NADP^+$) stimulated pregnenolone formation by these organelles (Simpson et al., 1975). These authors suggested that the respiration driven uptake of Ca^{2+} by adrenal mitochondria enhances the binding of substrate to cytochrome P-450 for cholesterol side-chain cleavage, thereby increasing the availability of substrate for pregnenolone formation (see Subsection VIII).

From *in vivo* studies utilizing the perfused cat adrenal, an interesting model has been proposed whereby ACTH-receptor interaction dissociates Ca^{2+} from adenylate cyclase, which is thereby activated, and concomitantly causing the redistribution of Ca^{2+} to some active site within the cell — possibly the mitochondria or endoplasmic reticulum — that couples steroid production and release (Rubin *et al.*, 1972).

If Ca^{2+} is indeed acting, like cyclic AMP, as a type of *secondary* (or tertiary?) *messenger* mediating the response to ACTH, then changes in the intracellular concentration of Ca^{2+} would be expected as a consequence of ACTH action. Studies on the uptake of $^{45}Ca^{2+}$ by adrenal glands stimulated by ACTH, dibutyryl cyclic AMP or theophylline have indeed demonstrated that the action of these stimulators is accompanied by a rapid, increased uptake of Ca^{2+} by the tissue (Leier and Jungmann, 1973). In this context, Rasmussen (1970) has emphasized that a virtually universal feature of stimulus-secretion coupling, is that Ca^{2+} uptake by cells is a parallel phenomenon to increased cyclic AMP production.

Studies in other tissues such as islets of Langerhans (Malaisse, 1973) have found that increased intracellular levels of cyclic AMP provoke an intracellular trans-location of Ca^{2+} from an organelle-bound pool to the cytosol — thereby increasing Ca^{2+} accumulation in the cytoplasm. Similarly, Borle (1974) from studies on isolated mitochondria from rat liver, heart and kidney has suggested that cyclic AMP brings about the efflux of Ca^{2+} from within the mitochondria. The vast majority of the cellular Ca^{2+} is stored within the mitochondria, and, particularly for the mitochondria-laden adrenal fasciculata cells, the idea that cyclic AMP acts within the cell to facilitate Ca^{2+} movement between mitochondria and cytoplasm (thereby activating some rate-limiting protein?) is an attractive hypothesis. It follows from this concept that studies involving large changes in medium Ca^{2+} concentrations and measurements of medium Ca^{2+} uptake might give a somewhat confusing picture of intracellular events.

If the role of calcium ions in the response to ACTH is unclear, the involvement of prostaglandins is even more so. Whereas for calcium ions there is agreement that they have a significant, and perhaps major, part to play in the ACTH mechanism, it is still far from certain that prostaglandins are involved. Measurements *in vitro* using superfused rat adrenal glands showed that prostaglandins could mimic the effect of ACTH in stimulating steroidogenesis, and Flack and Ramwell (1972) have reported a transient stimulation of corticoid synthesis by prostaglandin E_2, although it did not increase the cyclic AMP concentrations in the glands. Although the prosta-glandins have recently been implicated as playing a role in the mechanism of action of a variety of different hormones (Shaw and Tillson, 1974), data relating to their possible role in ACTH action is scanty at present. Prostaglandins may activate adrenocortical membrane-associated adenylate cyclase (Saruta and Kaplan, 1972), and localization studies utilizing autoradiography and [^{3}H]prostaglandin E_1 lend some support to this idea since some radioactivity was found in the plasma membrane (Penney *et al.*, 1973) — as well as in lipid droplets and many other cellular organelles. Gallant and Brownie (1973) have proposed that prostaglandins may play an allosteric role in the adrenal cell response to ACTH.

Prostaglandin E_1

Prostaglandin E_2

VIII. CHOLESTEROL METABOLISM

Mammalian adrenal tissue has a well documented ability to synthesize cholesterol from acetate as described in Chapter 4. Nevertheless, in some species (e.g. rat and dog) it is clear that blood-borne cholesterol (of hepatic or dietary origin) can play a major precursor role for corticosteroid biosynthesis. The major pathways and subcellular localization of the enzymes involved in the biosynthesis of adrenal corticosteroids from cholesterol are outlined in Figure 4.8 (see Simpson and Mason, 1975).

Cholesterol forms an important structural component of all membranes surrounding and inside the cell. However, up to 80% of the adrenal cholesterol is found esterified to unsaturated fatty acids (e.g. oleate, linoleate) within the lipid droplets. Whereas only small amounts of free cholesterol are found in the lipid droplets, most of the cholesterol found in the mitochondria and microsomes occurs as the free steroid. The numerous lipid droplet storage sites observed within adrenal fasciculata cells are often seen closely associated with the mitochondria (Figure 6.2c). Hydrolysis of the cholesterol esters within the lipid droplet is catalysed by cholesteryl esterase, and the activity of this enzyme in the adrenal was shown to increase following ACTH administration or stress-induced increases in endogenous ACTH (Trzeciak and Boyd, 1973). This increase was not inhibited by cyclo-heximide — indicating activation rather than new enzyme synthesis. Moreover, addition of cyclic AMP, theophylline and protein kinase to crude enzyme preparations increased cholesteryl esterase activity. Although the action of ACTH in enhancing cholesteryl esterase activity is not visualized as a rate-limiting step, it clearly plays an important (probably long-term) role in maintaining adequate supplies of free cholesterol to act as precursor for the subsequent steroidogenic pathway.

That the rate-limiting step in ACTH stimulated corticosteroidogenesis lies somewhere between the conversion of cholesterol into pregnenolone was first suggested by Stone and Hechter (1954). Although the exact identity of the intermediates involved in the conversion of cholesterol to pregnenolone is still somewhat uncertain, there is support for the scheme shown in Figure 4.6 (see Chapter 4.III), and in this regard Dixon et al., (1970) have described the isolation of crystalline 22R-hydroxycholesterol and 20α, 22R-dihydroxycholesterol (1.5 and 2.2 mg/kg of bovine adrenal, respectively). However, as discussed in Chapter 4.III,

188

it is possible that the intermediates involved in the conversion of cholesterol to pregnenolone are reactive transient complexes of the oxygenated steroid and a metalloenzyme, rather than isolatable, hydroxylated derivatives of cholesterol. Nevertheless, the locus of ACTH action on the steroidogenic pathway has now been well documented as lying somewhere in the conversion of cholesterol into pregnenolone (Farese, 1971a; Karaboyas and Koritz, 1965; Koritz and Kumar, 1970).

The cholesterol side-chain cleavage activity of the rat adrenal declines 7–9 days after hypophysectomy to about 10% of its normal activity. However, whereas the activity of the cholesterol side-chain cleavage enzyme falls by only 25% one day after hypophysectomy, the corticosteroid output rate declines rapidly – and even two hours after hypophysectomy it has fallen to about 10% of the ACTH stimulated rate. It follows that the side-chain cleavage enzyme itself is not the 'labile protein' postulated by Garren as mediating the ACTH response (see Section X).

As outlined in Figure 4.8, the cholesterol side-chain cleavage enzyme system and the 11β- and 18-hydroxylases are believed to reside within the mitochondria. These enzymes require NADPH and oxygen, and utilize cytochrome P-450 as a terminal oxidase (see Chapter 4.IV). The cytochrome P-450 associated with the side-chain cleavage system has been found to exist predominantly in a high-spin state which may be converted to a low-spin state by pregnenolone. The transfer of electrons via the NADPH-linked reductase system to the cytochrome P-450 associated with side-chain cleavage, induced a rapid change from high-spin to low-spin states, and this scheme is outlined in Figure 11.7.

Studies undertaken by Boyd, Simpson and co-workers have examined pregnenolone formation and the optical and electron paramagnetic resonance (e.p.r.) spectra of isolated adrenal mitochondria (for review see Simpson and Mason, 1975). It has been concluded from these studies that there is a limited amount of cholesterol within the mitochondria that is available for side-chain cleavage, and that this pool of cholesterol is bound to the cytochrome P-450 for side-chain cleavage in the form

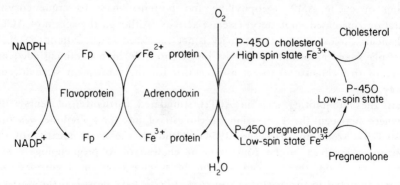

Figure 11.7   Possible role of cytochrome P-450 in the mitochondrial conversion of cholesterol to pregnenolone (see also Figures 4.10 and 4.11). Reproduced with permission from Schulster (1974a). Copyright by Academic Press Inc. (London) Ltd.

of a substrate: high-spin ferric complex. A biphasic rate of pregnenolone formation was observed for malate- or isocitrate-stimulated adrenal mitochondria, with a rapid initial phase lasting 2—5 min followed by a slower phase. Prior injection of the animals with ACTH or pretreatment with ether led to increased pregnenolone formation by the mitochondria, but no changes in 11-deoxycorticosterone conversion to corticosterone. This is again consistent with a locus for ACTH acting (via cyclic AMP) prior to pregnenolone on the steroidogenic pathway. Cyclo-heximide (see Subsection X) inhibited the effects of ACTH and ether stress on pregnenolone formation, and the ACTH-induced spectral changes. From the changes in spectral properties and cytochrome P-450 content, it has been concluded that cholesterol association with cytochrome P-450 in the adrenal mitochondria is the rate-limiting step for side-chain cleavage, and the effect of ACTH is to increase this association. This could be due either to enhanced availability of cholesterol within the mitochondria for binding to the cytochrome, or to removal by ACTH of some restraint from the enzyme which blocks its association with cholesterol.

These data imply a cycloheximide-sensitive mitochondrial locus for the primary site of action of ACTH on steroid synthesis. In this event, although the intramitochondrial supply of cholesterol that is suitable for steroidogenesis may not necessarily be rate-limiting initially, the amount of available cholesterol within the mitochondria is relatively small, and for continued steroid synthesis mobilization of cholesterol from extra-mitochondrial stores would be needed. As discussed earlier in this Subsection, ACTH activation (via cyclic AMP and protein kinase) of the cholesteryl esterase in the lipid droplet stores may be important in providing this continuing source of cholesterol.

The presence of a cholesterol-binding protein has been demonstrated in heated extracts of acetone-dried bovine adrenal mitochondria. Moreover, cholesterol side-chain cleavage in adrenal mitochondria was stimulated by this extract (Kan and Ungar, 1973). The hydrophobic character of cholesterol would imply that its movement from the lipid droplets into the mitochondria might be facilitated by a transport protein of some kind. Such a transport protein might be the cholesterol-binding protein reported by Kan and Ungar (1973). It is also conceivable that the labile protein factor proposed by Garren et al., (1965) from studies utilizing cycloheximide (see Subsection X) could fulfil this function both in transporting cholesterol into the mitochondria and facilitating cholesterol association with its mitochondrial cytochrome P-450 system.

Support for this concept has been provided by examination of the cholesterol accumulated in adrenal lipid droplets and mitochondria, following ACTH and cycloheximide treatment (Garren et al., 1971). Rats were hypophysectomized 8—12 hours before use and injected with either ACTH or cycloheximide or both; the adrenals were subsequently removed, homogenized and separated into subcellular fractions. Almost all of the cholesterol was found in the lipid droplet fraction (mostly in the esterified form) with less than 5% (predominantly as free cholesterol) in the combined mitochondrial, microsomal and soluble (lipid-free) cytoplasmic fractions. Following ACTH injection to the rats, the cholesterol ester content of the subsequently prepared lipid droplet fraction was considerably depleted, whereas the other subcellular fractions showed no substantial decrease in cholesterol content. Moreover, following injection of both cycloheximide and ACTH, a 4-fold increase in free cholesterol was found in the lipid droplet fraction with no significant changes in the other subcellular fractions. Thus ACTH stimulates the production of free cholesterol from the lipid droplet stores of esterified cholesterol by a process that is independent of continuing protein synthesis. Furthermore, Garren has suggested that because free cholesterol accumulates within the lipid droplets following cycloheximide treatment, then synthesis of a protein regulator (or some other cycloheximide-sensitive event) is required for the translocation of cholesterol from the lipid droplet into the mitochondrion.

Although the evidence supporting the above mechanism would appear convincing, studies by Mahaffee *et al.*, (1974) appear to conflict with this concept. In these experiments the cholesterol content of adrenal mitochondria prepared from rats, hypophysectomized 3 hours prior to killing, was determined. Following injection of cycloheximide and ACTH to the animals, a 2-fold increase in the cholesterol content of adrenal mitochondria was observed. Similar increases were observed following injection of aminoglutethimide (a drug that blocks the mitochondrial conversion of cholesterol to pregnenolone) and ACTH to the rats. These experiments support the concept that ACTH stimulates steroid by regulating the mitochondrial pool of cholesterol which acts as precursor for the adrenal steroids. This work moreover provides further evidence that cycloheximide inhibits the ACTH response at a mitochondrial locus. It also accords with the concept, discussed previously, that the event in the ACTH control system which is cycloheximide-sensitive involves an increase in the association of mitochondrial cholesterol with the cytochrome P-450 for side-chain cleavage to form an active enzyme-substrate complex.

Mechanical disruption of the mitochondrial membranes can alter the interaction of cytochrome P-450 with its substrate and activate cholesterol side-chain cleavage. Similarly, Ca^{2+} stimulates pregnenolone formation by isolated mitochondria (see Subsection VII), and it may be that Ca^{2+}-induced conformational changes in the mitochondrial membrane may participate in the regulation of cholesterol association with the mitochondrial side-chain cleavage system (Simpson and Mason, 1975).

IX. THE REGULATION OF PREGNENOLONE SYNTHESIS

In recent years the concept has gained support that ACTH controls steroidogenesis (via the intermediary action of cyclic AMP) by affecting the permeability of the mitochondrial membrane: either to enhance cholesterol entry (as discussed above) or to facilitate pregnenolone exit. The enzymes concerned in corticosteroid biosynthesis are found partly inside and partly outside the mitochondrion (see Figure 4.8). In particular, the enzymes involved in the conversion of cholesterol to pregnenolone are intramitochondrial, whereas those involved in the further conversion of pregnenolone to 11-deoxycortisol or 11-deoxycorticosterone are cytoplasmic. Hence, it would seem that pregnenolone synthesized inside the

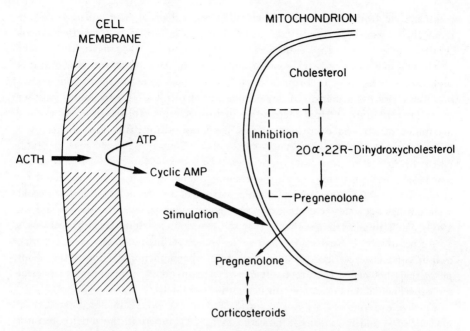

Figure 11.8   The Koritz—Hall model proposed to describe the steroidogenic action of ACTH via an effect on pregnenolone feedback inhibition. It was suggested that ACTH acting via cyclic AMP enhances the exit of pregnenolone from the mitochondria, thereby relieving the feedback inhibitory effect pregnenolone has on its own synthesis. For further details see text and Koritz (1968).

mitochondria must traverse the mitochondrial membrane before it can be further utilized as a corticosteroid precursor. From studies on isolated mitochondria, Koritz (1968) has suggested that ACTH has its effect (via cyclic AMP) at the level of the mitochondrial membrane to facilitate the exit of pregnenolone from within the mitochondria. A variety of agents, such as Ca^{2+}, myristic, oleic and palmitic acids, produced swelling of isolated mitochondria, and those agents capable of causing mitochondrial swelling also stimulated pregenolone synthesis. These results implied that a modification in mitochondrial membrane structure was a critical factor in the stimulation of pregenolone synthesis.

A change in the permeability properties of the mitochondrial membrane could affect pregnenolone synthesis in several ways, but from their studies Koritz and coworkers have proposed that such a permeability change could enhance the exit of pregnenolone formed inside the mitochondria. Using an acetone powder of adrenal mitochondria Koritz and Hall have shown that pregnenolone itself inhibits conversion of cholesterol to pregnenolone and that this inhibition by pregnenolone is allosteric in nature (see Koritz, 1968).

This observation, that pregnenolone can act as an end product inhibitor of its own synthesis, provided the basis for the Koritz and Hall model to describe the steroidogenic action of ACTH (Figure 11.8). It was postulated that ACTH, acting via cyclic AMP, affected the mitochondrial membrane in such a manner that exit of pregnenolone from within the mitochondria was enhanced. The increased rate of removal of pregnenolone would then relieve the feed-back inhibitory effect on its synthesis, and result in an overall increase in the rate of steroidogenesis.

The model proposed by Koritz and Hall for the ACTH mechanism was supported by the work of Urquhart and Li (1968) which established the dynamics of adrenocorticoid secretion of dog adrenals in vivo following continuous infusion of ACTH (2μU/ml). A rapid increase in cortisol secretion rate was observed up to a maximum which was over thirty times the basal output; this peak output rate subsequently declined to a steady-state level at about 60% of the maximal rate. When the ACTH infusion was stopped, cortisol secretion fell rapidly to a constant low basal rate. This characteristic overshoot phenomenon could be repeated by re-infusion of ACTH, and this dynamic pattern of in vivo adrenal corticosteroid secretion has been subjected to extensive mathematical analysis (Urquhart and Li, 1969). Such an analysis has shown that the Koritz and Hall model (Figure 11.8) is one type of model that can give rise to the experimentally observed dynamic output curve characterized by such an overshoot phenomenon. Of course this is not proof that the theory is correct — it merely demonstrates that rigorous analysis of the experimental data does not conflict with this model.

Further experiments, using a reconstituted system which included rat adrenal mitochondria and microsomes, indicated that ACTH increased the activity, but not the amount, of enzyme(s) involved in cholesterol conversion to pregnenolone (Koritz and Kumar, 1970). In this system, mitochondria from the adrenals of ACTH-treated rats had a 2—3 fold greater initial rate of steroidogenesis than those from the adrenals of animals not treated with ACTH. On the other hand, the microsomal fractions from ACTH treated and control animals were identical in their activity and, of the various enzymic steps involved in corticosterone synthesis, only the synthesis of pregnenolone was increased by ACTH (although it still remained the slowest step). From studies with mitochondria, obtained from adrenals of cycloheximide-treated rats and subjected to treatments designed to reduce permeability barriers, it was suggested (Koritz and Kumar, 1970) that the cycloheximide-sensitive step in the steroidogenic pathway was connected with the permeability properties of the mitochondrion, and that ACTH functioned by controlling the efflux of mitochondrial pregnenolone.

This model has stimulated further work in this field and was, until recently, an attractive concept, particularly because of evidence for the existence of a specific pregnenolone binding-protein in the adrenal cortex (Sauer, 1973) which could act as a regulator of pregnenolone exit from the mitochondria.

There are, however, a considerable amount of data which conflict with this concept. As discussed in Subsection VIII there is convincing evidence from several laboratories that ACTH acts to enhance the translocation of cholesterol from the lipid droplets and/or its association with the cytochrome P-450 system for side-chain cleavage (Garren et al., 1971; Simpson and Mason, 1975). In general these studies do not support a regulatory function for intramitochondrial pregnenolone. Several studies attempting to clarify the role of feed-back inhibition by pregnenolone in controlling its rate of synthesis have been unable to establish such a role. A central facet of the Koritz—Hall concept is that ACTH stimulates steroidogenesis by removing pregnenolone feedback inhibition. However, Farese (1971a) and Simpson *et al.*, (1972) have shown that the ACTH effect is not appreciably influenced by the total intra-adrenal pregnenolone concentration. Cyanoketone (2α-cyano-4,4,17α-trimethylandrost-5-en-17β-ol-3-one) inhibits the conversion of pregnenolone to progesterone, but the rate of cholesterol side-chain cleavage was the same in the presence or absence of cyanoketone even though pregnenolone accumulated in the presence of this inhibitor. Moreover, more endogenous pregnenolone was found in adrenal mitochondria from ether-stressed rats than in those from the control animals. If, as Koritz has suggested, ACTH acts to enhance the permeability of mitochondria to pregnenolone, then less (as opposed to more) pregnenolone should have been found in the mitochondria from the stimulated animals (Simpson *et al.*, 1972). Further evidence that ACTH does not affect the permeability of the mitochondria to pregnenolone stems from an examination of the intra- and extra-mitochondrial distribution of adrenal pregnenolone produced *in vitro* (Johnson *et al.*, 1973). Although the production of pregnenolone by mitochondria from ACTH-treated rats was four times greater than that of the non-stimulated control rats, there was no difference in the distribution of pregnenolone compared with the control.

It therefore appears that, although it is not at present possible to eliminate feedback inhibitory control by pregnenolone as a primary event in the ACTH mechanism, on balance the bulk of available evidence does not support this interesting idea as a physiological process. It would rather seem that adrenal steroidogenesis is controlled by ACTH regulation of cholesterol availability at a mitochondrial site.

X. THE ROLE OF PROTEIN AND RNA SYNTHESIS

A. Studies involving antibiotic inhibitors of protein synthesis

There is now a considerable amount of evidence that the mechanism by which ACTH stimulates adrenal corticosteroid synthesis involves the translation of stable messenger RNA (for review, see Wicks, 1974). The bulk of this evidence relies upon investigations in which antibiotic inhibitors of protein synthesis have been used. These studies are necessarily dependent upon the assumption that these inhibitors block steroidogenesis by their established effect on protein synthesis, rather than by some generalized toxic action or unknown side-effect.

The implication of a labile or short-lived protein in the ACTH response originated with the observation (Ferguson, 1962) that puromycin — an antibiotic known to inhibit protein synthesis — also inhibited the steroidogenic effect of ACTH on rat adrenals *in vitro*. The effect of cyclic AMP was similarly inhibited. Other antibiotics, such as chloramphenicol and cycloheximide (noted for their effectiveness as protein synthesis inhibitors), although structurally unrelated to puromycin, also inhibited the ACTH steroidogenic effect (cf. Ferguson, 1968). The idea that a short-lived protein was involved followed when Garren *et al.* (1965)

showed that there was a rapid decay in ACTH-stimulated steroidogenesis following cycloheximide injection. However, it was clearly recognized that these antibiotics, having a variety of effects on cells besides their established effect on protein synthesis, could not be used to *prove* a causal relationship between inhibition of protein synthesis by an antibiotic and its inhibition of the ACTH effect. For this reason, in an attempt to disprove an obligatory involvement of protein synthesis in the stimulation of steroidogenesis of ACTH, Ferguson undertook a series of experiments — all of which failed to dissociate these two processes. Thus structural analogues of puromycin were shown to correlate in their ability to inhibit both protein synthesis and the ACTH steroidogenic response. For example, the amino nucleoside derivative and the D-phenylalanyl derivative of puromycin inhibited neither amino acid incorporation into adrenal protein nor ACTH steroidogenic responsiveness. On the other hand L-phenylalanyl puromycin, an analogue which did inhibit amino acid incorporation, also blocked the ACTH response.

In further experiments it was shown that the effect of puromycin on protein synthesis was reversible and recovery required a finite time. Both the incorporation of radioactive amino acids and the steroidogenic responsiveness to ACTH were found to return at a similar slow rate after the removal of puromycin. Moreover, both inhibition of protein synthesis and inhibition of ACTH responsiveness were half maximal at the same dose of puromycin (about 10 μM). The effects of other antibiotics, chemically and structurally different from puromycin, have been similarly examined. Chloramphenicol is a potent inhibitor of protein synthesis in bacteria, but mammalian cells appear relatively resistant to it, and about 1 mM chloramphenicol was found to be required for half maximal inhibition of both adrenal [^{14}C]leucine incorporation into protein and ACTH steroidogenic responsiveness. Similarly, using an isolated adrenal cell suspension, it has been shown that cycloheximide at a dose (1 μM) that halved protein synthesis also halved the steroidogenic response for a range of ACTH concentrations (Schulster *et al.*, 1974).

If there had been a significant difference for any of these inhibitors in the concentration required to inhibit these two effects, then the existence of a causal relationship between them would have been dubious. Since *none* of these experiments were able to disprove the idea, Ferguson appears justified in suggesting that continued adrenal protein synthesis is necessary for the ACTH steroidogenic effect.

The effect of cycloheximide upon cyclic AMP concentrations in rat adrenal glands incubated *in vitro* with ACTH has also been studied, and doses of cycloheximide that were sufficient to block steroidogenesis did not inhibit the increase in adrenal cyclic AMP concentration induced by ACTH (Grahame-Smith *et al.*, 1967). It has been concluded that the cycloheximide-sensitive site on the ACTH steroidogenic pathway lies subsequent to the production of cyclic AMP (see Subsection V*c*).

The dynamics of corticosterone secretion *in vivo* after ACTH and cycloheximide injection have also been studied by Garren *et al.*, (1965). The intravenous injection of ACTH to hypophysectomized rats resulted in a rapid rise in corticosterone output which was maintained for at least 50 min. If cycloheximide was administered intraperitoneally 10 minutes after the injection of ACTH (when the corticosterone secretion rate was almost maximal), then there was an immediate and rapid decline in the rate of steroid synthesis. The half-life for this *in vivo* decay was 7—10 min. (Garren *et al.*, 1965; Rubin *et al.*, 1973). This compares with estimates, for the half-life of the key labile protein thus implicated, of 2—4 min in isolated adrenal cells (Schulster *et al.*, 1974; Schulster and Jenner, 1975) and 20—30 min in adrenal tumour cells (Kowal, 1970a).

These *in vivo* experiments have been confirmed and extended using an *in vitro* superfusion system in which adrenal glands from hypophysectomized rats were incubated in a flowing medium. Both ACTH and cycloheximide influence adrenal blood-flow rate, and the possibility that the *in vivo* observations for cycloheximide inhibition of ACTH induced steroidogenesis may be influenced by effects on adrenal blood-flow rate was eliminated by these *in vitro* superfusion studies (Schulster *et al.*, 1970). Cycloheximide was shown to have an immediate inhibitory effect on the steroidogenesis induced by either ACTH or cyclic AMP; this inhibition was reversible and the characteristics of the cycloheximide effect on both stimulators were very similar.

It is clear from these studies that a substantial part of such inhibitions by cycloheximide and puromycin (Ferguson, 1968) are not permanent effects and that, after the inhibitor is removed, the tissue is still responsive to ACTH or cyclic AMP. This inhibition of ACTH stimulated steroidogenesis can therefore not involve a mechanism that is solely dependent upon permanent damage to the steroid responsive cells. Moreover, the conversion of progesterone to corticosterone by superfused adrenal tissue was unaffected by 1 mM cycloheximide, thus again providing evidence that cycloheximide does not act via a general toxic effect on the tissue, since this would also affect the enzyme system that converts progesterone to corticosterone.

Evidence for the specificity of the inhibitory site of cycloheximide in the steroid biosynthetic route has been provided by the *in vivo* studies of Davis and Garren (1968), from which it was concluded that cycloheximide inhibits the ACTH response by preventing the conversion of cholesterol to pregnenolone. When 10 mg cycloheximide was injected into hypophysectomized rats, the incorporation of [^{3}H]acetate into adrenal cholesterol was stimulated, whereas the ACTH induced steroidogenic increase was inhibited. The data obtained showed that the antibiotic did not block a step in the pathway prior to cholesterol but rather at a site subsequent to this precursor of corticosterone. The locus of antibiotic action was more precisely determined when adrenals, endogenously labelled with [^{3}H]cholesterol, where incubated *in vitro* with [^{14}C]pregnenolone. The presence of ACTH in the incubation medium increased the conversion of endogenously labelled [^{3}H]cholesterol to [^{3}H]corticosterone, and cycloheximide added to the medium blocked this stimulation. On the other hand, the conversion of added [^{14}C]pregnenolone into [^{14}C]corticosterone was unaffected by the presence of either ACTH or cycloheximide.

These studies have further confirmed the previous reports (see Subsection VIII) that the rate-limiting step in the steroidogenic pathway stimulated by ACTH lies in the conversion of cholesterol to pregnenolone. Furthermore they have indicated that inhibitors of protein synthesis also inhibit steroid synthesis at this same site in the pathway.

Intact adrenal cells prepared by the trypsinization technique of Halkerston (1968) do not respond to NADPH, although they do respond to ACTH and this response is sensitive to cycloheximide. Garren and coworkers have demonstrated that when such cells were broken by sonication, they then responded to NADPH, and cycloheximide did not block this stimulation. It was therefore concluded that the enzymes involved in corticosterone synthesis were not themselves directly inhibited by cycloheximide. This observation is in keeping with the suggestion (see Section VIII) that a cycloheximide sensitive step, possibly synthesis of labile protein(s), is involved in the transport of cholesterol from its storage location in the lipid droplets to its site of further metabolism in the mitochondria.

Nevertheless the precise function of this labile protein is still obscure and alternative schemes remain possible.

The demonstration that ACTH can stimulate accumulation of free cholesterol within adrenal mitochondria despite cycloheximide inhibition (Mahaffee *et al.*, 1974) suggests that this labile protein is involved at a site subsequent to transport of free cholesterol into the mitochondria. Using the perfused cat adrenal, Rubin *et al.* (1973) have shown that it is possible to dissociate the effect of ACTH from that of cycloheximide. A 5 min pulse of ACTH elicited a high steroidogenic response that peaked after about 30 min and was maintained for a further 30 min. When cycloheximide infusion was started simultaneously with the brief pulse of ACTH and then continued for 15 min, the steroidogenic response was delayed (about 20 min) but was otherwise similar to that observed in the absence of cycloheximide. Moreover, a 10 min infusion of cycloheximide, started 25 min after a 5 min infusion of ACTH, rapidly inhibited steroidogenesis; however, continued perfusion washed out the cycloheximide and a further stimulation in the rate of steroidogenesis was observed. In these experiments ACTH had been absent since the initial brief pulse, indicating that it had elicited relatively stable changes, separate from the inhibitory effect of cycloheximide and which could be expressed upon restoration of protein synthesis. These data are in agreement with the concept, discussed earlier (see Subsection VIII) that ACTH regulates the supply of cholesterol to the mitochondrial side-chain cleavage system, and that the cycloheximide sensitive site in the ACTH mechanism involves the formation of an active enzyme—substrate complex by association of mitochondrial cholesterol with the cytochrome P-450 for side-chain cleavage.

B. Steroidogenesis and protein synthesis in the absence of antibiotics

Several valuable studies directed at this aspect of the problem have avoided the use of antibiotic inhibitors of protein synthesis. These studies are not subject to the criticisms levelled against the use of inhibitors, such as cycloheximide and puromycin, which may exert their action by some hitherto unidentified side-effect rather than via their established effect on protein synthesis.

In cultures of mouse adrenocortical tumour cells, Sato *et al.*, (1965) found that the omission of glutamine from the culture medium decreased both the steroidogenic response to ACTH and the rate of protein synthesis. Replacement of glutamine in the medium restored both these processes.

Two protein factors have been isolated from supernatant fractions of adrenal homogenates (Farese, 1967). One factor was induced in adrenal tissue by both ACTH and cyclic AMP, by a process that was blocked by puromycin; this factor enhanced steroid production as well as cholesterol side-chain cleavage by adrenal mitochondria. The other factor was isolated from control rat adrenal supernatant fractions and had the effect of inhibiting cholesterol side-chain cleavage by adrenal mitochondria. However, these factors have not been further defined.

Within 30 minutes of adding ACTH to cultures of Sato's mouse adrenal tumour cells, changes were evident in the amount and labelling of several protein fractions following acrylamide-gel electrophoresis (Grower and Bransome, 1970). These studies provide some further indication of a link between protein synthesis and the ACTH steroidogenic effect — although much more rapid changes in synthesis of specific protein need to be demonstrated before this is clearly established, and the likelihood remains that these changes are related to the trophic effects of the hormone.

Calcium ions have been shown to participate in the steroidogenic action of ACTH (see Subsection VII). Farese (1971b), using incubations of rat adrenal quarters, observed a marked dependence of adrenal protein synthesis on Ca^{2+}, and suggested that the maintenance of optimal adrenal protein synthesis conditions may be an explanation for the Ca^{2+} requirement during the ACTH and cyclic AMP response. Farese (1971b, c) has also demonstrated that Ca^{2+} directly stimulates protein synthesis in adrenal cell free systems. Moreover, in these studies, Ca^{2+} was found to mimic the effect of ACTH on adrenal protein synthesis by enhancing the transfer of amino acid from the amino acyl $\sim$ transfer RNA complex.

The studies discussed above have established that the continuous capability for protein synthesis is essential for expression of the adrenal steroidogenic response to ACTH. Two possibilities arise: either ACTH induces *de novo* synthesis of protein directly involved in the steroidogenic effect, or ACTH stimulates steroidogenesis by a mechanism that merely requires continuing synthesis of some labile protein factor. If the former of these alternatives is correct, then there must be sufficient time for the actual synthesis of new protein, and in order to distinguish between these alternatives, it is important to evaluate the rapidity with which ACTH can switch on steroidogenesis.

About 2–3 min elapse following ACTH addition and the discernible onset of steroidogenesis in *in vivo* perfusions (Beaven *et al.*, 1964; Urquhart and Li, 1968), *in vitro* using adrenal fragments (Grahame-Smith *et al.*, 1967; Pearlmutter *et al.*, 1973), and in static incubations using isolated adrenal cell suspensions (Beall and Sayers, 1972; Richardson and Schulster, 1972). However, technical limitations of the *in vivo* perfusion system detract from the accuracy of this estimation, and the static *in vitro* methodology only evaluates gross changes in accumulated product — fine changes in the rate of steroidogenesis are not discernible in this system. Further studies into the characteristics of this time-lag before onset of steroidogenesis, using static incubations of isolated adrenal cells (Schulster *et al.,* 1974), suggested that ACTH may bring about the rapid activation of pre-existing protein and indicated the necessity for an even more critical evaluation of the time-interval between ACTH addition and an observable steroidogenic effect.

Very rapid dynamic responses of isolated adrenal cells have recently been observed both in a column perfusion system of cells supported in a matrix of polyacrylamide beads (Lowry and McMartin, 1974) and in a superfusion system (Schulster and Jenner, 1975). In the latter study, at fast flow-rates, a large increase in the *rate* of steroidogenesis was apparent within 24 seconds of adding ACTH. The implication from these data is that there is insufficient time for ACTH to stimulate steroidogenesis by a mechanism involving direct induction of new protein (unless this protein contains exceptionally few amino acids). In a variety of eukaryotic cells, the average time taken for ribosomes, after attaching to a messenger RNA, to complete translation and release a finished polypeptide has been estimated to be at least 1–2 min, even for relatively small polypeptides (e.g. haemoglobin chains, mol. wt. 16,000).

Thus, although a role for protein synthesis is clearly implied in the ACTH effect by the data obtained using protein synthesis inhibitors, a translational control system for induction of new protein by ACTH, now appears most unlikely. An alternative scheme (Figure 11.9) has been proposed. In this concept ACTH (via

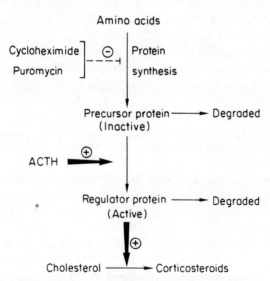

Figure 11.9   A model for the action of ACTH via activation of pre-formed labile protein. Reproduced with permission of *J. Steroid Biochem.* from Schulster and Jenner (1975).

cyclic AMP) may activate a labile 'precursor protein' — the activated 'regular protein' thus formed is also labile and facilitates the conversion of cholesterol to corticosteroids. Such an activation process (perhaps involving Ca^{2+} translocation) would be rapid and consistent with the rapidity of the ACTH effect. Protein synthesis inhibitors would block the production of 'precursor protein' and the ACTH response would then decay at a rate dependent upon the rate of depletion of 'regulator protein' within the cell. This would correspond to the decay rate assessed as having a half-life of 2—4 minutes in isolated cells or 7—10 minutes by *in vivo* perfusion studies.

C. RNA Synthesis

The role of RNA synthesis in the acute steroidogenic effect of ACTH has largely been studied with the aid of actinomycin D — a well documented inhibitor of RNA synthesis. Using rat adrenal quarters, Ferguson and Morita (1964) showed that addition of 10 μM actinomycin D had little or no effect on the ACTH steroidogenic response, although this dose of actinomycin D was sufficient to inhibit [^{14}C]-adenine and [^{14}C]uridine incorporation into adrenal RNA by about 95%. Similar observations have been made from *in vivo* studies on the effect of actinomycin D in the rat (Garren *et al.*, 1965; Ney *et al.*, 1966). From these data it has been concluded that ACTH initiates the stimulation of steroidogenesis by a mechanism that does not involve DNA synthesis.

It is however apparent that a considerable emphasis has been placed upon the ability of the adrenal to respond to ACTH after administration of actinomycin D over a narrow range of doses and time interval. Indeed there is a considerable amount of confusion as to the effects of this antibiotic on the adrenal. Actinomycin D has been reported to elevate, lower or not affect the basal production of corticosterone by the adrenal, and the ACTH response has been found to be prevented, potentiated as well as unaffected by this antibiotic (see Bransome, 1969).

Studies employing isolated adrenal cell suspensions have demonstrated that there are conditions under which actinomycin D does have a marked inhibitory effect on the ACTH and on the cyclic AMP response. Nevertheless, at low doses of actinomycin D (e.g. 1 μM) there is an inhibition of over 95% of adrenal incorporation of [^{3}H]uridine into acid-insoluble RNA, whereas the steroidogenic responses to various doses of ACTH and cyclic AMP are largely unaffected (Schulster, 1974c). The suggestion that the acute steroidogenic ACTH mechanism does not require newly synthesized RNA appears reasonably established from the studies described above. Using a superfusion system for continuous incubation of halved rat adrenals, Castells *et al.*, (1973) have demonstrated increased incorporation of radioactive precursor into total cytoplasmic RNA, as early as 15 min after exposure to ACTH. Nevertheless, this is not a rapid enough effect for it to be invoked in the steroidogenic response, and probably relates to the trophic effect of ACTH.

Mostafapour and Tchen (1971) have calculated that the ability of the adrenal to respond to ACTH after hypophysectomy, declines with a half-life of about 6–7 hours, and postulate that this might represent the slow decay of a RNA species involved in the synthesis of the labile protein invoked by Garren. Studies examining the effect of different actinomycin D concentrations on isolated adrenal cells (Schulster, 1974c) although eliminating the possibility that in stimulating steroidogenesis, ACTH acts via the synthesis of RNA, nevertheless are consistent with a permissive role for RNA synthesis. The small but distinct inhibition (20–40%) of both the ACTH and cyclic AMP responses by low concentrations (1 μM) of actinomycin D implies that continued synthesis of a relatively stable species of RNA (with a half-life of at least 70 min) is required for full continued expression of the ACTH response. Thus the available data would support the model outlined in Figure 11.10.

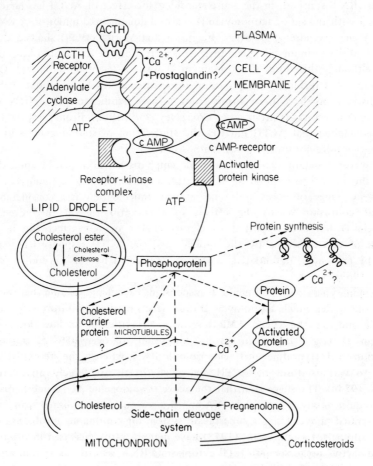

Figure 11.10 Summary of the mechanism by which ACTH may regulate steroidogenesis in adrenocortical cells. See text for discussion of the various steps shown in this hypothetical model. The intracellular role of the protein suggested to be phosphorylated by the action of ACTH is unknown; — — → indicates some of the possible sites of action.

XI. OTHER STIMULATORY AGENTS

A variety of agents have been found to stimulate adrenal steroidogenesis other than ACTH, cyclic AMP and prostaglandins. As discussed in Subsection VB) the methylxanthines (e.g. theophylline, caffeine) exert their effect by increasing intracellular cyclic AMP levels. However the antimicrotubular agents, colchicine, podophyllotoxin and vinblastine, stimulate steroidogenesis by cultures of adrenal tumour cells to the same extent as ACTH, by a mechanism which does not involve cyclic AMP (Temple and Wolff, 1973). These stimulatory agents act as a site between cholesterol and pregnenolone and are inhibited by cycloheximide and aminoglutethimide. From these studies it has been suggested that microtubules restrict transport of cholesterol into the mitochondria for interaction with the cholesterol side-chain cleavage system. Removal of this restriction by antimicrotubular reagents is postulated as the basis of the stimulation of steroidogenesis. It is feasible that ACTH, acting via cyclic AMP, might act in a similar way.

Angiotensin II also stimulates adrenal corticosteroid production and cyclic AMP output. Peytremann *et al.*, (1973b) have shown that this increase in cyclic AMP correlated with, and occurred prior to, the stimulation of steroidogenesis in isolated bovine fasciculata cells. Angiotensin has also been found to have an additive effect with prostaglandin E_1 in beef adrenal slices (Saruta and Kaplan, 1972). The role of angiotensin II is discussed further in Chapter 12.

The toxin produced by the *Cholera vibrio*, cholera toxin (or choleragen), is noted for its effect on the gut mucosa. However, in addition, it has been found to mimic the effect of many different hormones on their target tissues. The adrenal cortex is included in this wide range of tissues, and cholera toxin stimulates steroidogenesis in mouse adrenal tumour cells (Donta *et al.*, 1973) and isolated adrenal cells (Haksar *et al.*, 1975; Palfreyman and Schulster, 1975). The toxin is also thought to act via cyclic AMP, but there is a time-lag of at least 40 min between toxin addition and stimulation of steroidogenesis. This agent promises to be of considerable value in the study of the hormonal control system, particularly at the level of receptor mechanisms and the functioning of the adenylate cyclase system.

XII. SUMMARY

Although much is known about the ACTH control system, there are nevertheless many aspects that remain open to speculation. A summary of the overall scheme and the steps currently considered to be important in the regulation of adrenal steroidogenesis is depicted in Figure 11.10.

The rate-limiting step in the biosynthetic pathway lies between cholesterol and pregnenolone. Increased steroid biosynthesis is a consequence of increased intracellular pregnenolone production. All of the enzymes involved in corticosteroid biosynthesis are maintained by ACTH, and continued ACTH treatment results in adrenocortical growth and replication.

The initial interaction between ACTH and its specific cellular *receptors* occurs at the cell membrane. More than one type of *receptor* for ACTH exists, each with different binding characteristics; the activation of adenylate cyclase as a consequence of this specific binding, leads to increased amounts of intracellular cyclic AMP. Prostaglandins and Ca^{2+} may play a role in this process of binding and activation. Cyclic AMP inside the cell binds to its specific receptor protein, which exists as a unified regulatory complex with protein kinase, and causes the cyclic AMP receptor to release the kinase. The protein kinase is thus activated by cyclic AMP. The function of this cyclic AMP-dependent protein phosphokinase is to utilize ATP for the phosphorylation of proteins within the cell. This may have very broad effects on a variety of intracellular systems, and the protein phosphorylation of particular importance in controlling steroidogenesis is not yet clearly established.

Activation of cholesteryl esterase is mediated by cyclic AMP and protein kinase, and this produces free cholesterol in the lipid droplet stores. Free cholesterol is the precursor for steroidogenesis and control of its availability (to the mitochondrial enzyme complex that breaks it down) is believed to be the primary site by which hormonal control is exerted. Free cholesterol is believed to be transported, from the lipid droplet stores to the mitochondrial cholesterol side-chain cleavage complex by a cholesterol-binding protein, and this protein could function in a rate-limiting manner. Access of cholesterol to the mitochondria may also be affected by mitochondrial membrane permeability or microtubular disruption, and these could also be locations for hormonal control.

A role for protein synthesis in the ACTH response is accepted and a labile regulatory protein implicated, possibly acting at a mitochondrial locus to enhance cholesterol association with the cytochrome P-450 enzyme system for side-chain cleavage. It is possible that ACTH either directly induces the synthesis of this labile protein or that the hormonal response merely requires continuing protein for its effect. Current evidence suggests that ACTH generates this regulatory protein by activating a labile (inactive) precursor protein. Intracellular Ca^{2+} translocation may be involved in this aspect of the regulator sytem. The possibility that in the acute stimulation of steroidogenesis, ACTH acts via RNA synthesis has been eliminated.

XIII. REFERENCES (*indicates review or book)

Beall, R. J., and G. Sayers (1972). Isolated adrenal cells: steroidogenesis and cyclic AMP accumulation in response to ACTH. *Arch. Biochem. Biophys.*, 148, 70–76.

Beaven, D. W., E. A. Espiner and D. S. Hart (1964). The suppression of cortisol secretion by steroids and response to ACTH, in sheep with adrenal transplants. *J. Physiol. (London)*, 171, 216–230.

*Birnbaumer, L., S. L. Pohl and A. J. Kaumann (1974). Receptors and acceptors: A necessary distinction in hormone binding studies. In P. Greengard and G. A. Robison (Eds) *Advances in Cyclic Nucleotide Res.* Vol. 4. Raven Press, New York. pp. 239–281.

Borle, A. B. (1974). Cyclic AMP stimulation of calcium efflux from kidney, liver and heart mitochondria. *J. Membrane Biol.*, 16, 221–236.

Bowyer, F. and A. E. Kitabchi (1974). Dual role of calcium in steroidogenesis in the isolated adrenal cell of rat. *Bioch. Biophys. Res. Commun.*, 57, 100–105.

Bransome, E. D. (1969). Actinomycin D in vivo: Paradoxical and nonspecific effects on adrenal cortex. *Endocrinology*, **85**, 1114—1128.

Castells, S., N. Addo and K. Kwateng (1973). The relationship of rapidly labeled adrenal RNA synthesis to steroidogenesis in a superfusion system: effect of ACTH. *Endocrinology*, **93**, 285—291.

Davis, W. W., and L. D. Garren (1968). On the mechanism of action of ACTH. The inhibitory site of cycloheximide in the pathway of steroid biosynthesis. *J. Biol. Chem.*, **243**, 5153—5157.

De Haën, C. (1974). Adenylate Cyclase. A new kinetic analysis of the effects of hormones and fluoride ion. *J. Biol. Chem.*, **249**, 2756—2762.

Dixon, R., T. Furutachi and S. Lieberman (1970). The isolation of crystalline 22R-Hydroxycholesterol and 20α, 22R-Dihydroxycholesterol from bovine adrenals. *Biochem. Biophys. Res. Commun.*, **40**, 161—165.

Donta, S. T., M. King and K. Sloper (1973). Induction of steroidogenesis in tissue culture by cholera enterotoxin. *Nature New Biol.*, **243**, 246—247.

Farese, R. V. (1967). ACTH-induced changes in the steroidogenic activity of adrenal cell-free preparations. *Biochemistry*, **6**, 2052—2065.

Farese, R. V. (1971a). Stimulation of pregnenolone synthesis by ACTH in rat adrenal sections. *Endocrinology*, **89**, 958—962.

Farese, R. V. (1971b). On the requirement for calcium during the steroidogenic effect of ACTH. *Endocrinology*, **89**, 1057—1063 and 1064—1074.

Farese, R. V. (1971c). Calcium as a mediator of ACTH action on adrenal protein synthesis. *Science*, **173**, 447—450.

Ferguson, J. J. (1962). Puromycin and adrenal responsiveness to ACTH. *Biochim. Biophys. Acta*, **57**, 616—617.

Ferguson, J. J. (1968). Metabolic inhibitors and adrenal function. In K. W. McKerns (Ed.) 'Functions of the Adrenal Cortex' Vol. 1. Appleton-Century-Crofts, New York. pp. 463—478.

Ferguson, J. J., and Y. Morita (1964). RNA Synthesis and ACTH responsiveness. *Biochim. Biophys. Acta*, **87**, 348—350.

Finn, F. M., C. C. Widnell and K. Hofmann (1972). Localization of an ACTH receptor on bovine adrenal cortical membranes. *J. Biol. Chem.*, **247**, 5695—5702.

Flack, J. and P. Ramwell (1972). A comparison of the effects of ACTH, cyclic AMP, dibutyryl cyclic AMP and PGE_2 on corticosteroidogenesis in vitro. *Endocrinology*, **90**, 371—377.

Free, C. A., M. Chasin, V. S. Paik and S. M. Hess (1971). Steroidogenic and lipolytic activities of 8-substituted derivatives of cyclic AMP. *Biochemistry*, **10**, 3785—3789.

Gallant, S. and A. C. Brownie (1973). The in vivo effect of indomethacin and prostaglandin E_2 on ACTH and dbcAMP-induced steroidogenesis in hypophysectomized rats. *Biochem. Biophys. Res. Commun.*, **55**, 831—836.

*Garren, L. D., G. N. Gill, H. Masui and G. M. Walton (1971). On the mechanism of action of ACTH. *Recent Progr. Horm. Res.*, **27**, 433—478.

Garren, L. D., G. N. Gill, and G. M. Walton (1971). The isolation of a receptor for cyclic AMP from the adrenal cortex: the role of the receptor in the mechanism of action of cyclic AMP. *Ann. N.Y. Acad. Sci.*, **185**, 210—226.

Garren, L. D., R. L. Ney and W. W. Davis (1965). Studies on the role of protein synthesis in the regulation of corticosterone production by ACTH *in vivo. Proc. Natn. Acad. Sci. U.S.A.,* 53, 1443–1450.

*Gill, G. N. (1972). Mechanism of ACTH action. *Metabolism,* 21, 571–588.

*Gill, G. N. (1975). ACTH regulation of the adrenal cortex. In G. Gill (Ed.) *International Encyclopaedia of Pharmacology and Therapeutics:* Section on adrenal cortical hormones. Pergamon Press, in press.

Gill, G. N. and L. D. Garren (1970). A cyclic AMP-dependent protein kinase from the adrenal cortex: comparison with a cyclic AMP binding protein. *Biochem. Biophys. Res. Commun.,* 39, 335–343.

Gill, G. N. and L. D. Garren (1971). Role of the receptor in the mechanism of action of cyclic AMP. *Proc. Natn. Acad. Sci. U.S.A.,* 68, 786–790.

Grahame-Smith, D. G., R. W. Butcher, R. L. Ney and E. W. Sutherland (1967). Cyclic AMP as the intracellular mediator of the action of ACTH on the adrenal cortex. *J. Biol. Chem.,* 242, 5535–5541.

*Greengard, P., and G. A. Robison, (Eds) (1974). *Adv. in Cyclic Nucleotide Res.,* Vols. 1–4. Raven Press, New York.

Grower, M. R., and E. D. Bransome (1970). Cyclic AMP, ACTH and adrenocortical cytosol protein synthesis. *Science,* 168, 483–485.

Haksar, A., and F. G. Péron (1973). Role of calcium in the steroidogenic response of rat adrenal cells to ACTH. *Biochim. Biophys. Acta,* 313, 363–371.

Haksar, A., D. V. Maudsley and F. G. Péron (1975). Stimulation of cyclic AMP and corticosterone formation in isolated rat adrenal cells by cholera enterotoxin: comparison with the effects of ACTH. *Biochim. Biophys. Acta,* 381, 308–323.

*Halkerston, I. D. K. (1968). Heterogeneity of the response of adrenal cortex tissue slices to ACTH. In K. W. McKerns (Ed.) *Functions of the Adrenal Cortex* Vol. 1. Appleton-Century-Crofts, New York. pp. 399–461.

Johnson, L. R., A. Ruhmann-Weinhold and D. H. Nelson (1973). In vivo effect of ACTH on utilization of reducing energy for pregnenolone synthesis by adrenal mitochondria. *Ann. N.Y. Acad. Sci.,* 212, 307–318.

*Jost, J. P., and H. V. Rickenberg (1971). Cyclic AMP. *Ann. Rev. Biochem.,* 40, 741–774.

Kan, K. W. and F. Ungar (1973). Characterization of an adrenal activator for cholesterol side-chain cleavage. *J. Biol. Chem.,* 248, 2868–2875.

Karaboyas, G. C. and S. B. Koritz (1965). Identity of the site of action of cyclic AMP and ACTH in corticosteroidogenesis in rat adrenal and beef adrenal cortex slices. *Biochemistry* 4, 462–468.

Kelly, L A. and S. B. Koritz (1971). Bovine adrenal cortical adenyl cyclase and its stimulation by ACTH and NaF. *Biochim. Biophys. Acta,* 237, 141–155.

*Koritz, S. B. (1968). On the regulation of pregnenolone synthesis. In K. W. McKerns (Ed.) *Functions of the Adrenal Cortex,* Vol. 1. Appleton-Century-Crofts, New York. pp. 27–48.

Koritz, S. B. and A. M. Kumar (1970). On the mechanism of action of ACTH: The stimulation of the activity of enzymes involved in pregnenolone synthesis. *J. Biol. Chem.,* 245, 152–159.

Kowal, J. (1970a). Adrenal cells in tissue culture VII. Effect of inhibitors of protein synthesis on steroidogenesis and glycolysis. *Endocrinology,* 87, 951–965.

*Kowal, J. (1970b). ACTH and the metabolism of adrenal cell cultures. *Recent Progress in Hormone Research,* 26, 623–687.

Lefkowitz, R. J., J. Roth and I. Pastan (1970a). Effects of calcium on ACTH stimulation of the adrenal: Separation of hormone binding from adenyl cyclase activation. *Nature*, **228**, 864—866.

Lefkowitz, R. J., J. Roth, W. Pricer and I. Pastan (1970b). ACTH receptors in the adrenal: specific binding of ACTH-^{125}I and its relation to adenyl cyclase. *Proc. Natn. Acad. Sci. U.S.A.*, **65**, 745—752.

Lefkowitz, R. J., J. Roth and I. Pastan (1971). ACTH-receptor interaction in the adrenal: A model for the initial step in the action of hormones that stimulate adenyl cyclase. *Ann N.Y. Acad. Sci.*, **185**, 195—209.

Leier, D. J. and R. A. Jungmann (1971). Stimulation of adrenal cholesterol side-chain cleavage activity by theophylline. *Biochim. Biophys. Acta*, **239**, 320—328.

Leier, D. J. and R. A. Jungmann (1973). ACTH and dibutyryl cyclic AMP-mediated Ca^{2+} uptake by rat adrenal glands. *Biochim. Biophys. Acta*, **329**, 196—210.

Lowry, P. J., and C. McMartin (1974). Measurement of the dynamics of stimulation and inhibition of steroidogenesis in isolated rat adrenal cells by using column perfusion. *Biochem. J.*, **142**, 287—294.

Mackie, C., M. C. Richardson and D. Schulster (1972). Kinetics and dose-response characteristics of cyclic AMP production by isolated rat adrenal cells stimulated with ACTH. *FEBS Lett.*, **23**, 345—348.

Mackie, C., and D. Schulster (1973). Phosphodiesterase activity potentiation by theophylline of ACTH stimulated steroidogenesis and cyclic AMP levels in isolated rat adrenal cells. *Biochem. Biophys. Res. Comm.*, **53**, 545—551.

Mahaffee, D., R. C. Reitz and R. L. Ney (1974). The mechanism of action of ACTH. The role of mitochondrial cholesterol accumulation in the regulation of steroidogenesis. *J. Biol. Chem.*, **249**, 227—233.

*Malaisse, W. J. (1973). Insulin secretion: multifactorial regulation for a single process of release. *Diabetologia*, **9**, 167—173.

McIlhinney, R. A. J., and D. Schulster (1975). Studies on the binding of ^{125}I-labelled ACTH to isolated rat adrenocortical cells. *J. Endocr.*, **64**, 175—184.

Mostafapour, M. K., and T. T. Tchen (1971). Evidence for another factor in the regulation of corticosterone biosynthesis by ACTH. *Biochem. Biophys. Res. Commun.*, **44**, 774—785.

Moyle, W. R., Y. C. Kong and J. Ramachandran (1973). Steroidogenesis and cyclic AMP accumulation in rat adrenal cell. *J. Biol Chem.*, **248**, 2409—2417.

Ney, R. L., W. W. Davis and L. D. Garren (1966). Heterogeneity of template RNA in adrenal glands. *Science*, **153**, 896—897.

Palfreyman, J. W., and D. Schulster (1975). On the mechanism of action of cholera toxin on isolated rat adrenocortical cells: comparison with the effects of ACTH on steroidogenesis and cyclic AMP output. *Biochim. Biophys. Acta*, **404**, 221—230.

Pearlmutter, A. F., E. Rapino and M. Saffran (1971). ACTH and cyclic adenine nucleotides do not provoke identical adrenocortical responses. *Endocrinology*, **89**, 963—968.

Pearlmutter, A. F., E. Rapino and M. Saffran (1973). Comparison of steroidogenic effects of cAMP and dbcAMP in the rat adrenal gland. *Endocrinology*, **92**, 679—686.

Penney, D. P., J. Olson, G. V. Marinetti, S. Vaala and K. Averill (1973).

Localization of [^{3}H] Prostaglandin E$_1$ in rat adrenal cortices. *Z. Zellforsch.*, **146**, 309–317.

Peytremann, A., W. E. Nicholson, G. W. Liddle, J. G. Hardman and E. W. Sutherland (1973a). Effects of methylxanthines on cyclic AMP and corticosterone in the rat adrenal. *Endocrinology*, **92**, 525–530.

Peytremann, A., W. E. Nicholson, R. D. Brown, G. W. Liddle and J. G. Hardman (1973b). Comparative effects of angiotension and ACTH on cyclic AMP and steroidogenesis in isolated bovine adrenal cells. *J. Clin. Invest.*, **52**, 835–842.

Rasmussen, H. (1970). Cell communication, calcium ion, and cyclic AMP. *Science*, **170**, 404–412.

Richardson, M. C., and D. Schulster (1972). Corticosteroidogenesis in isolated adrenal cells: effect of ACTH, cyclic AMP and β^{1-24}ACTH diazotized to polyacrylamide. *J. Endocrinol.*, **55**, 127–139.

Richardson, M. C., and D. Schulster (1973). The role of protein kinase activation in the control of steroidogenesis by ACTH in the adrenal cortex. *Biochem. J.*, **136**, 993–998.

*Robison, G. A., R. W. Butcher and E. W. Sutherland (1971). *Cyclic AMP*. Academic Press, New York and London. 531 pages.

Rodbard, D. (1974). Apparent positive cooperative effects in cyclic AMP and corticosterone production by isolated adrenal cells in response to ACTH analogues. *Endocrinology*, **94**, 1427–1437.

Rubin, R. P., R. A. Carchman and S. D. Jaanus (1972). Role of calcium and cyclic AMP in action of ACTH. *Nature New Biol.*, **240**, 150–152.

Rubin, R. P., S. D. Jaanus, R. A. Carchman and M. Puig. (1973). Reversible inhibition of ACTH-induced corticosteroid release by cycloheximide: evidence for an unidentified cellular messenger. *Endocrinology*, **93**, 575–580.

Saruta, T., and N. M. Kaplan (1972). Adrenocortical steroidogenesis: the effect of prostaglandins. *J. Clin. Invest.*, **51**, 2246–2251.

Sato, G. H., T. Rossman, L. Edelstein, S. Holmes and V. Buonassisi (1965). Phenotypic alterations in adrenal tumor cultures. *Science*, **148**, 1733–1734.

Sauer, L. A. (1973). An NAD- and NADP-dependent malic enzyme with regulatory properties in rat liver and adrenal cortex mitochondrial fractions. *Biochem. Biophys. Res. Commun*, **50**, 524–531.

*Sayers, G. (1967). Adrenocorticotrophin. In C. H. Gray (Ed.), *Hormones in blood*, Vol. 1, Academic Press, New York and London. pp. 169–194.

Sayers, G., R. J. Beall and S. Seelig (1972). Isolated adrenal cells: ACTH, calcium, steroidogenesis and cyclic AMP. *Science*, **175**, 1131–1133.

*Schulster, D. (1974a). ACTH and the control of adrenal corticosteroidogenesis. In M. H. Briggs and G. A. Christie (Eds), *Advances in Steroid Biochem. and Pharmacol.* Vol. 4. Academic Press, London. pp. 233–295.

*Schulster, D. (1974b). Endocrine tissue receptors for radioligand-receptor assays. *Brit. Med. Bull.*, **30**, 28–31.

Schulster, D. (1974c). Corticosteroid and RNA synthesis in isolated adrenal cells: inhibition by actinomycin D. *Molecular and Cellular Endocr.*, **1**, 55–64.

Schulster, D., and C. Jenner (1975). A counter-streaming centrifugation technique for the superfusion of adrenocortical cell suspensions stimulated by ACTH. *J. Steroid Biochem.*, **6**, 389–394.

Schulster, D., M. C. Richardson and J. W. Palfreyman (1974). The role of protein synthesis in ACTH action: effects of cycloheximide and puromycin on the steroidogenic response of isolated adrenocortical cells. *Molecular and Cellular Endocr.*, 2, 17—29.

Schulster, D., S. A. S. Tait, J. F. Tait and J. Mrotek (1970). Production of steroids by *in vitro* superfusion of endocrine tissue III. Corticosterone output from rat adrenals stimulated by ACTH or cyclic AMP and the inhibitory effect of cycloheximide. *Endocrinology*, 86, 487—502.

Sharma, R. K. (1973). Regulation of steroidogenesis by ACTH in isolated adrenal cells of rat. *J. Biol. Chem.*, 248, 5473—5476.

*Shaw, J., and S. A. Tillson (1974). Interactions between the prostaglandins and steroid hormones. In M. H. Briggs and G. Christie (Eds), *Steroid Bioch. & Pharmacol.* Vol. 4. Academic Press, London. pp. 189—207.

Simpson, E. R., C. R. Jefcoate, A. C. Brownie and G. S. Boyd (1972). The effect of ether anaesthesia stress on cholesterol side-chain cleavage and cytochrome P450 in rat adrenal mitochondria. *European J. Biochem.*, 28, 442—450.

*Simpson, E. R., and J. I. Mason (1975). Molecular aspects of the biosynthesis of adrenal steroids. In G. Gill (Ed.), *International Encyclopaedia of Pharmacology and Therapeutics: Section on adrenal cortical hormones.* Pergamon Press, in press.

Simpson, E. R., J. Waters and D. Williams-Smith (1975). Effect of calcium on pregnenolone formation and cytochrome P-450 in rat adrenal mitochondria. *J. Steroid Biochem.*, 6, 395—400.

Stone, D., and O. Hechter (1954). Studies on ACTH action in perfused bovine adrenals: The site of action of ACTH in corticosteroidogenesis. *Arch. Biochem. Biophys.*, 51, 457—469.

Tait, J. F., S. A. S. Tait, R. P. Gould and M. S. R. Mee (1974). The properties of adrenal zona glomerulosa cells after purification by gravitational sedimentation. *Proc. Royal Society, London. B.*, 185, 375—407.

Temple, R., and J. Wolff (1973). Stimulation of steroid secretion by anti-microtubular agents. *J. Biol. Chem.*, 248, 2691—2698.

Trzeciak, W. H., an G. S. Boyd (1973). The effect of stress induced by ether anaesthesia on cholesterol content and cholesteryl-esterase activity in rat adrenal cortex. *Eur. J. Biochem.*, 37, 327—333; also *J. Steroid Biochem.* (1975) 6, 427—436.

Urquhart, J., and C. C. Li (1968). The dynamics of adrenocortical secretion. *Amer. J. Physiol.*, 214, 73—85.

Urquhart, J., and C. C. Li (1969). Dynamic testing and modeling of adrenocortical secretory function. *Ann. N.Y. Acad. Sci.*, 156, 756—778.

*Wicks, W. D. (1974). Regulation of protein synthesis by cyclic AMP. In P. Greengard and G. A. Robison (Eds), *Adv. in Cyclic Nucleotide Res.* Vol. 4. Raven Press, New York. pp. 335—438.

Wolfsen, A. R., H. B. McIntyre and W. D. Odell (1972). ACTH measurement by competitive binding receptor assay. *J. Clin. Endocr. Metab.*, 34, 684—689.

CHAPTER 12

Control of aldosterone synthesis

I. THE ADRENAL ZONA GLOMERULOSA AS THE ALDOSTERONE PRODUCTION SITE

Aldosterone is uniquely secreted by the cells in the glomerular layer of the adrenal gland (the zona glomerulosa: see Figure 6.1) and is the most potent mineralo-corticoid produced by the adrenal cortex. Its main physiological function is in regulating the metabolism of sodium and potassium ions. The concentrations of aldosterone, sodium and potassium ions normally found in human urine and blood are given in Table 12.1.

A cooperative effort between Simpson and Tait in London, Reichstein, von Euw and Schindler in Basel and Wettstein and Neher at the Ciba Laboratories, Basel, culminated with a publication (in 1953) reporting the isolation of active crystalline aldosterone. However, even before the isolation of aldosterone there were early indications that the zona glomerulosa was involved in the secretion of mineralo-corticoids. Thus only the inner zones of the adrenal cortex degenerated following

Table 12.1.
Sodium ion, potassium ion and aldosterone concentrations in man

	Normal Range*
Serum potassium	3.8—5.4 mEq/litre
Serum sodium	138—145 mEq/litre
Urinary sodium excretion	70—200 mEq/24 hr
Urinary potassium excretion	50—90 mEq/24 hr
Plasma aldosterone	1—12 ng/100 ml
Aldosterone secretion rate	70—250 μg/24 hr
Urinary aldosterone excretion rate	5—20 μg/24 hr
Plasma aldosterone metabolic clearance rate	1200—1600 litre/24 hr
Hepatic extraction ratio for aldosterone	85—95%

*For patients given Na$^+$ and K$^+$ ad libitum.

hypophysectomy, while the production of adrenal salt-retaining hormone remained virtually unaffected. Furthermore potassium deficiency or deoxycorticosterone acetate administration gave rise to cytological alterations indicative of zona glomerulosa inactivity. It was also found that potassium loading or sodium deficiency produced morphological and histochemical changes in the zona glomerulosa that were suggestive of increased secretory activity; for example, in sodium deficient rats, increased thickness of zona glomerulosa correlated with an increased aldosterone production (Eisenstein and Hartroft, 1957).

The actual separation of the glomerular layer from the other adrenal cell types was achieved by decapsulation of excised rat adrenal glands (Giroud et al., 1956) in which the outer capsule surrounding the gland was stripped off. This *capsular* portion of the adrenal contained all the zona glomerulosa with about 20% of the zona fasciculata, and produced amounts of aldosterone very similar to the output of the intact adrenal *in vitro*. The *decapsulated glands* on the other hand, comprising zona fasciculata, reticularis and medulla, produced undetectible amounts of aldosterone. Similar results were found by Ayres et al., (1956) using ox adrenal capsule strippings.

When aldosterone was first isolated, it was not then immediately recognized that its production was restricted to the zona glomerulosa, and the early *in vivo* studies were carried out without this knowledge. Although a considerable understanding of aldosterone biosynthesis and the factors regulating its cellular production has derived from *in vivo* studies and *in vitro* incubations using capsular adrenal tissue, the modes of action of the various stimulatory agents still remain obscure. This is partly due to the difficulties involved in interpreting results obtained using systems of mixed cell types. Many agents, including angiotensin II, serotonin, potassium ions, ACTH and cyclic AMP have been reported to stimulate aldosterone production *in vitro*. However, these effects have been largely obtained using preparations such as capsular strippings or outer slices of adrenals, which, although containing a high proportion of zona glomerulosa cells do also contain zona fasciculata cells in sufficient quantity to hinder interpretation of the results. Corticosterone, the major precursor for aldosterone, is produced by both zones, and when produced as a result of zona fasciculata stimulation under conventional *in vitro* incubation conditions, it can act as precursor for conversion to aldosterone by zona glomerulosa. This does not happen *in vivo* since the blood flow through the gland is from the glomerulosa to the fasciculata, and the fascicular products are metabolized peripherally before recirculation. Studies *in vivo*, however, have not allowed the detailed examination of the control mechanisms operating at the cellular and subcellular level for aldosterone production.

Partially purified glomerulosa cells have been obtained from rat adrenals chronically stimulated by a low salt diet (Boyd *et al.*, 1973). Under these circumstances the adrenal cortex largely comprises zona glomerulosa. Although the capsule strippings obtained from such glands contain very few zona fasciculata cells, the degree of fasciculata contamination is uncertain and the glomerulosa cells so derived may differ from normal glomerulosa cells in their responses to steroidogenic stimuli. However, important information on the characteristics of glomerulosa cells derives from these studies and Boyd *et al.* (1973) have demonstrated that the potassium concentration in the glomerulosa (17 mEq K^+/100 g tissue) was significantly higher than that in the inner zones of the adrenal cortex (13 mEq K^+/100 g tissue). Similarly, the glomerulosa cells had a higher activity of sodium-potassium ATPase than inner zone tissue. These results indicate that glomerulosa cells are biochemically constituted to be susceptible to fluctuations in the concentration of extracellular and/or intracellular K^+ ions.

The development of methods for the preparation of isolated cells (see Chapter 3.IV) from capsular adrenal tissue (e.g. Haning *et al.*, 1970) has allowed the further refinement of fractionating these isolated (or dispersed) cells into discrete cell types, using unit gravity sedimentation to purify zona glomerulosa cells free from contaminating zona fasciculata cells (Tait *et al.*, 1974b). In particular ACTH, cyclic AMP and angiotensin II all stimulate steroidogenesis by zona fasciculata cells (see Chapter 11), and therefore for reasons discussed above, studies on the detailed mode of action of these stimuli on glomerulosa cell steroidogenesis will be greatly aided by the use of purified glomerulosa cell systems.

On the other hand, serotonin and changes in K^+ ions are without effect on the *in vitro* steroidogenesis of zona fasciculata (Kaplan, 1965; Müller, 1971; Haning, 1970). It must therefore follow that previous studies which have demonstrated the stimulation of aldosterone production from zona glomerulosa by both K^+ ions and serotonin – have done so indisputably, even though these studies utilized mixed cell preparations. A useful aid in the evaluation of cell purification procedures is the selectivity of the serotonin and K^+ ion effects coupled with the stimulatory effects of other agents (e.g. ACTH) that affect both cell types. Thus, with removal of fasciculata from glomerulosa cells, the serotonin response remains constant (at about 2-fold: see later) while the ACTH response diminishes (to about 2-fold).

In order to elucidate the mode of action of all the various stimulatory agents for glomerulosa cells, it is necessary to measure not only steroidogenesis, but also cyclic AMP production and intracellular changes in cations (such as Ca^{2+}, K^+, Na^+) and to correlate these effects under a variety of circumstances. It is clear that purified glomerulosa cell systems are important for these studies, since the different cell types each respond differently to the various stimuli.

II. BIOSYNTHETIC PATHWAY FOR ALDOSTERONE

The biosynthesis of aldosterone has been discussed in Chapter 4.IV and the generally accepted scheme is that depicted in Figure 4.7. Normally cholesterol is converted via pregnenolone, progesterone and 11-deoxycorticosterone to corticosterone as outlined in Figure 12.1. The mechanism whereby the C-18 angular methyl group of corticosterone is converted to an aldehyde is less well established. The intermediary role of 18-hydroxycorticosterone now appears most likely in normal adrenal tissue (Müller, 1971).

Examination of the ultrastructure of the rat adrenal zona glomerulosa using the electron microscope suggests that different stages of aldosterone biosynthesis occur in different mitochondria of these cells (Wassermann, 1974).

18-Hydroxy-11-deoxycorticosterone has also been shown to be secreted by both zona glomerulosa and fasciculata. However, secretion of this relatively weak mineralocorticoid in man is influenced by those stimuli which regulate cortisol production, but not by agents or conditions which affect secretion of both aldosterone and 18-hydroxycorticosterone (Ulick, 1973). Using superfused rat adrenal tissue, both 18-hydroxycorticosterone and 18-hydroxy-11-deoxy-corticosterone were shown to be produced by both glomerulosa (capsular) and fasciculata (decapsulated) tissue, and the outputs of these steroids were compared with those of corticosterone and aldosterone (Tait et al., 1970). It was concluded that most of the 18-hydroxycorticosterone and all of the aldosterone derive from zona glomerulosa, whereas the 18-hydroxy-11-deoxycorticosterone and corticosterone (the corticoid secreted in the largest quantity by the rat adrenal) derive mainly from zona fasciculata. The intermediary role of 18-hydroxy-11-deoxycorticosterone in the biosynthesis of aldosterone may, nevertheless, pertain under certain circumstances (see Chapter 4.IV).

The detailed mechanism whereby the 18-methyl group of corticosterone is converted to an aldehyde is still under active discussion. Evidence has been provided for the involvement of a mitochondrial cytochrome P-450 and mixed function oxidase system in the 18-hydroxylation of corticosterone, and it now appears likely that the further conversion of the 18-hydroxyl group to the aldehyde function in aldosterone also involves a mitochondrial oxidase mechanism (Ulick, 1973).

Currently, two different sites on the steroidogenic pathway are believed to be rate-limiting in the control of aldosterone biosynthesis. One site occurs at an *early stage* in the pathway, between the conversion of cholesterol to pregnenolone (cf. Chapters 11 and 13 for the site of action of ACTH, LH and FSH). Another site is believed to occur at a *late stage* in the pathway, probably lying somewhere between the conversion of corticosterone to aldosterone (see Figure 12.1).

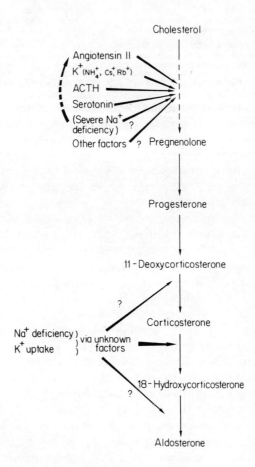

Figure 12.1 Regulation of aldosterone biosynthesis. The pathway for biosynthesis of aldosterone in the zona glomerulosa showing the sites of action of stimulatory agents.

III. THE REGULATION, BY SODIUM AND POTASSIUM IONS, OF ALDOSTERONE BIOSYNTHESIS

A. Sodium ions

The correlation between sodium ion balance and aldosterone secretion, first observed in man (Leutscher and Axelrad, 1954), has now been established in a wide variety of animals. It is now clear that limiting Na^+ ion intake or enhancing the loss of Na^+ ions from the body (e.g. via sweating, diuresis or salivation) has the effect of increasing aldosterone output, whereas increasing the Na^+ ion intake results in a decreased aldosterone secretion. This regulation of aldosterone secretion by Na^+ ions is undoubtedly a fundamentally important physiological control system in view of the principal effect of aldosterone itself on Na^+ ion retention, (see Chapter 15).

Nevertheless, despite considerable experimental effort, this mechanism is poorly understood. The complexity of the system has hampered progress. For example the manifold physiological effects of Na^+ ion depletion include:

decreased extracellular fluid volume
decreased total and circulating plasma volume
decreased arterial blood pressure and flow rate
potassium ion retention
changes in intracellular and extracellular concentrations of electrolytes
and modulation of the renin—angiotensin system.

The diversity of these effects contributes to the difficulties in determining their relative importance in the mechanism whereby Na^+ ion loss stimulates aldosterone production.

In vivo studies on sheep with adrenal autotransplants to the neck have shown that increases of K^+ and decreases of Na^+ ion concentrations (within the physiological range) in the adrenal arterial blood, stimulated aldosterone secretion (Blair-West *et al.*, 1963). Although independent changes in the concentration of either cation were effective, the greatest stimulus arose from an increase in K^+ ion concentration coupled to a decrease in Na^+ ion concentration. However, they clearly showed that Na^+ ion depletion does not act by a direct effect on the adrenal.

Extensive studies in man, dog, sheep and recently in the rat (see Spielman and Davis, 1974) have shown a parallel activation by Na^+ ion depletion of the renin—angiotensin system (see later; Subsection IV) and aldosterone secretion. From these studies it has been suggested that the primary effect of Na^+ ion depletion is to activate the renin—angiotensin system, which is then responsible for the stimulation of aldosterone secretion. In the dog the renin—angiotensin system is established as the primary mediatory mechanism for the control of aldosterone secretion during Na^+ ion depletion with the pituitary gland playing an important supportive role. Other factors are also believed to be involved in the stimulation of aldosterone during Na^+ ion depletion in the rabbit (Braverman and Davis, 1973) and in the sheep (Blair-West *et al.*, 1972). In the latter, angiotensin is suggested to play a permissive role, since it will not maintain aldosterone hypersecretion for more than about 12 hours and it is ineffective in mildly Na^+ ion depleted sheep (see also McCaa *et al.*, 1975).

That Na^+ ion depletion does not operate to stimulate aldosterone secretion solely by an effect on the renin—angiotensin system has been suggested from many studies (cf. Müller, 1971). For example, the Na^+ ion status and the renin—angiotensin system do not always change in equivalent amounts following severe Na^+ ion depletion and during some disease conditions. Thus severe Na^+ ion depletion can stimulate aldosterone secretion to a far greater extent than infusions of angiotensin II to intact animals. Moreover, *in vitro* studies using outer slices of beef adrenal have demonstrated increased aldosterone synthesis in the presence of lowered Na$^+$ ion concentrations in the incubation medium — with simultaneous decreases in corticosterone synthesis (Saruta et al., 1972), although very large changes in Na$^+$ ion concentration were required to show this effect.

From various studies in which a decreased corticosterone production coupled with an increased aldosterone production has been observed following Na$^+$ ion depletion, it has been suggested (Davis et al., 1968; Tait et al., 1970) that Na$^+$ ion restriction also stimulates aldosterone biosynthesis at a step lying between corticosterone and aldosterone (in addition to an effect between cholesterol and pregnenolone; see Figure 12.1).

B. Potassium ions

That potassium ions exert a stimulatory effect on aldosterone biosynthesis was first demonstrated by Giroud and coworkers twenty years ago using in vitro rat adrenals — although this was found only using grossly non-physiological ionic changes. K$^+$ ions are now known to act exclusively on the zona glomerulosa cells of the rat adrenal. In capsular regions of the gland (containing zona glomerulosa) K$^+$ ions stimulated output of aldosterone, corticosterone and deoxycorticosterone, but in decapsulated glands (zona fasciculata/reticularis) they did not affect corticosteroid biosynthesis (Müller, 1971). In further studies with this system, increases in K$^+$ ion concentration (up to 8.4 mM) did not further increase aldosterone biosynthesis by tissue maximally stimulated by serotonin — indicating that K$^+$ ions and serotonin may act on the same cells. (This contrasts with the effect of K$^+$ ions on beef adrenal tissue, observed by Kaplan in 1965, in which the aldosterone-stimulating effect of angiotensin was potentiated.)

This aspect has now been examined in detail using isolated rat glomerulosa cells functioning in response to varying K$^+$ ion concentrations (Haning et al., 1970; Tait et al., 1972) and, like the response of capsular tissue (Müller, 1971), in both these and purified glomerulosa cells (Tait et al., 1974a,b) it was found that maximal steroidogenic responses were obtained at 8.4 mM K$^+$. Higher and lower K$^+$ ion concentrations than this considerably reduced the response by these cells — thus with 8.4 mM K$^+$, corticosterone output was 3-fold and aldosterone output was 6-fold that obtained with 2 mM K$^+$. It was shown that increasing K$^+$ ion concentrations, in the presence of a maximally stimulating dose of serotonin (10^{-4} M), further increased the outputs of both corticosterone and aldosterone to reach maximal outputs at 5.9 mM K$^+$. At high K$^+$ ion concentrations (8.4–13 mM), serotonin was ineffective. It was suggested that at low K$^+$ ion concentrations, K$^+$ and serotonin both act (possibly by the same mechanism) to stimulate steroidogenesis, but that at high concentrations K$^+$ ions inhibit steroidogenesis whereas serotonin does not.

Considerable interest has arisen from the suggestion that changes in intracellular K$^+$ concentrations could be the common denominator in the actions of the various known stimuli for aldosterone secretion (Baumber et al., 1971). Recent studies (Mendelsohn and Mackie, 1975) have however demonstrated that under certain conditions changes in the intracellular K$^+$ ion content do not correlate with alterations in steroidogenesis by isolated glomerulosa cells.

Stimulation of aldosterone output by K^+ ions can be inhibited by ouabain (an inhibitor of the Na^+/K^+-ATPase, or exchange pump which transports cations across cell membranes). Cycloheximide (a protein synthesis inhibitor) and the absence of Ca^{2+} ions from the incubation medium also inhibit the K^+ ion effect.

Solutions of CsCl or RbCl infused *in vivo* to isolated dog adrenals have also been shown to stimulate aldosterone and corticosterone secretion (Bartter *et al.*, 1964), and NH_4Cl stimulated aldosterone secretion by perfused sheep adrenals to an extent similar to that observed in Na^+-deficient sheep (Blair-West *et al.*, 1968).

Similar stimulatory effects of these ions have been observed on aldosterone production *in vitro* by adrenal tissue from Na^+-deficient rats, with maximal effects at concentrations of about 7 mEq/litre (Müller, 1971). These cations all mimic K^+ ions in their effects on the plasma membrane Na^+/K^+-ATPase.

IV. THE RENIN—ANGIOTENSIN SYSTEM

The renin—angiotensin system is one — and in some species perhaps the principal — mechanism that regulates aldosterone biosynthesis *in vivo*. It is initiated by the release of the enzyme renin from the kidney. The output of renin increases both when the renal blood supply is reduced and following Na^+ ion depletion. Renin has a relatively long half-life (about 15 min), and is degraded largely by the liver after recirculating several times.

In the blood, angiotensin I is formed by the action of renin which cleaves this N-terminal decapeptide from a plasma α_2-globulin known as angiotensinogen (or renin substrate) (see Figure 12.2). Angiotensin I is biologically inactive in most systems. A 'converting enzyme', found in lung, plasma and other tissues, cleaves two amino acid residues from the C-terminal end to form the short-lived octapeptide angiotensin II, noted for its powerful hypertensive effect. The role of the renin—angiotensin II system in regulating blood pressure is currently an intense field for research (e.g. Davies *et al.*, 1973).

Angiotensin has a wide variety of physiological and pharmacological effects (Gross, 1971). Besides increasing aldosterone secretion from the adrenal cortex, it also stimulates the adrenal medulla to release catecholamines and may modulate the action of noradrenalin in adrenergic neurons. Pharmacological studies have centred on its effects on blood pressure using isolated smooth muscle (e.g. uterus, intestine, artery) preparations. Synthetic angiotensin and many of its analogues (synthesized, with the object of finding antagonists or peptides with higher or different activities) have been assayed using this pressor response; plasma angiotensin levels have also been determined using radioimmunoassay, and by an assay based on stimulation of the rat colon. Other reported effects of angiotensin II include stimulation of the plasma membrane Na^+/K^+-ATPase and effects on cellular ion fluxes, stimulation of protein synthesis and enhancement of mitochondrial energy-producing reactions. For a comprehensive survey of the angiotensin field see Page and Bumpus (1974).

Angiotensin II infusions in rabbit, sheep, dog and man (e.g. Urquhart *et al.*, 1963; Braverman and Davis, 1973; Ames *et al.*, 1965) have resulted in 2—6 fold increases in aldosterone levels. This steroidogenic effect has been obtained at very

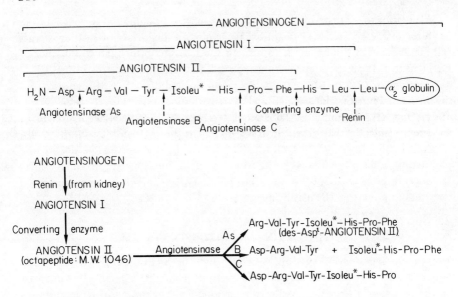

All forms of angiotensin II isolated so far are either isoleucine -5- angiotensin II or valine -5- angiotensin II.

Figure 12.2   Biosynthesis and degradation of Angiotensin II.

low doses of the peptide (e.g. 10—40 ng/min). Although the rat adrenal, using a variety of different experimental preparations, has traditionally shown little or no response to angiotensin II, recent studies have demonstrated that following 20 min infusions of the peptide into conscious rats, plasma concentrations of aldosterone increased up to 8-fold above control values (Coleman *et al.*, 1974). This response was severely reduced by anaesthesia and surgical preparation. However, it has not been shown that angiotensin II can maintain high increases in aldosterone output over a long period.

A. Angiotensin II receptors

Monoiodinated angiotensin II has been used to examine the characteristics and distribution of cellular receptors for angiotensin. Its binding to adrenal particulate fractions was first demonstrated by Goodfriend and Lin (1970). The preparation of [H^3]angiotensin of high specific radioactivity and biological activity has further allowed the study of various characteristics of angiotensin binding. Thus, in vascular smooth muscle clear evidence has been presented for the presence of angiotensin II receptors in the cell membrane (Meyer *et al.*, 1972), and rabbit aortic microsomes have been subfractionated using Ficoll gradients with the demonstration of specific binding to a fraction containing adenylate cyclase activity (Devynck *et al.*, 1973).

The specific binding of angiotensin II to a particulate cell fraction derived from rat adrenal zona glomerulosa has been demonstrated (Brecher *et al.*, 1974). The binding activity was saturable and markedly reduced by heating or preincubation with proteolytic enzymes (but not by DNase, RNase or neuraminidase) and at least two orders of binding sites were suggested by the binding data.

Similar studies on the binding of monoiodinated and tritiated angiotensin II to an adrenal microsomal membrane fraction suggested a plasma membrane location for angiotensin II receptors and further attempts to characterize them were made (Glossman *et al.*, 1974); however these studies were performed on decapsulated bovine adrenal cortex (as opposed to glomerulosa tissue) and are therefore difficult to evaluate in relation to aldosterone biosynthesis. It is of interest that guanyl nucleotides (e.g. GTP) were found to inhibit the angiotensin II binding in this system, and this may relate to the suggestion by Rodbell and coworkers (1974) regarding the ability of hormones to modulate the affinity of a guanyl nucleotide binding site (and *vice versa*) in the hepatic cell membrane.

The heptapeptide, des-Asp[1]-angiotensin II, produced from angiotensin II via aminopeptidase action (angiotensinase As; see Figure 12.2) has also been shown to have aldosterone stimulating activity. On a molar basis, the heptapeptide was more potent, and exerted a more immediate effect than angiotensin II *in vitro*, in stimulating aldosterone biosynthesis. Chiu and Peach (1974) have also reported that this heptapeptide has a much higher affinity for the angiotensin receptor of isolated rabbit adrenal capsular cells than angiotensin II itself. A possible physiological role for the heptapeptide metabolite of angiotensin II is thus implicated in the regulation of aldosterone biosynthesis (Goodfriend and Peach, 1975).

B. Site of action of angiotensin II

That angiotensin stimulates biosynthesis of aldosterone rather than inducing release of preformed steroid is indicated from measurements of adrenal aldosterone content (0.22 µg/sheep adrenal) and the very much greater amounts secreted in response to angiotensin infusions (0.54 µg aldosterone/hr secreted by sodium-replete sheep increased several times during angiotensin infusions over several hours, see Müller, 1971).

In vitro stimulation of aldosterone biosynthesis from endogenous precursors has been observed in studies with beef adrenal. In response to angiotensin II (0.1 − 1.0 µg/g), outer slices (glomerulosa) of beef adrenal cortex produced more aldosterone and corticosterone, whereas inner slices (fasciculata-reticularis) produced more corticosterone and cortisol (Kaplan, 1965). It was suggested from these studies that angiotensin stimulates steroidogenesis early in the biogenic pathway, before the conversion of corticosterone to aldosterone. Superfused capsular glands from hypophysectomized-nephrectomized rats also responded to high concentrations of angiotensin II (2.8 µg/min) with slightly stimulated outputs of aldosterone, 18-hydroxycorticosterone and corticosterone (Tait *et al.*, 1970).

Presently available evidence indicates that angiotensin II acts at an early point in the aldosterone biosynthetic pathway (see Figure 12.1). Thus angiotensin II stimulated beef adrenal aldosterone production in the presence of exogenous cholesterol, but not in the presence of exogenous progesterone or corticosterone. Again in sheep adrenal perfusion studies although angiotensin II stimulated aldosterone production from endogenous precursors, it did not stimulate conversion of [H^3]corticosterone to aldosterone (Blair-West *et al.*, 1972). Similarly in rat adrenal, angiotensin II stimulated conversion of [H^3]cholesterol to aldosterone, but not the incorporation of [H^3]pregnenolone, [H^3]progesterone, [H^3]deoxycorticosterone or [H^3]corticosterone into aldosterone (Müller, 1971). In addition to the effect at an early stage in the pathway, an effect of angiotensin on the activity of the late pathway of aldosterone biosynthesis had been indicated by, for example, the studies of Haning *et al.* (1970) using isolated rat glomerulosa cells, in which an increased conversion of [H^3]corticosterone to aldosterone was found. This has been confirmed by the work of Williams *et al.* (1972) using rat glomerulosa tissue, but these workers suggested that the acute effect on the late pathway is mediated (at least in part) by increased corticosterone produced in response to an action on the early pathway of aldosterone biosynthesis. An effect of angiotensin II on the late pathway has been found *in vivo* in the dog (Aguilera and Marusic, 1971) and this effect was similar to that observed with Na$^+$ ion depletion.

Angiotensin II has also been demonstrated to stimulate corticosteroid production by isolated fasciculata cells from bovine adrenals; a maximal steroidogenic response was obtained with 1 μg angiotensin/ml (Peytremann *et al.*, 1973). Most studies in this field have been performed on preparations containing a mixture of cell types, and because of the established effect of angiotensin on both glomerulosa and fasciculata cells, these results are difficult to interpret quantitatively and mechanistically. It is particularly difficult to select a dose of angiotensin that will have a maximal effect on glomerulosa cells and a minimal effect on fasciculata cells, and this dose has been exceeded in most published reports. However, studies with isolated rat glomerulosa cells (Williams *et al.*, 1974) have shown aldosterone stimulation at 0.25 ng angiotensin/ml, with maximal responses achieved at about 250 ng angiotensin/ml. Further studies are necessary using 'physiological levels' of angiotensin in the region of this former low concentration.

V. ACTH

The control of adrenal *glucocorticoid* synthesis is almost exclusively the domain of ACTH and the details of this mechanism have been discussed in Chapter 11. Although the short-term stimulation of aldosterone secretion by ACTH has been established for over 20 years in both animals and man (see Müller, 1971), this effect is not maintained in the long-term and aldosterone secretion falls to basal levels, or below, after about 6 days of exogenous ACTH administration. Moreover, whereas hypophysectomy reduces glucocorticoid secretion by almost 99%, the secretion of aldosterone is only halved compared with that of intact animals. The hypophysectomized animal still responds to other aldosterone-stimulatory agents (albeit to a diminished extent) and ACTH administration returns aldosterone secretion to normal. In superfused capsular adrenals of normal and of acutely hypophysectomized rats, ACTH (at high concentration) stimulated by about 2-fold the initial outputs of aldosterone, 18-hydroxycorticosterone, corticosterone and

18-hydroxydeoxycorticosterone (Tait *et al.*, 1970). Several-fold increases in production of aldosterone and other corticosteroids have also been reported using capsular adrenals of normal and sodium-deficient rats incubated with high concentrations of ACTH (Müller, 1971).

Studies with radioactive steriod precursors have indicated that ACTH acts at a locus on the steroidogenic pathway for aldosterone, similar to that in which it promotes glucocorticoid synthesis — i.e. between cholesterol and pregnenolone (see Chapters 11.VIII, 11.IX). It would appear that ACTH acts in a 'permissive' fashion, presumably by regulating the supply of precursors, particularly corticosterone, for aldosterone synthesis. The studies of Baumann and Müller (1974) indicate that in the rat (in which the pituitary is believed to play a more important aldosterone-regulating role than in other species) the activity of enzymes converting corticosterone to aldosterone are largely independent of a functioning pituitary. Thus within 6 days, hypophysectomy without replacement therapy decreased neither the normal nor the elevated rates of [H^3]corticosterone conversion to 18-hydroxycorticosterone and aldosterone by capsular adrenals of rats on normal or sodium-deficient diets, respectively. In experiments with isolated glomerulosa cells (Haning *et al.*, 1970) and rat capsular tissue (Williams *et al.*, 1972), ACTH was found to increase the conversion of [H^3]corticosterone to aldosterone, and (at maximal concentrations) to a greater extent than other stimulators (angiotensin, K^+ ions and serotonin). But these workers have concluded that this was due to the use of non-purified cells and that the effect on [H^3]corticosterone conversion to aldosterone was primarily due to alterations in endogenous corticosterone production (partly originating from contaminating fasciculata cells); however some direct effect on the late pathway could not be completely excluded.

VI. SEROTONIN

The steroidogenic effect of serotonin (5 hydroxytryptamine; see Figure 16.6) was first reported by Rosenkrantz and coworkers, and its specific aldosterone-stimulating effect has since been confirmed in *in vitro* studies using adrenals from a variety of species.

In vitro, serotonin is one of the most potent aldosterone-stimulatory factors and is effective at 10^{-8} M on quartered adrenals from sodium-deficient rats; corticosterone production was not affected by concentrations even as high as 10^{-3} M (Müller, 1971). The effect of serotonin and of changes in K^+ ion concentration on corticosteroid output by isolated rat glomerulosa cells has also been examined (Tait *et al.*, 1972; see above, Subsection IIIB). A maximal stimulation of aldosterone (8-fold basal value) and corticosterone (twice basal value) was obtained at 10^{-6} M serotonin.

Serotonin, like K^+ ions, acts specifically on the zona glomerulosa at an early stage on the biosynthetic pathway and generates cyclic AMP within the cell. It acts mainly on the conversion of cholesterol to pregnenolone and has only a small effect on the later stages of the pathway (Müller, 1971).

In vivo evidence for a corticosteroid stimulating action for serotonin is lacking,

Table 12.2.

Aldosterone stimulating activity of serotonin (5-hydroxytryptamine) and related compounds.
(For further details see Müller, 1971.)

Active in Stimulating Aldosterone (conc. effective in doubling basal production of rat adrenal quarters)	Aldosterone production stimulated by less than 20% at 10^{-5} M, using rat adrenal quarters
Serotonin (10^{-7} M)	Melatonin
Bufotenine (10^{-6} M)	Histamine
5-Methoxytryptamine (10^{-6} M)	Adrenalin
L-5-Hydroxytryptophan (10^{-5} M)	Noradrenalin
	L-Thyroxine
	Tryptamine
	L-Tryptophan

however, and for example in sodium-replete sheep, Blair-West *et al.* (1973) have reported that it did not stimulate aldosterone, corticosterone or cortisol secretion. It is not considered as a physiological stimulatory agent, but nevertheless is a useful biochemical tool for the elucidation of the aldosterone control mechanism. Thus in conjunction with ACTH, serotonin is useful in assessing the purity of glomerulosa cell preparations (as discussed above, Subsection I) and it may be used to generate cyclic AMP in experiments designed to evaluate the role of this nucleotide in the regulation of aldosterone synthesis.

A variety of indole derivatives related to serotonin also have the ability to stimulate aldosterone synthesis (Table 12.2) and may also prove of value in biochemical studies.

VII. THE ROLE OF CYCLIC AMP

The functioning of adenylate cyclase and the intermediary role of cyclic AMP in the control of adrenal steroidogenesis by ACTH has been discussed at length in Chapter 11.V. A similar involvement for cyclic AMP in the peptide hormone stimulation of aldosterone production by the glomerulosa cell has been indicated, although the details are less well established.

The stimulatory effect of exogenously added cyclic AMP on aldosterone production was demonstrated in beef adrenal slices (Kaplan, 1965) and rat capsular adrenals (Müller, 1971). Studies on the effect of angiotensin II on isolated bovine fasciculata cells (Peytremann *et al.*, 1973) have established that, in these cells, angiotensin elicits a small, but rapid, increase in cyclic AMP output that precedes the stimulation of steroidogenesis. The effect of angiotensin II on these fasciculata cells was considered to be consistent with an intermediary role for cyclic AMP in the corticosteroidogenic mechanism.

The effect of the various stimulatory factors for aldosterone synthesis on cyclic AMP concentrations in separated rat fasciculata and glomerulosa cells has been determined, and compared with corticosteroid synthesis by these cell types (Albano *et al.*, 1974). These studies have confirmed the stimulation by angiotensin II of cyclic AMP output by fasciculata cells; on the other hand serotonin and increased

K^+ ion concentration had no effect on cyclic AMP output by fasciculata cells. Purified and unpurified glomerulosa cells responded equally to serotonin and increased K^+ ions with increased outputs of cyclic AMP of about 2-fold. Cyclic AMP outputs by unpurified glomerulosa cells were stimulated by ACTH (about 5-fold) and by angiotensin II (about 3-fold), but following purification (and the virtual elimination of fasciculata contamination) the responses to both these agents were reduced to stimulations of about 2-fold. Similar 2-fold stimulations of corticosteroidogenesis were observed for these purified glomerulosa cells. From their studies, these workers suggest a link between steroidogenesis and cyclic AMP production by the adrenal glomerulosa.

In further studies with purified rat glomerulosa cells, Tait *et al.* (1974a) have observed that there were submaximal concentrations of angiotensin II, serotonin and K^+ ions which markedly increased steroidogenesis, but which had no detectable increase on cyclic AMP output. It was considered possible that this could have been due to kinetic considerations, in that the increase in the effective cyclic AMP concentration might occur at a different time from the consequent increase in steroidogenesis. Examination of the kinetics of cyclic AMP output at increased K^+ ion concentration, however, showed this to be an unlikely explanation for the stimulatory effect of K^+ ions – although it remains a possibility for the other stimulatory agents. In an alternative explanation compartmental effects of cyclic AMP concentrations within the cell might account for the lack of correlation between cyclic AMP output and steroidogenesis. To examine these aspects further, a maximally steroidogenic-effective amount of cyclic AMP was added (either to the medium or internally to the cells by the action of serotonin). Under these circumstances the steroid output was found to vary markedly at different K^+ ion concentrations and it was concluded that either the activity of cyclic AMP varies with K^+ ion concentration, or there is a mechanism for controlling steroidogenesis independent of cyclic AMP, but responsive to K^+ ion alterations. Nevertheless, these studies in no way preclude an intermediary role for cyclic AMP in the aldosterone-stimulating mechanism of the peptide hormones, angiotensin II and ACTH in the glomerulosa cell.

The phosphodiesterase activities have been found to be 10-fold higher in the zona glomerulosa than in the fasciculata—reticularis regions of the adrenal gland (Gallant *et al.*, 1974). This compares with the similar adenylate cyclase activities in these zones; these studies suggested the presence of multiple forms of adrenal phosphodiesterase and a possible role for this enzyme in the different responsiveness to peptide hormone stimulation for the various cell types.

VIII. OTHER FACTORS INVOLVED IN THE STIMULATION OF ALDOSTERONE PRODUCTION

The effects of various prostaglandins have been studied using beef adrenal tissue slices; prostaglandins E_1 and E_2 (1 μg/g adrenal tissue; p. 187) consistently and significantly stimulated aldosterone biosynthesis (Kaplan, 1973). Prostaglandin E_1 stimulated steroidogenesis in a manner similar to that of ACTH, and on a molar basis was about as potent as angiotensin II in this system. Prostaglandins A, $F_{1\alpha}$ and $F_{2\alpha}$ were ineffective (Saruta and Kaplan, 1972).

The presence of Ca^{2+} ions is required for the steroidogenic effect of aldosterone-stimulatory factors (confer Chapter 11.VII). Thus the *in vitro* response of rat adrenal tissue to stimulation by increases in angiotensin II or K^+ ion was completely abolished in a Ca^{2+}-free medium (Müller, 1971). Similarly in beef adrenal tissue slices in the absence of Ca^{2+} ions, angiotensin did not significantly stimulate aldosterone production (Kaplan, 1973). However, short-term infusions of $CaCl_2$ into the adrenal arterial blood supply of sheep with autotransplanted adrenals (giving rise to increases in local Ca^{2+} ion concentrations of up to 9 mEq/litre) did not affect aldosterone secretion (Blair-West *et al.*, 1968).

The effect of protein synthesis inhibitors such as cycloheximide and puromycin have been examined and found to block the action of aldosterone-stimulatory factors such as serotonin, K^+ ions, ACTH and prostaglandin E_1 (confer Müller, 1971; Saruta and Kaplan, 1972). Cycloheximide inhibition at an early stage of the pathway was indicated — at a point preceding pregnenolone formation (confer Chapter 11.X). Inhibition of RNA synthesis by actinomycin D, however, has little effect on aldosterone biosynthesis.

Other, as yet unidentified, factors have also been implicated in the aldosterone control system, and for example from their studies Abraham *et al.* (1973) and Blair-West *et al.* (1973) have suggested the existence of an unidentified humoral factor controlling aldosterone — perhaps an inhibitor substance from the brain, or possibly the cessation of secretion of a stimulator.

IX. FEEDBACK MECHANISMS FOR THE REGULATION OF ALDOSTERONE BIOSYNTHESIS

It is important to note that not only is aldosterone biosynthesis by the glomerulosa cell affected by Na^+ and K^+ ion concentrations as discussed in Subsection III above, but also that aldosterone itself regulates the retention of Na^+ and K^+ ions by the body (see Chapter 15). There is therefore a physiologically important feedback-loop operating whereby Na^+ ions (probably acting via the renin-angiotensin system) and K^+ ions influence the circulating level of aldosterone, which in turn increases the retention of Na^+ (and excretion of K^+) ions. This is illustrated in Figure 12.3.

In the normal, healthy animal the osmotic activity of the extracellular fluid equals that of the intracellular fluid, and whenever the osmotic activity of the extracellular fluid alters there is a movement of fluid tending to maintain osmotic equilibrium. The osmolarity of the extracellular fluid is determined very largely by the sodium ion content, since it contains this cation in by far the greatest concentration (the plasma Na^+ concentration is 140 mEq/litre, whereas that of K^+ is only 4 mEq/litre; see Figure 12.4 and Table 12.1). Moreover, living cells have systems (the Na^+/K^+-ATPase or exchange pump localized in the plasma membrane) for maintaining relatively low intracellular Na^+ concentrations (about 10 mEq/litre). It is because Na^+ ions are excluded from within the cell to such an extent and are also the main regulator of osmotic activity outside the cell, that Na^+ ions play

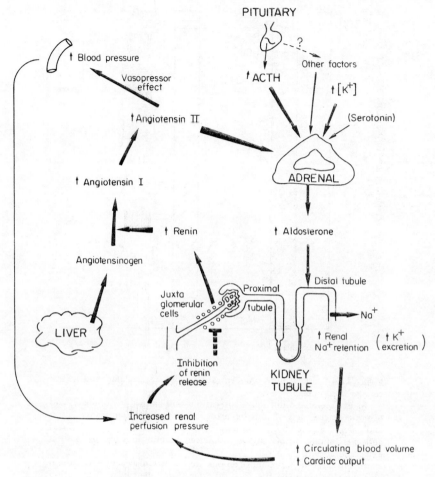

Figure 12.3 The renin-angiotensin system and the multifactorial control of aldosterone synthesis.

such a fundamental role in maintaining water balance. Any change in Na^+ ion concentration in the extracellular fluid has the immediate consequence of a fluid movement involving the intracellular compartment.

A. The regulation by aldosterone of sodium ion distribution

Aldosterone is one of three major factors regulating how much Na^+ is retained by an animal and its primary site of action is at the distal convoluted tubules of the kidney (as well as other glandular epithelial cells such as those in the bowel mucosa, the salivary and sweat gland). Sodium ions are reabsorbed back into the body by transport across these epithelial cells in response to aldosterone (for a discussion of this mechanism, see Chapter 15). In the kidney this is followed by the secretion and

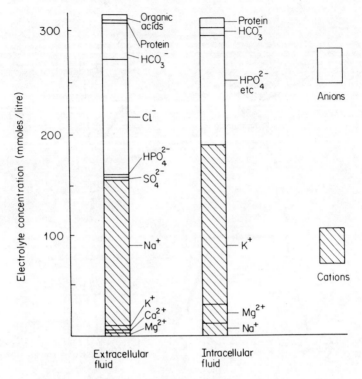

Figure 12.4 Electrolyte concentrations of intracellular and extra-cellular fluid in man.

In extracellular fluid univalent cations and anions predominate, and osmotic inactivation of ions by protein binding is insignificant. Cation and anion concentrations are thus very similar (at 150—160 mmole/litre) and exert similar total osmotic influences. Sodium ions predominate in extracellular fluid.

In intracellular fluid, most anions are bi- or multivalent and protein binding robs some of the ions of their osmotic activity. The cation concentration (190 mmole/litre) is thus considerably greater than the anion concentration (110 mmole/litre) and cations exert a proportion-ately greater osmotic influence. Potassium ions predominate in the intracellular fluid.

Nevertheless the total intracellular and extracellular ion concen-trations are equal and thus the osmotic activities inside and outside the cell are the same.

loss of K^+ and/or H^+ ions into the tubular lumen in an effort to maintain the balance of ionic electrical charges. Increased blood levels of aldosterone result in an increased rate of reabsorption of Na^+ ions taken from the urine passing through the tubular lumen and transported across the tubular epithelial cells of the kidney. In the body, water movement follows this uptake of Na^+ ions to maintain the osmolarity. Water and Na^+ ions both move into the interstitial fluid compartment of the kidney and from there equilibrate with the blood system.

If an excess of Na^+ ions and water is reabsorbed by the kidney (as for example under the influence of an abnormally high aldosterone production), then the salt and water pass into the blood system and increase the blood volume, the capillary hydrostatic pressure and the fluid movement from the vascular to the interstitial fluid compartment.

In some forms of hypertension, an imbalance in sodium ion retention has been well documented (Lebel *et al.*, 1974). Since aldosterone has a major role in controlling Na^+ ion retention, it is thought to have a definitive influence on the development of the hypertension evident in Conn's syndrome. Disturbances in aldosterone regulation and metabolism have been described in other forms of hypertensive disease, but precisely how aldosterone is involved in hypertension is not yet clear.

B. The regulation by aldosterone of potassium ion distribution

The effect of aldosterone at its renal distal tubular site of action is to operate a Na^+-K^+ 'exchange process'. Aldosterone thereby also determines the amount of K^+ ions retained or excreted by the animal. Potassium ions are reabsorbed by the proximal tubules and secreted by the distal tubules. The two principal factors regulating potassium loss in the urine are aldosterone concentration and the amount of Na^+ ions available at the distal tubule Na^+-K^+ exchange site. Thus, following increases in aldosterone production there will be a more efficient or accelerated exchange of Na^+ ions for K^+ and H^+ ions, with increased amounts of K^+ ions lost in the urine. Similarly, if for any reason increased amounts of Na^+ ions arrive at the distal tubule of the kidney, then more K^+ ions will be involved in the exchange process and again urinary K^+ ion levels will rise.

Whereas Na^+ ion concentration is the main determinant of the extracellular fluid volume, the principal defining agent of intracellular osmolarity is the K^+ ion concentration (see Figure 12.4). Clearly any alteration in intracellular K^+ ion concentration affects intracellular osmolarity with consequent changes in cell water movement.

X. MULTIFACTORIAL CONTROL OF ALDOSTERONE BIOSYNTHESIS: A SUMMARY

The biosynthesis of aldosterone occurs in the adrenal glomerulosa cell and is controlled by a very complex regulatory system. A number of known stimulators including angiotensin II, ACTH, K^+ ions, serotonin, prostaglandins and cyclic AMP act directly on glomerulosa tissue and enhance the conversion of cholesterol to pregnenolone, and hence the production of aldosterone.

Perhaps the most important physiological control is exerted via the renin–angiotensin system. Na^+-depletion (an important stimulus for aldosterone production) is thought to operate via activation of this system, with the pituitary gland (ACTH secretion, plus other unknown factors?) playing a largely supportive role (see Figure 12.3).

A further regulatory site on the biosynthetic pathway exists between corticosterone conversion to aldosterone. This late stage is also believed to be under the control of aldosterone-stimulatory agents such as Na^+ ion depletion and K^+ ion uptake (and perhaps by the other stimulatory agents) as well as by unknown factors. These unknown factors may hold a key position in the regulation of aldosterone biosynthesis and are the subject of considerable current research interest.

XI. REFERENCES (*indicates review or book)

Abraham, S. F., E. H. Blaine, J. R. Blair-West, J. P. Coghlan, D. A. Denton, D. R. Mouw, B. A. Scoggins and R. D. Wright (1973). New factors in control of aldosterone secretion. In R. O. Scow, (Ed.) Endocrinology *Excerpta Medica*, Amsterdam, American Elsevier Pub. Co. New York. pp. 733—739.

Aguilera, G., and E. T. Marusic (1971). Role of the renin—angiotensin system in the biosynthesis of aldosterone. *Endocrinology, 89*, 1524—1529.

Albano, J. D. M., B. L. Brown, R. P. Ekins, S. A. S. Tait and J. F. Tait (1974). The effects of potassium, 5-hydroxytryptamine, ACTH and angiotensin II on the concentration of cyclic AMP in suspensions of dispersed rat adrenal zona glomerulosa and fasciculata cells. *Biochem. J., 142*, 391—400.

Ames, R. P., A. J. Borkowski, A. M. Sicinski and J. H. Laragh (1965). Prolonged infusions of angiotensin II and norepinephrine and blood pressure, electrolyte balance, aldosterone and cortisol secretion in normal man and cirrhosis with ascites. *J. clin. Invest., 44*, 1171—1186.

Ayres, P. J., R. P. Gould, S. A. S. Simpson and J. F. Tait (1956). The *in vitro* demonstration of different corticosteroid production within the ox adrenal gland. *Biochem. J., 63*, 19P.

*Bartter, F. C., B. H. Barbour, A. A. Carr and C. S. Delea (1964). On the role of potassium and of the central nervous system in the regulation of aldosterone secretion. In E. E. Baulieu and P. Robel, (Eds) *Aldosterone*. Blackwell, Oxford. pp. 221—242.

Baumann, K., and J. Müller (1974). Effects of hypophysectomy with or without ACTH maintenance therapy on the final steps of aldosterone biosynthesis in the rat. *Acta Endocr., 76*, 102—116.

Baumber, J. S., J. O. Davis, J. A. Johnson and R. T. Witty (1971). Increased adrenocortical potassium in association with increased biosynthesis of aldosterone. *Amer. J. Physiol., 220*, 1094—1099.

Blair-West, J. R., J. P. Coghlan, D. A. Denton, J. W. Funder, C. J. Oddie and B. A. Scoggins (1973). Current concepts in aldosterone control. In R. O. Scow, (Ed.) *Endocrinology. Excerpta Medica*, Amsterdam, American Elsevier Pub. Co. N.Y. pp. 768—773

*Blair-West, J. R., J. P. Coghlan, D. A. Denton, J. W. Funder and B. A. Scoggins (1972). Role of the renin—angiotensin system in the control of aldosterone secretion. In T. A. Assaykeen, (Ed.) *Control of renin secretion*. Plenum Press, New York. pp. 167—187.

Blair-West, J. R., J. P. Coghlan, D. A. Denton, J. R. Goding, M. Wintour and R. D. Wright (1968). The local action of ammonium, calcium and magnesium on adrenocortical secretion. *Aust. J. exp. Biol. med. Sci., 46*, 371.

*Blair-West, J. R., M. Wintour and R. D. Wright (1963). The control of aldosterone secretion. *Recent Progress Hormone Research,* **19**, 311.

*Boyd, J., L. Manuelidis and P. J. Mulrow (1973). The importance of potassium in the regulation of aldosterone biosynthesis. In R. O. Scow, (Ed.) *Endocrinology. Excerpta Medica,* Amsterdam, American Elsevier Pub. Co. N.Y. pp. 785–789.

Braverman, B., and J. O. Davis (1973). Adrenal steroid secretion in the rabbit: sodium depletion, angiotensin II and ACTH. *Amer. J. Physiol.,* **225**, 1306–1310.

Brecher, P. I., H. Y. Pyun and A. V. Chobanian (1974). Studies on the angiotensin II receptor in the zona glomerulosa of the rat adrenal gland. *Endocrinology,* **95**, 1026–1033.

Chiu, A. T., and M. J. Peach (1974). Inhibition of induced aldosterone biosynthesis with a specific antagonist of angiotensin II. *Proc. Nat. Acad. Sci.,* **71**, 341–344.

Coleman, T. G., R. E. McCaa and C. S. McCaa (1974). Effect of angiotensin II on aldosterone secretion in the conscious rat. *J. Endocrinol.,* **60**, 421–427.

*Davies, D. L., D. G. Beevers, J. J. Brown, R. Fraser, J. B. Ferriss, A. F. Lever, A. Medina, J. J. Morton and J. I. S. Robertson (1973). Sodium and the renin–angiotensin system in patients with hypertension. In R. O. Scow, (Ed.) *Endocrinology. Excerpta Medica,* Amsterdam, American Elsevier Pub. Co. N.Y. pp. 693–698.

Davis, W. W., L. R. Burwell, A. G. T. Casper and F. C. Bartter (1968). Sites of action of sodium depletion on aldosterone biosynthesis in the dog. *J. Clin. Invest.,* **47**, 1425–1434.

Devynck, M., M. Pernollet, P. Meyer, S. Fermandjian and P. Fromageot (1973). Angiotensin receptors in smooth muscle cell membranes. *Nature New Biol.,* **245**, 55–57.

Eisenstein, A. B., and P. M. Hartroft (1957). Alterations in the rat adrenal cortex induced by sodium deficiency: a) steroid hormone secretion; b) correlation of histological changes with steroid hormone secretion. *Endocrinology,* **60**, 634 and 641.

Gallant, S., F. C. Kauffman and A. C. Brownie (1974). Cyclic nucleotide phosphodiesterase activity in rat adrenal gland zones. *Life Sciences,* **14**, 937–944.

Giroud, C. J. P., J. Stachenko and E. H. Kenning (1956). Secretion of aldosterone by the zona glomerulosa of rat adrenal glands incubated *in vitro. Proc. Soc. Exp. Biol. (N.Y.),* **92**, 154–158.

Glossman, H., A. J. Baukal and K. J. Catt (1974). Properties of angiotensin II receptors in the bovine and rat adrenal cortex. *J. Biol. Chem.,* **249**, 664–666 and 825–834.

Goodfriend, T. L., and S. Y. Lin (1970). Receptors for angiotensin I and II. *Circulation Res.,* **26** and **27** (Suppl. 1), 163–174.

Goodfriend, T. L. and M. J. Peach (1975). Angiotensin III: (Des-aspartic acid[1])–angiotensin II. Evidence and speculation for its role as an important agonist in the renin–angiotensin system. *Circulation Res.* **36** and **37** (Suppl. 1), 1–38.

*Gross, F. (1971). Angiotensin. In *Int. Encycl. Pharmacol. & Therap.* Section 72, Vol. 1. Pergamon Press, New York. pp. 73–286.

Haning, R., S. A. S. Tait and J. F. Tait (1970). *In vitro* effects of ACTH, angiotensins, serotonin and potassium on steroid output and conversion of corticosterone to aldosterone by isolated adrenal cells. *Endocrinology,* **87**, 1147–1167.

228

Kaplan, N. M. (1965). The biosynthesis of adrenal steroids; effects of angiotensin II, ACTH and potassium. *J. clin. Invest.,* **44,** 2029—2039.

Kaplan, N. M. (1973). Effects of prostaglandins, angiotensin and electrolytes on cyclic AMP and steroid synthesis in beef adrenal tissue. In R. O. Scow, (Ed) *Endocrinology. Excerpta Medica,* Amsterdam; American Elsevier Pub. Co. N.Y. pp. 795—800.

Lebel, M., M. A. Schalekamp, D. G. Beevers, J. J. Brown, D. L. Davies, R. Fraser, D. Kremer, A. F. Lever, J. J. Morton, J. I. S. Robertson, M. Tree and A. Wilson (1974). Sodium and the renin-angiotensin system in essential hypertension and mineralocorticoid excess. *Lancet,* ii, 308—310.

Leutscher, J. A. and B. J. Axelrad (1954). Increased aldosterone output during sodium deprivation in normal men. *Proc. Soc. Exp. Biol. (N.Y.),* **87,** 650.

McCaa, R. E., C. S. McCaa and A. C. Guyton (1975). Role of angiotensin II and potassium in the long-term regulation of aldosterone secretion in intact conscious dogs. *Circulation Res.,* **36,** Suppl. 1. I-57—I-67.

Mendelsohn, F. A., and C. Mackie (1975). Relationships of intracellular potassium and steroidogenesis in isolated adrenal zona glomerulosa and fasciculata cells. *Clinical Science & Mol. Med.* **49,** 13—26.

*Meyer, P., M. Baudouin, S. Fermandjian, M. Worcel, J. L. Morgat and P. Fromageot (1972). In J. Genest and E. Koiw, (Eds) *Hypertension 1972,* Springer-Verlag, Berlin. pp. 495—505.

*Müller, J. (1971). Regulation of aldosterone biosynthesis. *Monographs on Endocrinology,* **5,** Springer-Verlag, Berlin, 137 pages.

*Page, I. H., and F. M. Bumpus (1974). Angiotensin. *Handbook of Experimental Pharmacology,* **37,** Springer-Verlag, Berlin, 680 pages.

Peytremann, A., W. E. Nicholson, R. D. Brown, G. W. Liddle and J. G. Hardman (1973). Comparative effects of angiotensin and ACTH on cyclic AMP and steroidogenesis in isolated bovine adrenal cells. *J. Clin. Invest.,* **52,** 835—841.

Rodbell, M., M. C. Lin and Y. J. Salomon (1974). Evidence for interdependent action of glucagon and nucleotides on the hepatic adenylate cyclase system. *J. Biol. Chem.,* **249,** 59—65. [also: (1975) *J. Biol. Chem.,* **250,** 4239—4245; 4246—4252 and 4253—4260.]

Saruta, T., R. Cook and N. M. Kaplan (1972). Adrenocortical Steroidogenesis, Studies on the mechanism of action of angiotensin and electrolytes. *J. Clin Invest.,* **51,** 2239—2245.

Saruta, T., and N. M. Kaplan (1972). Adrenocortical steroidogenesis: the effects of prostaglandins. *J. Clin. Invest.,* **51,** 2246—2251.

Simpson, S. A., J. F. Tait, A. Wettstein, R. Neher, J. von Euw and T. Reichstein (1953). Isolierung eines neuen kristallisierten hormons aus nebennieren mit besonders hoher wierksamkeit auf den mineralstofwechsel. *Experientia (Basel),* **9,** 333.

Spielman, W. S., and J. O. Davis (1974). The renin-angiotensin system and aldosterone secretion during sodium depletion in the rat. *Circulation Res.,* **35,** 615—624.

Tait, S. A. S., D. Schulster, M. Okamoto, C. Flood and J. F. Tait (1970). Production of steroids by *in vitro* superfusion of endocrine tissue II. Steroid output from bisected whole capsular and decapsulated adrenals of normal intact, hypophysectomized and hypophysectomized-nephrectomized rats as a function of time of superfusion. *Endocrinology,* **86,** 360—382.

Tait, S. A. S., J. F. Tait and J. E. S. Bradley (1972). The effect of serotonin and potassium on corticosterone and aldosterone production by isolated zona glomerulosa cells of the rat adrenal cortex. *Aust. J. Exp. Biol. med. Sci.,* **50**, 833–846.

Tait, S. A. S., J. F. Tait, R. P. Gould, B. L. Brown and J. D. M. Albano (1974a). The preparation and use of purified and unpurified dispersed adrenal cells and a study of the relationship of their cAMP and steroid output. *J. Steroid Biochem.,* **5**, 775–787.

*Tait, J. F., S. A. S. Tait, R. P. Gould and M. S. R. Mee (1974b). The properties of adrenal zona glomerulosa cells after purification by gravitational sedimentation. *Proc. Royal Soc. London B.,* **185**, 375–407.

Ulick, S. (1973). Normal and alternate pathways in aldosterone biosynthesis. In R. O. Scow, (Ed.) *Endocrinology. Excerpta Medica*, Amsterdam, American Elsevier Pub. Co. N.Y. pp. 761–767.

Urquhart, J., J. O. Davis and J. T. Higgins (1963). Effects of prolonged infusion of angiotensin II in normal dogs. *Am. J. Physiol.,* **205**, 1241–1246.

Wassermann, D., and M. Wassermann (1974). The fine structure of adrenal zona glomerulosa in the adult rat. *Cell Tissue Res.,* **149**, 235–243.

Williams, G. H., L. M. McDonell, M. C. Raux and N. K. Hollenberg (1974). Evidence for different angiotensin receptors in rat adrenal glomerulosa and rabbit vascular smooth muscle cells. *Circulation Res.,* **34**, 384–390.

Williams, G. H., L. M. McDonnell, S. A. S. Tait and J. F. Tait (1972). The effect of medium composition and *in vitro* stimuli on the conversion of corticosterone to aldosterone in rat glomerulosa tissue. *Endocrinology,* **91**, 948–960.

CHAPTER 13

Control of gonadal steroidogenesis by FSH and LH

I. INTRODUCTION

The main trophic hormones secreted by the pituitary in the male and female mammal involved in the control of growth, steroid biosynthesis and formation of spermatozoa in the male and ova in the female are: luteinizing hormone (LH) (also referred to as interstitial cell stimulating hormone (ICSH) in the male) and follicle stimulating hormone (FSH). The effects of these hormones, expecially LH, can be clearly shown by classical methods of removal of the hormones by hypophysectomy, resulting in atrophy of the glands, cessation of steroidogenesis and gametogenesis. These functions can be restored by administration of the two hormones. For a long time it was difficult to obtain pure preparations of FSH and LH and thus difficult to attribute the observed effects solely to one hormone. Very pure preparations are now available together with very sensitive radioimmunoassays for their determination in plasma and tissues. In spite of recent intensive research there is still little known about their mechanism of action. The present evidence indicates that like many other hormones, they act through the activation of adenylate cyclase to form cyclic AMP (see Chapter 11). However, the way in which their different actions on growth, steroidogenesis and gametogenesis are distinguished is difficult to understand if they are all mediated by cyclic AMP.

The following discussion on the mechanisms of action of FSH and LH is divided into sections dealing with the sequence of events in which they are thought to occur.

II. BINDING STUDIES

It has been demonstrated by binding and radioautography studies with ^{131}I- and ^{3}H-labelled hormones that specific binding sites exist for trophic hormones in

Table 13.1.
Specific Binding Sites Demonstrated for Trophic Hormones in the Testes and Ovaries

Hormone	Organ	Cell or tissue	References
LH	Testis	Leydig cells ⎫	Rommerts et al., (1974)
FSH	Testis	Seminiferous tubules ⎬	(review)
LH/hCG	Ovary	Corpus luteum	Danzo et al., (1972)
		Granulosa cells	Kammerman et al., (1972)
		(in tissue culture)	
		Theca cells	Lee and Ryan (1971)
			Rajaniemi and Vanha-
			Perttula (1972)

the testes and ovaries. LH binds specifically to Leydig cells of the interstitial tissue and FSH binds to cells (possibly Sertoli cells) in the seminiferous tubules of the rat testis (Table 13.1). In addition, immunofluorescence studies have shown that LH may also bind to the peritubular myoid cells of the seminiferous tubules.

In the ovary it has been found that LH or hCG, but not FSH, specifically bind to the corpus luteum and theca cells and also to granulosa cells grown in cell culture (Table 13.1). hCG and LH compete for binding sites in the ovary and the testis thus suggesting that they bind at the same site. The subunits of both these hormones show negligible binding with ovarian or testicular cells.

hCG-LH receptors from rat testis, rat ovary and bovine corpus luteum have now been solubilized by treatment of cell fractions with non-ionic detergents (Dufau et al., 1973, 1974; Haour and Saxena, 1974). From the characterization studies so far carried out it appears that the receptors from all three tissues are very similar with respect to size, hormone affinity and hormone specificity. Furthermore using appropriate enzymes and separation techniques, it has been shown that the receptors are mainly protein in nature but contain a small but essential lipid component. The availability of these soluble receptors obviously opens up the way for the full structural analysis of the hormone binding site.

III. TROPHIC HORMONE ACTIVATION OF ADENYLATE CYCLASE AND STEROIDOGENESIS

For the ovary it was originally shown by Marsh and his colleagues in 1966 that the corpus luteum contains cyclic AMP and that the addition of LH *in vitro* to slices of this tissue markedly increased the levels of this nucleotide. It was further shown that the increases in cyclic AMP stimulated by LH occurred before the increases in progesterone synthesis were detectable. These data were consistent with cyclic AMP being an intracellular mediator of LH action on steroidogenesis in the corpus luteum. Further experiments have confirmed these earlier results using corpora lutea from different species (humans, cows, sheep and rats). The found evidence indicates that cyclic AMP is also the mediator of LH action on steroidogenesis in the Graafian follicle, granulosa cells in tissue culture and total ovarian cell suspensions. The effect of LH on cyclic AMP and steroidogenesis is apparently specific, no effect was found with other trophic hormones including FSH. In agreement with work on the action of ACTH on the adrenal gland, LH apparently stimulates plasma membrane bound adenylate cyclase.

For the testis the data obtained so far indicate that cyclic AMP may be a second messenger of LH action on steroidogenesis in the testis (Rommerts *et al.*, 1974). It has been shown in various species and tissue preparations that LH activates testicular adenylate cyclase and that cyclic AMP and dibutyryl cyclic AMP stimulate testicular steroidogenesis. Furthermore, in studies carried out with separated testis tissues, it has shown that LH specifically stimulates cyclic AMP production in interstitial tissue (the main site of testosterone formation in the testis) and that FSH specifically stimulates cyclic AMP production in the seminiferous tubules (Cooke *et al.*, 1972, 1974; Dorrington, Vernon and Fritz, 1972; Moyle and Ramachandran, 1973; Dorrington and Fritz, 1974). These specific sites of action of the trophic hormones on testicular adenylate cyclase coincide with their specific binding sites. A simple scheme for the action of LH and FSH on the testis is given in Figure 13.1.

A discrepancy has been found between the amounts of trophic hormone required to stimulate testosterone and cyclic AMP production in testis tissues. Several groups have reported that approximately ten times more LH is required to detect changes in cyclic AMP production compared with that required to stimulate testosterone production (Catt and Dufau, 1973; Moyle and Ramachandran, 1973; Rommerts *et al.*, 1973). This may, of course, imply that with low levels of LH, cyclic AMP is not involved in the intracellular action of this hormone. It is also possible that small changes in cyclic AMP occurring with low levels of gonadotrophins were not detected; that the latter may be true is indicated by the stimulatory effect of theophylline on testosterone release (but not on *detectable* cyclic AMP) produced by low levels of hCG (Catt and Dufau, 1973).

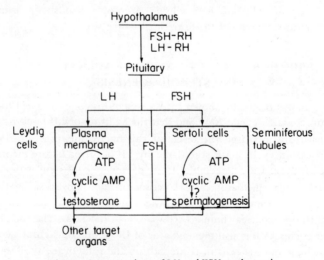

Figure 13.1   Actions of LH and FSH on the testis.

IV. ROLE OF PROSTAGLANDINS

It has been shown by several workers that certain prostaglandins (particularly the E series) will stimulate both cyclic AMP and steroidogenesis in ovarian preparations. It has therefore been proposed that prostaglandins mimic the action of LH on steroidogenesis in the ovary. However, the results obtained are equivocal; they vary according to the species, ovarian preparation and the amount and nature of prostaglandin used.

It has been shown (mainly by Marsh and Kuehl and coworkers) that prostaglandins increase cyclic AMP production in ovarian preparations from the mouse, rat and bovine and that they also enhance ovarian progesterone synthesis in the rat and the bovine. In contrast, Armstrong et al., (1972) found that an inhibitor of prostaglandin synthesis, indomethacin, blocked LH induced ovulation in the rabbit but had no effect on steroidogenesis. It has been proposed by Kuehl and coworkers that the prostaglandins are obligatory mediators of LH action on the ovary. These workers found that a prostaglandin antagonist inhibited the action of LH on cyclic AMP production and steroidogenesis in the mouse ovary in vitro. However, Lamprecht et al., (1973) were not able to confirm these findings in the rat ovary. Furthermore, Marsh (1971) and coworkers demonstrated an additive effect of LH and prostaglandin E_2 on bovine ovarian adenylate cyclase, thus suggesting that LH and prostaglandins act by different mechanisms.

Very little information is available on the role of prostaglandins in cyclic AMP and steroid synthesis in the testis. A small stimulation of rat testis adenylate cyclase by prostaglandins have been shown by Kuehl et al., (1972) and Cooke et al., (1974). In contrast to the stimulatory effects of prostaglandins on ovarian steroidogenesis, Bartke et al., (1973) found that administration of $PGF_{2\alpha}$ to male mice for 3 days lowered plasma testosterone levels and raised the concentration of esterified cholesterol in the testes. It can be concluded from the foregoing discussion that the role of prostaglandins in ovarian and testicular steroidogenesis remains uncertain.

V. ROLE OF PROTEIN KINASE, PROTEIN RNA AND DNA SYNTHESIS

The cyclic AMP-dependence of protein kinase(s) has been demonstrated both in the testis and ovary (Reddi et al., 1971; Menon, 1973). LH has been found to stimulate both cyclic AMP production and protein kinase activity during in vitro incubation of rat ovarian tissue (Lamprecht et al., 1973). In accordance with the separate sites of action of the male trophic hormones, FSH stimulates cyclic AMP production and protein kinase activity in rat testis seminiferous tubules (Means et al., 1974), whereas LH stimulates cyclic AMP production and protein kinase activity in rat testis interstitial tissue (Cooke and van der Kemp, 1976). It has not yet been established that activation of protein kinase(s) is an obligatory step in the intracellular action of LH on steroidogenesis in the ovary and testis or of FSH action on the seminiferous tubules.

Inhibitors of cytoplasmic protein synthesis have been shown to inhibit the stimulation of steroidogenesis by trophic hormones both in the ovary (Hermier *et al.*, 1971; Tsafriri *et al.*, 1973; Arthur and Boyd, 1974) and the testis (Hall and Eik-Nes, 1962; Moyle *et al.*, 1971; Cooke *et al.*, 1975). The inhibition is very rapid, with a half-life of decrease in steroidogenesis of 8 to 13 min (Hermier *et al*, 1971; Cooke *et al.*, 1975) and hence in similarity with the adrenal gland, it has been suggested that a protein with a short half-life is required for the increase in steroidogenesis in the presence of trophic hormones. The testis appears to be different from the adrenal gland and ovary in that the basal testosterone production is independent of protein synthesis.

LH has no detectable effect on total protein synthesis in the interstitial tissue and Leydig cell preparations *in vitro*. This suggests, therefore, that LH may be stimulating the synthesis of a small amount of a specific protein(s) without making a quantitatively important overall contribution to protein synthesis during *in vitro* incubation of this tissue. Whether LH actually stimulates the complete synthesis of this protein regulator(s) or merely activates an existing precursor as has been suggested for the steroidogenic action of ACTH (see Chapter 11) has yet to be determined. Irby and Hall (1971) found that little or no increase in protein synthesis occurred in rat testis Leydig cell preparations isolated from animals treated *in vivo* with LH. They did, however, find that 5 days after hypophysectomy LH increased protein synthesis in these cells 5 hours after injection of the hormone, indicating that LH does have a long-term effect on protein synthesis. These results suggest, therefore, that LH has at least two effects on protein synthesis in the Leydig cell; an acute one on the synthesis of rapidly turning over protein(s) involved in steroidogenesis and a chronic effect on general protein synthesis.

Jungman and Schweppe (1972) have studied the molecular action of hCG on ovaries from immature rats. They found in agreement with Reel and Gorski (1968) that hCG stimulates ovarian nuclear RNA synthesis *in vivo* within 10 minutes of administration of the hormone. They also demonstrated that the synthesis of certain nuclear proteins and the phosphorylation and acetylation of various histone and acidic proteins also occurred within 10 minutes. These authors suggested that their data are compatible with the idea that modification of ovarian nuclear protein metabolism is an early event in the action of hCG.

FSH has been shown to stimulate testicular protein synthesis in rat testis within 1 hour following administration to immature (20-day old) or mature hypophysectomized rats. The stimulation obtained in immature rats continued for at least 12 hours and occurred independent of amino acid transport or activation. An earlier effect of FSH was found on RNA synthesis; the testicular incorporation of ^{3}H-cytidine into rapidly labelled nuclear RNA occurred within 15 min and was inhibited by actinomycin D (see review Means, 1974). FSH has also been shown to induce the production of an androgen binding protein (ABP) in the testis (Hansson *et al.*, 1974; Vernon *et al.*, 1974) which is secreted into the testicular fluid and concentrated in the caput epididymis. The protein is produced within the seminiferous tubules, since it is present in efferent duct fluid and completely absent from testicular lymph. The present evidence indicates that it is formed in the Sertoli cells and may have important functions in spermatogenesis.

The significance of all these observations of the actions of the trophic hormones in relation to the action of cyclic AMP and steroidogenesis remains to be determined. It is apparent, however, that there is a rapid sequence of events following stimulation making it a difficult task to determine the pathways specifically involved in trophic hormone action on the endocrine and germinal processes in the ovary and testis.

VI. EFFECT OF TROPHIC HORMONES ON CHOLESTEROL ESTERS

One of the postulated control sites in the stimulation of steroidogenesis by trophic hormones in the ovary and testis is activation of cholesterol esterase. It is suggested that this takes place in the lipid droplets and that the free cholesterol released is transported to the mitochondria where it is converted to pregnenolone. This postulated scheme is depicted in Figure 13.2 for the testis Leydig cell.

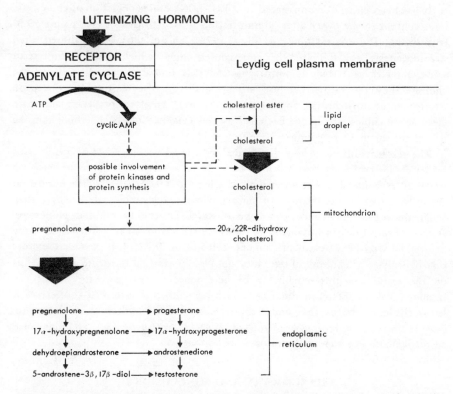

Figure 13.2   Control of testis Leydig cell steroidogenesis (from Cooke *et al.*, 1973). Reproduced by permission of IPPF.

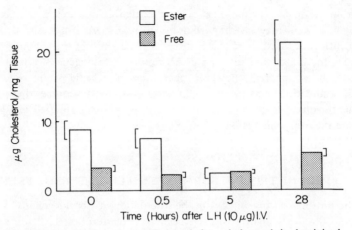

Figure 13.3 Levels on esterified and free cholesterol in luteinized ovaries of rats 6–7 days after hCG priming, and at varying intervals after intravenous injections of LH (5–10 µg NIH–LH–B1 or B4) (from Armstrong, 1968). Reproduced by permission of Academic Press.

It has been clearly demonstrated that LH (hCG) causes depletion of cholesterol ester content in the ovary after administration *in vivo* to the rat (see Figure 13.3) (Armstrong, 1968; Armstrong and Flint, 1973). This effect was not altered when steroidogenesis was inhibited by aminoglutethimide (which inhibits cholesterol side-chain cleavage) thus demonstrating that LH probably acts directly on the cholesterol esterase rather than just causing a depletion of cholesterol by conversion to pregnenolone (Behrman and Armstrong, 1969). An effect of LH on side-chain cleavage of cholesterol is not excluded by this evidence and is still thought to be one, if not the main, rate-limiting step in steroidogenesis.

The testis is different from the ovary and the adrenal gland in having a much higher cholesterol to cholesterol ester ratio. In rat testis interstitial tissue this ratio is 10–20 in contrast to the adrenal gland where it is 0.05–0.10. In the normal rat there is a high concentration of mitochondrial cholesterol (50–100 µg/testis). Furthermore no difference could be observed in cholesterol and cholesterol ester concentrations in homogenates of whole testis and isolated interstitial tissue before and after hCG treatment (van der Molen *et al.*, 1972). It is possible therefore that hydrolysis of cholesterol ester may not be important in the acute action of LH on the testis, but this remains to be determined. In studies with Leydig cell tumours, which contain an abnormally high percentage of esterified cholesterol, it has been demonstrated that under the influence of LH hydrolysis of cholesterol ester to cholesterol does occur (Moyle *et al.*, 1973a,b) (Figure 13.4) and that this is accompanied by an increase in testosterone formation.

VII. SUMMARY AND CONCLUSIONS

Knowledge of the biochemical mechanism of action of trophic hormones on the testis and ovary is more limited compared with that of the adrenal gland. This may

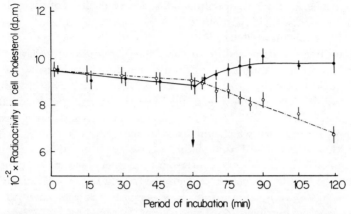

Figure 13.4   Effect of LH on Leydig cell cholesterol. 1,2-^{3} H-Cholesterol (50 μ Ci) was injected intravenously into a Leydig tumour-bearing C57B1/6J mouse. Cell suspensions were then incubated with (vertical arrow) LH (5 μg/ml) as indicated and the changes in cholesterol (——) and esterified cholesterol (—·—·) measured (from Moyle *et al.*, 1973a). Reproduced by permission of the *Biochemical Journal.*

well reflect the more complex nature of these two organs with their multiple cell types and tissue compartments. However, it has been demonstrated that specific trophic hormone receptors are present and that adenylate cyclase is specifically stimulated in different ovarian and testis cell types. For example for LH, specific binding and stimulation of adenylate cyclase and steroidogenesis occurs in the testis

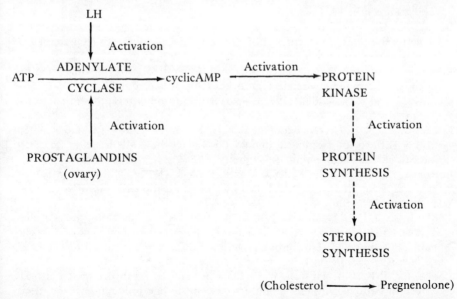

Figure 13.5   Proposed mechanisms for control of steroidogenesis in the ovary and testis.

238

Leydig cell, whereas for FSH specific binding and stimulation of adenylate cyclase occurs in the testis seminiferous tubules. The evidence obtained so far indicates that cyclic AMP is the intracellular mediator of trophic hormone action on steroidogenesis in both ovarian and testicular tissue. Prostaglandins have also been implicated in trophic hormone action on the ovary, but their precise role still remains to be determined.

There is also evidence to suggest that like the adrenal gland, stimulation of protein kinase by cyclic AMP occurs in the ovary and testis and that subsequently a specific protein is formed which stimulates steroidogenesis (Figure 13.5). It is also probable that activation of cholesterol esterase occurs in the fat droplet thus making cholesterol available for conversion to pregnenolone in the mitochondria. This activation has been demonstrated in the ovary and Leydig cell tumours but not yet in the testis from normal animals. A summary of the pathways of testis steroidogenesis and possible control mechanisms is given in Figure 13.2.

VIII. REFERENCES (*indicates review article)

*Armstrong, D. T. (1968). Gonadotrophins, ovarian metabolism and steroid biosynthesis. *Recent Progress in Horm. Res.,* 24, 255—319.
*Armstrong, D. T., Y. S. Moon and D. L. Grinwich (1972). Possible role of prostaglandins in ovulation. In *Advances in the Biosciences*, No. 9. International Conference on Prostaglandins. p. 709.
Armstrong, D. T., and A. P. F. Flint (1973). Isolation and properties of cholesterol ester storage granules from ovarian tissues. *Biochem. J.,* 134, 399—406.
Arthur, J. R., and G. S. Boyd (1974). The effect of inhibitors of protein synthesis on cholesterol side-chain cleavage in the mitochondria of luteinized rat ovaries. *Eur. J. Biochem.,* 49, 117—127.
Bartke, A., N. Musto, B. V. Caldwell and H. R. Behrman (1973). Effects of a cholesterol esterase inhibitor and of prostaglandin $F_{2\alpha}$ on testis cholesterol and on plasma testosterone in mice. *Prostaglandins,* 3, 97—104.
Berhman, H. R., and D. T. Armstrong (1969). Cholesterol esterase stimulation by luteinizing hormone in luteinized rat ovaries. *Endocrinology,* 85, 474—480.
Catt, K. J., and M. L. Dufau (1973). Spare gonadotrophin receptors in rat testis. *Nature New Biology,* 244, 219—221.
Cooke, B. A., W. M. O. van Beurden, F. F. G. Rommerts and H. J. van der Molen (1972). Effects of trophic hormones on 3',5'-cyclic AMP levels in rat testis interstitial tissue and seminiferous tubules. *FEBS Letters,* 25, 83—86.
Cooke, B. A., H. J. van der Molen and B. P. Setchell (1973). The Testis (Map). In *Research in Reproduction*. Published by The International Planned Parenthood Federation, 5, No. 6.
Cooke, B. A., F. F. G. Rommerts, J. W. C. M. van der Kemp, and H. J. van der Molen (1974). Effects of LH, FSH, PGE₁ and other hormones on adenosine, 3:5'-cyclic monophosphate and testosterone production in rat testis tissues. *Molecular and Cellular Endocrinology,* 1, 99—111.
Cooke, B. A., F. H. A. Janszen, W. F. Clotscher and H. J. van der Molen (1975). Effect of protein-synthesis inhibitors on testosterone production in rat testis interstitial tissue and Leydig-cell preparations. *Biochem. J.* 150, 413—418.

Cooke, B. A. and J. W. C. M van der Kemp (1976). Protein kinase in rat interstitial tissue. Effect of luteinizing hormones and other factors. *Biochem. J.,* **154,** 371–378.

Danzo, B. J., A. R. Midgley and L. J. Kleinsmith (1972). Human chorionic gonadotrophin binding to rat ovarian tissue in vitro. *Proc. Soc. Exp. Biol. Med.,* **139,** 88–92.

Dorrington, J. H., R. G. Vernon and I. B. Fritz (1972). The effect of gonadotrophins on the $3',5'$-AMP levels of seminiferous tubules. *Biochem. Biophys. Res. Comm.,* 46, 1523–1528.

Dorrington, J. H., and I. B. Fritz (1974). Effects of gonadotrophins on cyclic AMP production by isolated seminiferous tubules and interstitial cell preparations. *Endocrinology,* **94,** 395–403.

Dufau, M. L., E. H. Charreau and K. J. Catt (1973). Characteristics of a soluble gonadotrophin receptor from the rat testis. *J. Biol. Chem.,* **248,** 6973–6982.

Dufau, M. L., E. H. Charreau, D. Ryan and K. J. Catt (1974). Soluble gonadotropin receptors of the rat ovary. *FEBS letters,* **39,** 149–153.

Hall, P. F., and K. B. Eik-Nes (1962). The action of gonadotropic hormones upon rabbit testis *in vitro. Biochemica Biophysica Acta,* **63,** 411–422.

Hansson, V., O. Trygstad, F. S. French, W. S. McLean, A. A. Smith, D. J. Tindall, S. C. Weddington, P. Petruoz, S. N. Nayfeh and E. M. Ritzen (1974). Androgen transport and receptor mechanisms in testis and epididymis. *Nature,* **250,** 387–391.

Haour, F., and B. B. Saxena (1974). Characterization and solubilization of gonadotropin receptor of bovine corpus luteum. *J. Biol. Chem.,* **249,** 2195–2205.

Hermier, C., Y. Combarnous and M. Jutisz (1971). Role of a regulating protein and molecular oxygen in the mechanism of action of luteinizing hormone. *Biochemica Biophysica Acta,* **244,** 625–633.

Irby, D. C., and P. F. Hall (1971). Stimulation by ICSH of protein synthesis in isolated Leydig cells from hypophysectomized rats. *Endocrinology,* **89,** 1367–1375.

Jungman, R. A., and J. S. Schweppe (1972). Mechanism of action of gonadotropin I. Evidence of gonadotrophin-induced modification of ovarian nuclear basic and acidic protein biosynthesis, phosphorylation and acetylation II. Control of ovarian nuclear ribonucleic acid polymerase activity and chromatin template capacity. *J. Biol. Chem.,* **247,** 5535–5542 and 5543–5548.

Kammerman, S., R. E. Canfield, J. Kolena and C. P. Channing (1972). The binding of iodinated HCG to porcine granulosa cells. *Endocrinology,* **91,** 65–74.

*Kuehl, F. A., J. L. Humes, E. A. Ham and V. J. Cirillo (1972). Cyclic AMP and prostaglandins in hormone action. *Intra-Science Chem. Rept.,* **6,** 85–95.

Lamprecht, S. A., U. Zor, A. Tsafriri and H. R. Lindner (1973). Action of prostaglandin E_2 of luteinizing hormone on ovarian adenylate cyclase, protein kinase and ornithine decarboxylase activity during postnatal development and maturity in the rat. *J. Endocr.,* **57,** 217–233.

Lee, C. C., and R. J. Ryan (1971). The uptake of human luteinizing hormone (LH) by slices of luteinized rat ovaries. *Endocrinology,* **89,** 1515–1523.

Marsh, J. M., R. W. Butcher, K. Savard and E. W. Sutherland (1966). The stimulatory effect of luteinizing hormone on adenosine $3',5'$-monophosphate accumulation in corpus luteum slices. *J. Biol. Chem.,* **241,** 5436–5440.

*Marsh, J. (1971). The effect of prostaglandins on the adenyl cyclase of the bovine corpus luteum. *Ann. New York Academy of Sciences,* **180**, 416—425.

*Means, A. R. (1974). Mini Review. Early sequence of biochemical events in the action of follicle stimulating hormone on the testis. *Life Sciences,* 15, 371—389.

Means, A. R., E. MacDougall, T. R. Soderling and J. D. Corbin (1974). Testicular adenine 3':5'-monophosphate-dependent protein kinase regulation by follicle stimulating hormone. *J. Biol. Chem.,* **249**, 1231—1238.

Menon, K. M. J. (1973). Purification and properties of a protein kinase from bovine corpus luteum that is stimulated by cyclic adenosine 3',5'-monophosphate and luteinizing hormone. *J. Biol. Chem.,* **248**, 494—501.

Moyle, W. R., N. R. Moudgal and R. O. Greep (1971). Cessation of steroidogenesis in Leydig cell tumours after removal of luteinizing hormone and adenosine cyclic 3'-5'-monophosphate. *J. Biol. Chem.,* **246**, 4978—4982.

Moyle, W. R., and J. Ramachandran (1973). Effect of LH on steroidogenesis and cyclic AMP accumulation in rat Leydig cell preparations and mouse tumor Leydig cells. *Endocrinology,* 93, 127—134.

Moyle, W. R., R. L. Jungas and R. O. Greep (1973a). Influence of luteinizing hormone and adenosine 3':5'-cyclic monophosphate on the metabolism of free and esterified cholesterol in mouse Leydig-cell tumours. *Biochem. J.,* **134**, 407—413.

Moyle, W. R., R. L. Jungas and R. O. Greep (1973b). Metabolism of free and esterified cholesterol by Leydig cell tumour mitochondria. *Biochem. J.,* **134**, 415—424.

Rajaniemi, H., and T. Vanha-Perttula, (1972). Specific receptor for LH in the ovary: evidence by autoradiography and tissue fractionation. *Endocrinology,* **90**, 1—9.

Reddi, A. H., L. L. Ewing and H. G. Williams-Ashman (1971). Protein phosphokinase reactions in mammalian testis. Stimulatory effects of adenosine 3':5'-cyclic monophosphate on the phosphorylation of basic proteins. *Biochem. J.,* **122**, 333—345.

Reel, J. R., and J. Gorski (1968). Gonadotrophin regulation of precursor incorporation into ovarian RNA, protein and acid-soluble fractions. II. Changes in nucleotide labeling, nuclear RNA synthesis, and effects of RNA and protein synthesis inhibitors. *Endocrinology,* 83, 1092—1100.

Rommerts, F. F. G., B. A. Cooke, J. W. C. M. van der Kemp and H. J. van der Molen (1973). Effect of luteinizing hormone on 3',5'-cyclic AMP and testosterone production in isolated interstitial tissue of rat testis. *FEBS letters,* **33**, 114—118.

*Rommerts, F. F. G., B. A. Cooke and H. J. van der Molen (1974). The role of cyclic AMP in the regulation of steroid biosynthesis in testis tissue. *J. Steroid Biochem.,* **5**, 279—285.

Tsafriri, A., M. E. Lieberman, A. Barnea, S. Bauminger and H. R. Lindner (1973). Induction by luteinizing hormone of ovum maturation and of steroidogenesis in isolated graafian follicles of the rat: Role of RNA and protein synthesis. *Endocrinology,* 93, 1378—1386.

Van der Molen, H. J., M. H. Bijleveld, G. J. van der Vusse and B. A. Cooke (1972). Effect of gonadotrophins on cholesterol esters as precursors of steroid production in the testis. *J. Endocrinology,* **57**, vi—vii.

Vernon, R. G., B. Kopec and I. B. Fritz (1974). Observations on the bindings of androgens by rat testis seminiferous tubules and testis extracts. *Molecular and Cellular Endocrinology*, 1, 167–187.

SECTION IV
Mode of Action of Steroid Hormones

CHAPTER 14

Mode of action of estrogens, progesterone and androgens

I. INTRODUCTION

The elucidation of the molecular mode of steroid hormone action is one of the most challenging areas of present day research. One of the main problems is to determine the first biochemical events which occur at a molecular level and which ultimately result in the observed physiological effects of the steroid hormones. As can be seen from Table 14.1, these effects are many and diverse.

Initial work concentrated on studying the effects of steroid hormones injected *in vivo* in terms of changes in enzyme activities, uptake of small molecules and synthesis of macromolecules such as protein, phospholipids and nucleic acids in cells of target organs. These studies helped to elucidate the biochemical events and sequence of these events brought about by the hormone (Figure 14.8). However, a different approach was required in order to look at the molecular interaction of the hormone itself with its target cell. With the introduction of tritiated steroid hormones of high specific activity, it became possible to localize the hormone at a tissue, cellular and intracellular level. It was quickly realized that very specific *intracellular* binding of the hormone occurred in its target cells, and that this was most probably the first event which occurred in the molecular action of the hormone. The specific interaction of the steroid hormones with the particular

Table 14.1.

Hormone	Effects
Estradiol	Stimulates growth of female reproductive tract and mammary glands; controls estrous and menstrual cycles; inhibits gonadotrophin secretion; increases plasma lipids, lipoproteins and calcium. Increases protein and RNA synthesis in avian liver and oviduct.
Testosterone	Stimulates (*a*) differentiation of male reproductive organs *in utero* and adult development, (*b*) development of male secondary sexual characteristics in mammals, birds, fish, amphibia and reptiles, (*c*) spermatogenesis, fructose and citrate formation in vesicular glands, (*d*) nitrogen retention (anabolic effects).
Progesterone	Acts synergistically with estradiol in maintaining uterine growth; inhibits gonadotrophin production by the pituitary; stimulates galactose metabolism in rabbit liver; may affect central nervous system.

macromolecules in their target cells was then examined *in vitro* and the knowledge gained by this work has been formulated into a RECEPTOR theory. This concept attempts to unify all the diverse effects of the hormones in terms of one general initial mechanism which is followed by events determined genetically or environmentally for that particular cell and tissue. The extensive work in this field has recently been documented by King and Mainwaring (1974).

II. THE RECEPTOR THEORY

Baulieu *et al.* (1971) have described the action of the hormones in target organs by the model illustrated in Figure 14.1. The interaction, i.e. binding of the hormone at a specific ('receptive') site (r), produces a specific regulatory signal and this information is transferred to the executive site (e). This causes the cellular

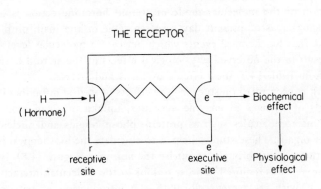

Figure 14.1 The RECEPTOR model for interaction of a hormone with its receptor site. The resultant effect on the executive site may not take place within the same molecule; a concerted effect on a series of molecules may be involved (from E.-E. Baulieu *et al.*, 1971). Reproduced by permission of Academic Press.

machinery to be switched on to perform specific biochemical reactions. The hormone itself plays no further part in these reactions apart from its removal from the system (e.g. by metabolism or exit from the active site). The receptor need not be a single entity; there may be a variety of complex combinations of concerted receptor systems.

It is now well established that binding of high specificity and high affinity occurs both extracellularly and intracellularly between hormones and specific macro-molecules (a prerequisite of the receptor theory). In addition, metabolism of the steroid hormones takes place within their target cells. Both binding and metabolism play an important role in the action of the steroid hormones, and will now be discussed in more detail.

III. LOCALIZATION AND METABOLISM OF HORMONES AT THEIR ACTIVE SITE

An important aspect of the study of hormone action is to determine the fate of the hormone in terms of metabolism and retention by tissues after *in vivo* administration of physiological amounts of the hormone. One of the first hormones to be investigated in this way was estradiol (Jensen and Jacobson, 1962). It was found that when tritiated estradiol was injected subcutaneously into young female rats the subsequent distribution of radioactivity was as shown in Figure 14.2. Those tissues which were not responsive to estradiol, such as liver, kidney, muscle and blood, showed a pattern of radioactive uptake and retention which varied with time in a characteristic fashion quite different from that exhibited by target tissues such as the uterus and vagina. The former non-responsive tissues attained their maximum radioactive content very early with a rapid decrease thereafter; whereas the uterus and vagina continued to incorporate and retain radioactive steroid for a much longer period. The nature of the retained radioactive material has been investigated, and it has been shown that in the uterus and vagina most of the labelled steroid is present as estradiol, whereas other tissues contain a mixture of metabolites consisting of conjugated (water soluble) and unconjugated steroids. Further studies have shown that a small amount of metabolism of estradiol-17β to estrone can occur in uterine tissue particularly in other species, but it is generally accepted that estradiol-17β itself is the active hormone and not estrone. Similar early experiments designed to study the uptake of tritiated progesterone by target organs were unsuccessful: retention of radioactivity similar to that obtained with estradiol was not observed. However, it was discovered that the incorporation of locally administered progesterone was greatly increased in guinea pig vagina if the animals were pretreated with estrogen. Subsequent experiments have shown that retention of progesterone by target organs such as uterus and vagina depend on the presence of estradiol.

Progesterone is more quickly and extensively metabolized after *in vivo* administration than estradiol. Metabolism also occurs in its target organs to 5α-pregnane-3,20-dione and to 20-dihydro products. However, the steroid taken up

248

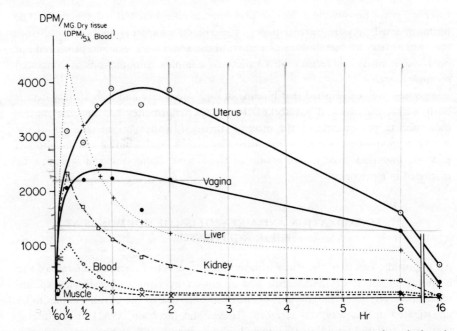

Figure 14.2 Concentration of radioactivity in tissues of immature rats after single sub-cutaneous injection of estradiol-6,7-^{3}H (0.1 μg, 11.5 μCi). Total radioactivity expressed as dpm/mg of dry tissue or per 5 μl of blood. Because blood contains a mixture of radioactive metabolites, but uterus and vagina incorporate only estradiol, the ratio of estradiol concentration between uterus and blood is about 500 to 1 (from E. V. Jensen and H. K. Jacobson, 1962). Reproduced by permission of Academic Press.

and bound by the target organs is mainly progesterone itself. Present evidence from *in vitro* binding studies and progesterone—receptor interaction suggests that, like estradiol, progesterone is the active hormone.

Testosterone is extensively metabolized in many tissues including not only the normal main site of steroid metabolism, the liver, but also target organs such as the ventral prostate. Unlike estradiol and progesterone, some of the metabolic products of testosterone are hormonally active, the most potent being 5α-dihydro-

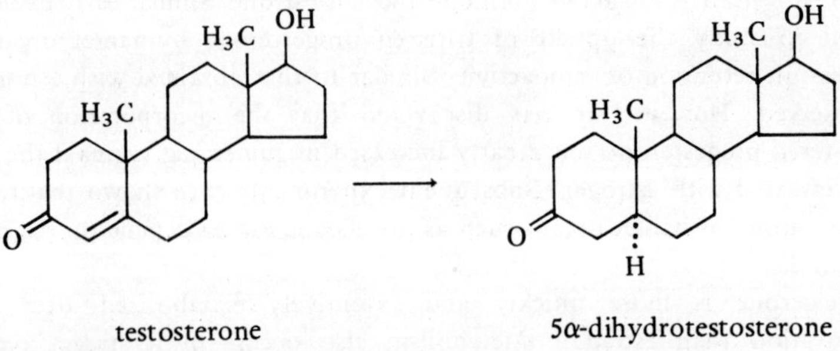

testosterone   5α-dihydrotestosterone

Figure 14.3 Conversion of testosterone to the biologically active androgen 5α-dihydrotestosterone.

testosterone (Figure 14.3). The latter is the main compound formed in ventral prostate nuclei from testosterone (>75% of the radioactivity) following administration of the tritiated parent compound (see section on Androgen Receptors for further details). Baulieu and coworkers have studied the effects of testosterone and its metabolites on the growth and secretory activity of explants of prostatic tissue in organ culture. Many of the metabolites were active (mainly ring A reduced 17β-hydroxysteroids) and exhibited different hormonal properties. It was concluded from this study that testosterone acts through the metabolites formed in the target organ. However in some target tissues e.g. *levator ani* muscle, testosterone itself may be the active hormone as no metabolites could be detected (Baulieu, 1975).

IV. STEROID HORMONE RECEPTORS

The observation that steroid hormones (and/or their metabolites) are selectively retained by their target organs opened up a whole new era of steroid biochemical investigation. It became of the utmost importance to determine the nature, intracellular localization and kinetics of steroid macromolecular interactions.

A. Methods of measuring steroid—macromolecular interactions

There are many ways of studying the non-covalent reversible binding of steroids which occur in their target organs. The most commonly used parameters (e.g. affinity of binding and number of binding sites) are derived from simple kinetics applied to the following equation:

$$S + P \underset{K_2}{\overset{K_1}{\rightleftharpoons}} SP \tag{1}$$

where S = steroid

P = protein

SP = steroid bound to protein

K_1 = velocity constant for formation of SP

K_2 = velocity constant for breakdown of SP

According to the law of mass action, at equilibrium the velocity of the forward reaction is equal to the velocity of the reverse reaction, thus

$$K_1 [U][N_m - B] = K_2 [B] \tag{2}$$

where [U] = concentration of unbound steroid

[N_m] = the concentration of one set of m, independent identical binding sites on the macromolecules

[B] = concentration of bound steroid

Rearranging equation (2)

$$\frac{K_1}{K_2} = \frac{[B]}{[U][N_m - B]} = K_a \tag{3}$$

where K_a = the *association constant* or *affinity constant*.

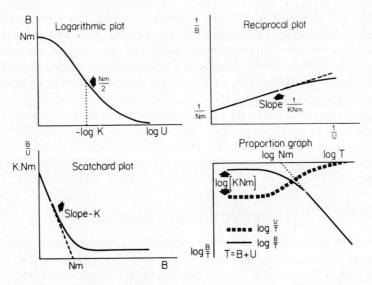

Figure 14.4 Different graphical representations of steroid-macromolecular binding (Brinkman, 1972).

It has the units of litres/mole and is a measure of the affinity of the steroid for the protein. The reciprocal of the affinity constant is K_d, the *dissociation constant*, and has the units of moles/litre. Both these constants are frequently used. Equation (3) can be rearranged into several convenient forms so that the K_a and N_m can be determined graphically knowing B and U for different concentrations of steroid e.g.

$$\frac{B}{U} = K_a \cdot [N_m] - K_a \cdot [B] \tag{4}$$

or

$$B = \frac{[N_m] \cdot [U]}{\frac{1}{K_a} + [U]} \tag{5}$$

In Figure 14.4 are given typical graphical results using the above equations. The most extensively used is the so-called Scatchard plot where B/U is plotted against B (Equation 4), the slope of the line gives $-K_a$ and the intercept on the x-axis, N_m, the number of binding sites. Using this plot, different classes of binding sites can be distinguished; the steep slope represents high affinity binding and a low number of binding sites, whereas the almost horizontal line represents low affinity binding and a very high number of binding sites. For a discussion of other graphical representations, especially the proportional graph (which can be used for a wide range of steroid concentrations and complex binding systems), the reader is referred to Baulieu and Raynaud (1970), Westphal (1971) and King and Mainwaring (1974).

When studying steroid–macromolecular interactions, it is important to distinguish between specific (i.e. binding to a 'receptor') and non-specific binding. Because the number of receptor binding sites are usually very limited, they will be easily saturated with a very small amount of steroid and therefore non-specific binding will also occur in the presence of excess steroid. The amount of binding to ← the two types of binding sites can be measured by incubating, in parallel, the receptor preparation with labelled steroid, and also labelled steroid in the presence of a 100-fold excess of the same unlabelled steroid. The difference between the two measurements will give the steroid bound to specific receptor sites. In the first incubation, providing enough labelled steroid is added, binding will occur at specific and non-specific sites. In the second incubation the binding of the labelled steroid to the specific sites will be so diluted by the binding to the non-specific sites (present in comparatively large quantities) that non-specific binding will be mainly measured.

In order to determine K_a and N_m by any of the above methods the amount of bound and free steroid must be determined. There are various ways of doing this depending on the nature of the steroid protein complex (e.g. its stability) and the amount of information required (e.g. the number and types of binding proteins present). Most methods measure either the amount of unbound labelled steroid or the amount of bound labelled steroid. Methods which give information not only on the amount of free and bound steroid, but also the nature of the binding systems present, include gel chromatography, sucrose gradient centrifugation and acrylamide gel electrophoresis. A good example of the use of different methods to investigate specific binding has been published by van Beurden-Lamers et al. (1974).

Equilibrium dialysis: this is a technique where equilibrium is maintained during dialysis. Essentially the binding system is kept in one compartment and the free unbound steroid in another. The concentration of bound steroid can be obtained by subtracting the amount of unbound steroid from the total amount added to the system.

Charcoal adsorption: At equilibrium the unbound steroid is removed by shaking with charcoal. After centrifugation the amount of bound steroid can be measured in the supernatant.

Gel chromatography: Column chromatography using, for example, Sephadex G-25 of a previously equilibrated steroid—protein mixture gives a separation of free and bound steroid. The bound steroid is eluted without retention; the free steroid is eluted in subsequent fractions.

Sucrose-gradient centrifugation: The equilibrated mixture is layered on a linear sucrose gradient and is then centrifuged. Macromolecules are separated according to their size. Steroid bound to these macromolecules is separated in the same way (see Figure 14.9), whereas the unbound steroid remains at the top of the tube.

The behaviour of macromolecules during sucrose density centrifugation is usually expressed in terms of their sedimentation constants which are given in Svedberg (S) units which correspond to the size of the molecule — the higher the S value the larger the molecule.

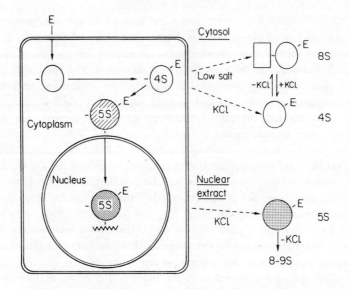

Figure 14.5 Schematic representation of interaction pathway of estradiol (E) in uterine cell. Diagram on the left indicates uterine cell with extranuclear estradiol-receptor complex undergoing transformation and entering nucleus to bind to chromatin. Diagrams on the right indicate ultracentrifuge sedimentation properties of complexes extracted from the cell (from E. V. Jensen and E. R. DeSombre, *Science*, **182**, pp. 126–134 (1973). Copyright © 1973 by the American Association for the Advancement of Science).

Acrylamide gel electrophoresis: Electrophoresis of steroid bound to macromolecules on acrylamide gels has the advantage of giving very high resolution, and hence gives a good resolution of mixtures of more than one binding system.

B. Estradiol receptors

It is currently believed that estradiol (E) enters its target cell and combines non-covalently and specifically with a receptor protein present in the cytoplasm region of the cell. This receptor protein—estradiol complex then moves into the nucleus where it is thought to affect specific transcription processes at the level of the gene. This has been referred to as a two-step process, i.e. first step, entry of estradiol into the cytoplasm and combination with the receptor, and second step, entry into the nucleus of the receptor bound estradiol (Figure 14.5). The physical nature of the receptor complex, particularly with regard to the effect of different salt concentrations on its size, has been, and still is being, intensely investigated (Jensen and DeSombre, 1972; Mueller *et al.* 1972; O'Malley and Means, 1974).

It appears that when estradiol enters the cell it interacts with a macromolecular component which, when isolated in a low ionic strength media, sediments at 8–9S in the ultracentrifuge. This 8–9S receptor was found to be sensitive to conditions liable to denature proteins (e.g. pH changes and reagents capable of reacting with

—SH groups), and only proteolytic enzymes such as trypsin or pronase were effective in liberating tritiated estradiol from the 8—9S component. The protein nature of the receptor was thus established. It was shown that the 8—9S receptor could be reversibly dissociated to 4—5S forms in the presence of 0.3—0.4 M KCl.

The estradiol—receptor extracted from the nucleus by 0.3 M KCl has been shown to be a 5S protein. When the binding studies of estradiol and uterine tissue are carried out at $4°C$, the estradiol—receptor complex remains mainly in the cytoplasm region of the cell and is only slowly transferred to the nucleus. However, when the temperature is increased to $37°C$ the transfer of the complex to the nucleus is rapid. The cytoplasmic estradiol—receptor complex can be formed directly by mixing the hormone with preparations of the cytoplasmic fraction of different target tissues, but the nuclear estradiol-receptor complex can only be demonstrated after incubation of hormone with both cytoplasm and nuclei. The binding and intracellular transfer of estradiol is not blocked by inhibitors of RNA and protein synthesis, whereas the subsequent effects of estradiol have been found to be inhibited by these agents.

There is still some discussion as to the physiological forms of the receptor—estradiol complex in the cytoplasm and the nucleus. Jensen and other workers have proposed that the physiological form of the complex in the cytoplasm is the 4S unit and not the 8—9S form. Furthermore it has been shown that the 4S unit can be transformed into the nuclear 5S form in the cytoplasm (Figure 14.5). This can be demonstrated by warming uterine cytosol in the presence of estradiol; the resulting hormone—receptor complex sediments in sucrose-density gradients containing salt at approximately the same rate as the nuclear complex (5S). It has also been observed that ammonium sulphate precipitation of the estradiol—receptor complex of calf uterine cytosol, prepared in the absence of EDTA, yields a complex that sediments at approximately 5S. In contrast to the temperature-dependent transformation in uterine cytosol, which takes place only in the presence of estradiol, the alteration that accompanies ammonium sulphate precipitation proceeds rapidly in the cold and does *not* require estradiol. The significance of these findings remain to be determined.

The requirement of conversion of the estradiol-4S receptor to estradiol-5S receptor before transfer to the nucleus can be demonstrated by uptake studies *in vitro*. When purified uterine nuclei are incubated at $0°C$ with uterine cytosol containing estradiol—receptor complex, little or no transfer of the complex takes place. It does occur, however, if the system is warmed to $37°C$ or if the cytosol is prewarmed to $37°C$ before addition of nuclei. In both the latter circumstances transformation of the 4S to the 5S complex occurs.

C. Progesterone receptors

Attempts to demonstrate progesterone binding in uterine tissue were not very successful until it was found that priming with estrogens enhanced the binding nearly tenfold. Estradiol was later found to increase the progesterone receptor concentration. Subsequent studies, especially by O'Malley and coworkers (1974), with the chick oviduct have shown that in estrogen primed tissue, progesterone specifically binds with a protein receptor in the cytoplasm which is subsequently transferred to the nucleus by a process that is more rapid at 37°C than at lower temperatures. The characteristics of the progesterone receptor with regard to size and distribution in the nucleus and cytoplasm are similar to those previously described for estradiol. However, prior treatment with estrogen apparently has an effect on the progesterone receptor size; the 4S binding unit is partly or wholly converted to a unit which sediments more rapidly in low salt gradients.

D. Androgen receptors

The prostate, one of the main target organs for testosterone, has received most attention with regard to the mechanism of androgen action. The original observation by Bruckovsky and Wilson (1968) that ^{3}H-testosterone was transformed in target organs to [3]H-5α-dihydrotestosterone (5α-DHT) was demonstrated with this tissue. It was further shown that transformation to this metabolite not only occurs in the cytoplasm but also in the nucleus. The latter transformation was demonstrated to be a characteristic feature of accessory sexual glands (see King and Mainwaring, 1974, p. 58). The 5α-DHT binds to high affinity receptor molecules both in the cytoplasm and nucleus of the prostate gland. Like the binding of estradiol to the uterine nuclear receptor, the binding of 5α-DHT to the prostate nucleus has been found to be a temperature-dependent step; significant binding only occurs when the incubations are carried out at 30°C or 37°C, but not at 4°C. The exact size of the receptor is not yet certain, but a complex of 3.5−5S size is found in the nucleus where it is bound to the chromatin (the protein−DNA complex derived from lysed nuclei). The proposed overall scheme is as shown in Figure 14.6 (Wilson, 1972). Testosterone is not only transformed into 5α-DHT, but

Androgen target cell

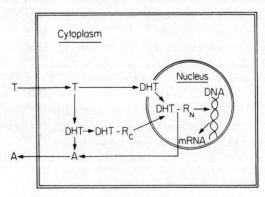

Figure 14.6 Proposed mechanism of testosterone action on its target cell. (T = testosterone, DHT = 5α-dihydrotestosterone, R_C = cytoplasmic receptor, R_N = nuclear receptor, A = 5α-dihydroandrostane-3β,17β-diol or 5α-dihydroandrostane-3α,17β-diol.)

further reduction by the 3α- and 3β-hydroxy reducing enzymes can occur; these enzymes are only present in the cytoplasm and not in the nucleus.

V. THE JACOB–MONOD THEORY IN RELATION TO THE MECHANISM OF HORMONE ACTION

A. The Jacob–Monod theory

The original concept of Jacob–Monod for the induction of enzymes in bacteria cells has been used as a basic hypothesis for the mechanism of hormone action. Briefly what Jacob and Monod (1961) proposed was that the *structure* of an enzyme is specified by one gene, called a *structural gene*, and that the *rate of synthesis* is determined by another gene, called a *regulator gene* (Figure 14.7).

The product of a structural gene is a short-lived messenger RNA (mRNA) which moves to the ribosomes to initiate the production of the enzyme molecules. The regulator gene itself produces mRNA molecules which code for a protein *repressor* molecule which binds with the operator gene to *inhibit* the production of mRNA molecules from the structural gene(s). When induction of enzyme synthesis occurs in bacteria a substance, for example a regulating metabolite or an 'effector', combines with the repressor and neutralizes its effect, and thus initiates mRNA

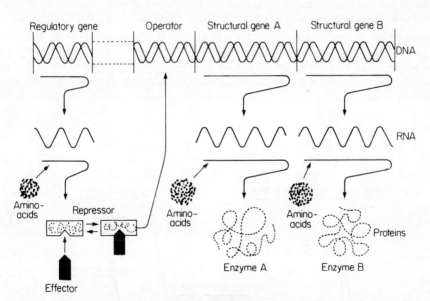

Figure 14.7   Control of protein synthesis by genetic 'repressor' as proposed by Jacob and Monod for bacteria. A regulatory gene directs the synthesis of a molecule, the repressor, which binds with the operator. When an effector is added, it binds with the repressor which then dissociates from the operator causing the genes to be 'switched on' to produce mRNA molecules which code for the synthesis of specific proteins (from 'The Control of Biochemical Reactions', J-P. Changeux, *Scientific American*, April 1975. Copyright © 1965 by Scientific American, Inc. All rights reserved.)

synthesis from the structural gene. Because the mRNA's produced are short-lived, the production of the enzyme depends on the continuing presence of the effector. Another substance which is required for mRNA synthesis is DNA dependent RNA polymerase.

It is apparent that a similar sort of mechanism could be put forward for the action of steroids on their target organs. The steroids could play the role of the effector in derepressing the gene and causing induction of mRNA molecules for protein synthesis. From the evidence already discussed, it is apparent that the situation in hormonally responsive mammalian cells is not so simple as in bacterial cells. A specific cytoplasmic receptor is involved which undergoes transformation before entering the nucleus (the site of mRNA synthesis). What happens there is undoubtedly also more complicated than in the prokaryotic bacterial cells because of the much more complicated and multiple DNA's present in eukaryotic cells. However, the following discussion on the effect of steroids on RNA and protein synthesis illustrates that the same basic mechanisms may be involved.

B. The role of specific RNA and protein synthesis in estrogen action

As stated earlier, estrogen (E) administration to immature rats dramatically stimulates the development of the uterus and causes a rapid increase in protein, RNA and phospholipid synthesis. The time sequence of events is depicted in Figure 14.8. It can be seen that changes in protein synthesis are not detectable until 3 hours after E administration. However, Gorski and coworkers found that cycloheximide (an inhibitor of protein synthesis — see Figure 15.3) blocked the earlier changes in RNA synthesis. These workers therefore suggested that the early effects of estrogen depended on changes in the synthesis of one or a few proteins,

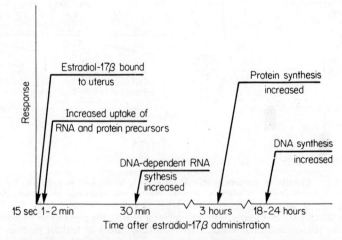

Figure 14.8 Time sequence of induced biochemical events in rat uterus after estradiol-17β administration *in vivo*.

which were not detectable by measuring the change in the overall rate of protein synthesis.

Subsequently, it was demonstrated by Gorski and coworkers and independently by Baulieu and coworkers that estradiol specifically stimulates the accumulation of specific protein(s). These elegant experiments employed a double-labelling technique in which the incorporation into protein of ^{3}H-leucine by the uteri of control animals was compared with the incorporation of ^{14}C-leucine into protein by the uteri of estradiol-treated animals. Cytoplasmic fractions prepared from both control

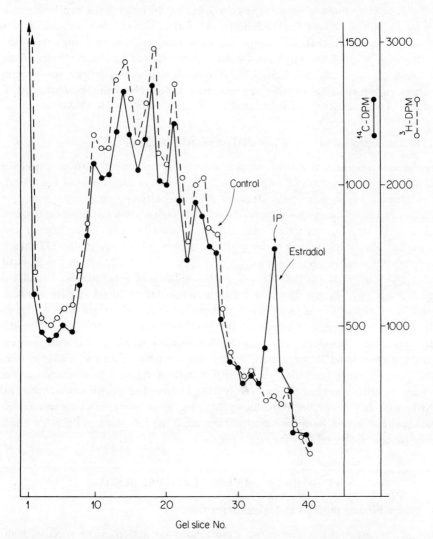

Figure 14.9 The electrophoretic distribution of soluble proteins, isolated from uteri incubated *in vitro* with either ^{14}C-leucine and estradiol (———) or ^{3}H-leucine (–––). (Reprinted with permission from A. Barnea and J. Gorski (1970), *Biochemistry*, **9**, p. 1899. Copyright by the American Chemical Society.)

and estradiol-treated tissue were combined, and then subjected to polyacrylamide gel electrophoresis in order to fractionate the protein products. Subsequent examination of the gel for ^{3}H- and ^{14}C-labelled products demonstrated the presence of a peak of radioactivity present only in the ^{14}C-labelled material (i.e. that derived from the estradiol-treated tissue) (Figure 14.9). The protein nature of this new 'induced protein' (IP) was further indicated by the observation that cycloheximide blocked this effect of estradiol — no IP peak was discerned in the presence of this inhibitor of protein synthesis.

It was later shown that actinomycin D (an inhibitor of RNA synthesis — see Figure 15.3) also blocks the accumulation of the 'induced protein', and it was therefore suggested that the early action of estrogen was to bring about the synthesis of the mRNA which subsequently was required for the synthesis of the 'induced protein'. The synthesis of this mRNA also occurs before any general increase in the synthesis of RNA can be detected. The role of the 'induced protein' remains to be elucidated, and so far it has only been demonstrated in the uterus.

C. Effect of progesterone and estradiol on protein synthesis

In the estrogen primed chick oviduct, subsequent treatment with progesterone stimulates the production of a specific protein, avidin (a component of egg white). This stimulation is detectable 10 hours after progesterone treatment *in vivo* or 6 hours *in vitro*. During this time no change in overall protein synthesis occurs, and there is no increase in other major oviduct proteins such as ovalbumin and lysozyme. Direct evidence that the synthesis of new mRNA for avidin was caused by progesterone has been obtained by O'Malley *et al.* (1972). RNA was isolated from the ribosomal fraction derived from oviducts of progesterone stimulated chicks, and purified by filtration through nitrocellulose filters. Under the very specific conditions of the experiment, these filters selectively retain mRNA (due to the binding of the poly A region of the mRNA to the nitrocellulose). When the purified mRNA obtained was added to an *in vitro* rabbit reticulocyte protein synthesizing system, it specifically caused the synthesis of an avidin-like protein. The same workers have also shown that a mRNA fraction from chick oviduct pretreated with estrogens directed the synthesis of another specific oviduct protein, ovalbumin, in the rabbit reticulocyte system. Thus these results support the concept that steroid hormones act by stimulating the formation of mRNA's which code for specific proteins in the target organs.

VI. SOME OF THE UNSOLVED PROBLEMS

A. Plasma binding proteins and receptor proteins

One of the main characteristics of steroid hormone action is the specific, high affinity, intracellular binding which occurs between the hormone and macromolecule(s) situated within their target cells. In plasma there are also proteins which specifically bind certain steroids. The precise physiological functions of these

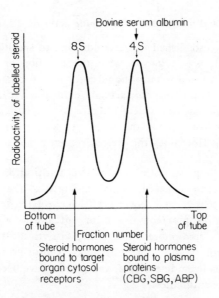

Figure 14.10 Sucrose gradient centrifugation sedimentation pattern of steroids bound to plasma and receptor protein-complexes carried out in low salt media.

plasma binding proteins are unclear. It has been suggested that they may act as carrier proteins for entry of steroids into cells. However, unconjugated steroids (but not steroid sulphates) are freely permeable to cells and so apparently do not require the plasma proteins for this process. They may of course regulate the amount of steroid which is available to its target organ, i.e. steroid which is bound to the plasma protein is not free to enter tissue cells (see Chapter 6.V). It is curious, however, that if one binding site per molecule is assumed, the levels of two of the plasma binding proteins SBG* and CBG* are normally 2- or 3-fold greater than the physiological levels of their respective steroid hormones, i.e. testosterone and cortisol. It is not generally accepted that CBG and SBG enter tissue cells. However, Baulieu and coworkers have found a CBG-like substance in rat uterus which was identical in all respects (specificity of binding, physical properties, and so on) to plasma CBG. In the rabbit an androgen binding protein (ABP) in testis and epididymis with a high affinity for testosterone and 5α-dihydrotesterone has also been found. This protein only differs from SBG in its isoelectric point (SBG: pH 5.4—5.8; ABP: pH 4.5—5.8, rabbit). In general the androgen, estrogen and progesterone cytosol receptors are found in the 8S region of sucrose density gradients in low salt media, whereas the plasma binding proteins are in the 4S region (Figure 14.10).

*Sex steroid binding globulin and corticosteroid binding globulin (or transcortin).

B. Steroid receptors and mechanism of hormone action

Although it is clearly established that steroids bind to specific macromolecules in their target organs, it is not known what the function of this steroid protein complex is. Does the steroid require the receptor to get it into the nucleus or vice versa? Does the cytoplasmic receptor actually enter the nucleus or does it merely 'hand over' the steroid to the nuclear receptor at the nuclear membrane? Is the receptor and/or steroid required in the nucleus to set in motion the transcriptional events which follow? How does the steroid/receptor molecule interact with the chromatin?

The answer to these questions may come after purification and identification of the receptors have been achieved. Rapid progress is now being made in this direction. Already Jensen and coworkers have reported the isolation of a transformed estrogen receptor complex from calf uterine nuclei which is homogeneous both on gel electrophoresis and during analytical ultracentrifugation; the amino acid composition of this apparently pure receptor protein, which they have named estrophilin, has been determined, and rabbits have been immunized for the preparation of specific antibodies.

VII. REFERENCES (*denotes review or book)

Barnea, A., and J. Gorski (1970). Estrogen-induced protein. Time course of synthesis. *Biochemistry*, 9, 1899–1904; also *J. Steroid Biochem.* (1975) 6, 459–461.

*Baulieu, E. E. (1975). Some aspects of the mechanism of action of steroid hormones. *Molec. Cell Boichem.*, 7, 157–174.

*Baulieu, E. E., A. Alberga, I. Jung, M. C. Lebeau, C. Mercier-Bodard, E. Milgrom, J. P. Raynaud, C. Raynaud-Jammet, H. Rochefort, H. Truong and P. Robel (1971). Metabolism and protein binding of sex steroids in target organs: An approach to the mechanism of hormone action. *Recent Progress in Horm. Res.*, 27, 351–412.

Baulieu, E. E., and J. P. Raynaud (1970). A 'proportional graph' method for measuring binding systems. *Eur. J. Biochem.*, 13, 293–304.

van Beurden-Lamers, W. M. O., A. O. Brinkmann, E. Mulder and H. J. van der Molen (1974). High affinity binding of estradiol by cytosols of different tissues in the male rat: Specific binding macromolecules in testis interstitial tissue, pituitary, adrenal, liver and sex accessory glands. *Biochem. J.*, 140, 495–502.

Brinkmann, A. O. (1972). Cellular uptake of steroids. *M.D. thesis.* Erasmus University, Rotterdam.

Bruckovsky, N., and J. D. Wilson (1968). The conversion of testosterone to 5α-androstan-17β-ol-3-one by rat prostate *in vivo* and *in vitro*. *J. Biol. Chem.*, 243, 2012–2021.

*Changeux, J. P. (1965). The control of biochemical reactions. *Sci Am.*, 212, 36–46.

Jacob, F., and F. Monod (1961). Genetic regulator mechanisms in the synthesis of proteins. *J. Mol. Biol.*, 3, 318–330.

*Jensen, E. V., and E. R. DeSombre (1972). Mechanism of action of the female sex hormones. *Ann. Review of Biochemistry*, 41, 203–230; also *J. Steroid Biochem.* (1975) 6, 469–474.

*Jensen, E. V., and H. I. Jacobson (1962). Basic guides to the mechanism of estrogen action. *Recent Progress in Horm. Res.*, 18, 387–414.

*King, R. J. B., and W. I. P. Mainwaring (1974). *Steroid-cell interactions.* Butterworth, London.

*McKerns, K. W. (Ed.) (1972). *The Sex Steroids-Molecular Mechanisms.* Pub. Appleton-Century-Crofts, Ed. Div. Meridith Corp., N.Y.

Mueller, G. C., B. Vonderhaar, U. H. Kim and M. Le Mahieu (1972). Estrogen action: an inroad to cell biology. *Recent Progress in Horm. Res.*, 28, 1–45.

O'Malley, B. W., G. C. Rosenfeld, J. P. Constock and A. R. Means (1972). Steroid hormone induction of a specific translatable messenger RNA. *Nature New Biology*, 240, 45–48.

*O'Malley, B. W., and A. R. Means (1974). Female steroid hormones and target cell nuclei. *Science*, 183, 610–620.

*Westphal, U. (1971). *Steroid-Protein Interactions.* Springer Verlag, Berlin, Heidelberg, New York.

*Wilson, J. D. (1972). Recent studies on the mechanism of action of testosterone. *New England J. of Medicine*, 287, 1284–1291.

CHAPTER 15

Mode of action of aldosterone

I. INTRODUCTION

The prime example of a mineralocorticoid hormone is aldosterone (Figure 4.7) secreted solely by the zona glomerulosa of the adrenal cortex (see Chapter 6). Other natural steroids showing mineralocorticoid activity are 11-deoxy-corticosterone and corticosterone, but, although they are produced by the adrenal in much greater quantities, they are respectively about thirty-fold and three-hundred-fold less active in this respect than aldosterone (Table 6.2). The action of corticosteroids on the metabolism of electrolytes is essentially to conserve Na^+ in the body and eliminate K^+. This effect is an overall result of the complex action of these hormones on many different tissues and organs and these vary widely with different cell types. The action of aldosterone on the Na^+-K^+ exchange process by the kidney has been discussed in Chapter 12.IX. However the kidney is very complex and it is only by the exploitation of simpler systems that an understanding of the mechanism of action of mineralocorticoids is emerging. Gaunt (1971) has provided an excellent general survey of the effect of corticosteroids on electrolyte and water metabolism and several comprehensive reviews on aldosterone mechanism of action have been written (Sharp and Leaf, 1966; Edelman, 1968; Edelman and Fimognari, 1968; Fanestil, 1969; Edelman and Fanestil, 1970; Fraser, 1971).

   The mineralocorticoids regulate salt transport across *epithelial structures*: the cells forming the outer layer of a mucous membrane. It is important at this point to distinguish between epithelial cells and other tissues which transport sodium ions. The sodium ion pump in skeletal muscle, red cells and brain neurons operates to evacuate the intracellular space of Na^+ and to accumulate K^+ — the effect is not to produce a net transport of salt, but to maintain the intracellular composition and osmotic pressure within the cell at an optimum level. Epithelial cells on the other hand – such as the cells which line the gut, the proximal and distal tubules of the kidney, the salivary glands and the sweat glands – are all specialized to carry out salt transport from one side of the cell to the other; all these cells respond to mineralocorticoids with the same kind of response – namely increased Na^+ transport from the various tubules or ducts back into the body. In this way aldosterone decreases Na^+ excretion by these epithelial cells.

II. THE TOAD BLADDER SYSTEM AND SHORT CIRCUIT CURRENT MEASUREMENTS

In mammals the mineralocorticoids exert their effect on sodium and potassium ion balance primarily at the level of tubular transport processes in the kidney. However, the difficulties of working with an organ as intricate as the mammalian kidney precluded any early development in our understanding of the biochemical mechanism of mineralocorticoid action. It was not until the introduction, by Ussing and Zerahn in 1951, of the short circuit current method of measuring active transport of ions across isolated tissues that it became possible to study the regulation of ion transport continuously and accurately in *in vitro* systems. Little progress was made until such an *in vitro* system was exploited using simple epithelial structures, such as that of the urinary bladder of the toad, *Bufo marinus*.

Toads in particular have to have an efficient water storage mechanism since they depend for their survival on maintaining their hydration, and, when necessary, they can reabsorb the water stored in their urinary bladder. Operating from the inside of the toad bladder, there is a constant pumping system for transporting sodium chloride from the urine into the sub-epithelial space where the salt is assimilated via capillaries and returned to the circulation. In addition to this salt conserving system in the bladder, there is another important salt conserving system in the skin. Both the skin and the urinary bladder systems show their effects on salt conservation under the influence of aldosterone, and a great deal of our present understanding of the aldosterone mechanism stems from studies using these tissues. Of course, important observations have also been made using other tissues, for example the rat kidney – although this organ has proved less amenable to study.

Early experiments using the isolated toad bladder and toad or frog skin showed stimulation of active sodium ion transport in the isolated system after addition of aldosterone directly to the bathing medium. Given this starting impetus both Edelman and Leaf independently developed the toad bladder system. The basic technique they employed was to place the tissue as a diaphragm between the ground glass surfaces of two tubes bent at right angles – a device known as the 'Ussing–Zerahn Chamber' (Figure 15.1). Each side of the hemi-bladder is bathed by a simple medium – one bathes the epithelial cells on the urine side of the bladder (the side that is actually involved in the transport of sodium ions), while the medium in the other tube bathes the serosal side of the bladder containing the blood vessels. Salt transport then occurs across the bladder diaphragm from the mucosal to the serosal side. As salt transport occurs, the *short circuit current* in the bladder tissue changes. Thus by measuring scc_t/scc_o (the ratio of the short circuit

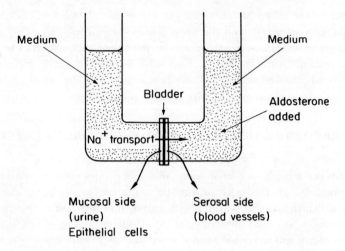

Figure 15.1 Chamber (Ussing and Zerahn, 1951) for measuring short circuit current (scc) in the isolated toad bladder. As sodium ion transport occurs, so the scc in the bladder tissue changes.

current at any time, t, to the short circuit current at time zero) a measure of the rate of active sodium transport may be obtained.

III. THE LATENT PERIOD IN THE ALDOSTERONE RESPONSE

Using these techniques a dynamic study of the aldosterone response was possible, and showed that when aldosterone was added to the medium on the serosal side of the bladder, then 60—90 minutes later there was a marked rise in active sodium ion transport. After this initial latent period, a linear increase in sodium ion transport over a period of about 6 hours was observed. This latent period of up to 90 minutes was not influenced by the concentration of aldosterone in the medium, and although at lower aldosterone concentrations the actual rate of sodium ion transport was ·lowered, the latent period remained the same. It follows that the delay in onset of the effect does not result from a slow rate of penetration of aldosterone to its site of action — but instead it suggested that aldosterone activates the synthesis of a substance involved in sodium ion transport. The 90 minute latent period is envisaged as the time involved in this process, and this has been likened to a biological clock set in motion by aldosterone.

A considerable body of evidence has accumulated over recent years to support the concept that aldosterone acts by stimulating the production of an intermediate, and that the latent period is the time required for its synthesis. Thus for example if the latent period is indeed the time required to synthesize an intermediate, there should be no relationship between the time course of tissue uptake of aldosterone and the time course of active sodium ion transport. It has been shown using the toad bladder system that there is in fact no such relationship (see Edelman, 1968).

After 30 minutes the uptake of [H^3]aldosterone was at the maximum level, whereas it was not until 90 minutes after the addition of aldosterone that any effect on sodium ion transport could be observed. There is, therefore, no diffusion delay in uptake of aldosterone into the system, and, regardless of how it penetrates the tissue, the actual quantity in the tissue does not seem decisive with regard to its time of action.

Subsequent experiments with the isolated toad bladder showed that aldosterone exhibited a trigger-like action (see Sharp and Leaf, 1966). Firstly, aldosterone was added to the medium, then at various times afterwards the medium was removed and the tissue washed with steroid-free medium. No significant effect was observed on either the duration of the latent period or the magnitude of the subsequent increase in sodium ion transport rate. From this it was concluded that the quantity of aldosterone which had to be present in the medium is not important once the process has been initiated. However, it is possible that washing the tissue with fresh medium does not remove all the aldosterone, and that it is the steroid left behind after washing that accounts for this continued response. It is likely that it is this aldosterone which is tightly bound to its receptor that accounts for this trigger-like action.

IV. NUCLEAR AND CYTOPLASMIC RECEPTORS FOR ALDOSTERONE

It became clear that one of the first problems to elucidate, if this concept was correct, was what was the initial receptor or binding site for aldosterone. Then it was necessary to establish whether this receptor has any specific role in the mechanism of action on sodium ion transport. Some of the first information that was obtained about the site of aldosterone binding came from high resolution radioautographs. These showed that [H^3]aldosterone in the isolated toad bladder was selectively localized in the nuclei and regions surrounding the nuclei of the mucosal, epithelial cells. These are the particular cells which have been shown by other studies to be responsible for active sodium ion transport in the toad bladder. In contrast [H^3]progesterone — a steroid which has no mineralocorticoid activity in the toad bladder system — was found to be evenly distributed throughout the cell, and showed no sign of being concentrated in the nucleus (see Edelman, 1968). Similarly, epithelial cell nuclei isolated from toad bladder were shown to have associated with them about 60% of the aldosterone binding capacity of the tissue (Ausiello and Sharp, 1968).

Unlike the isolated toad bladder, the intact animal of course metabolizes steroid hormones to physiologically inactive metabolites, and therefore localizing receptor sites for aldosterone in mammalian systems such as kidney presented an altogether more difficult problem. However, the difficulties have been circumvented (Fanestil, 1969) and following injection of [H^3]aldosterone into adrenalectomized rats, it was found that the radioactive aldosterone was associated very largely with the nuclear fraction rather than any other cell fraction prepared from the kidney.

The release of this bound aldosterone was accelerated only by proteolytic

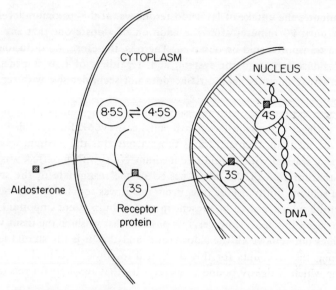

Figure 15.2   Overall scheme for the binding of aldosterone to the mineralocorticoid receptors of the kidney. The sedimentation constants are given in Svedburg units (S).

enzymes (e.g. pronase, chymotrypsin) and was unaffected by DN-ase, RN-ase, lipase, phospholipase or neuraminidase. These studies indicated that this receptor molecule is protein, located in or on the nuclei of epithelial cells.

Further progress was made (Herman *et al.*, 1968) following the isolation and characterization of aldosterone-binding proteins from both the cytosol and nuclear fractions of rat kidney cells. The receptor system is now understood to be considerably more complex than was originally envisaged and the nuclear binding system has itself been resolved into two different components: a 3S complex that can be solubilized and a 4S complex that is tightly bound to chromatin. A model has been constructed (Edelman, 1972) on the basis of studies with kidney slices and reconstituted cytosol and nuclear fractions that invokes a three-step hypothesis, and the scheme is depicted in Figure 15.2. This envisages aldosterone binding initially with a cytosol receptor (size 8.5S or 4.5S) to produce a cytosol complex which can then give rise to the 3 S soluble nuclear complex. This in turn results in the formation of the 4 S complex that is chromatin-bound. The detailed involvement of these different aldosterone receptors is still unclear but an up-to-date account of the evidence relating to the general binding mechanisms involved in aldosterone action is provided in the recent book by King and Mainwaring (1974).

V. STIMULATION OF RNA AND PROTEIN SYNTHESIS BY ALDOSTERONE

The next question that arises is how does the complex of aldosterone-protein regulate active Na^+ transport? From the prolific studies that have been undertaken

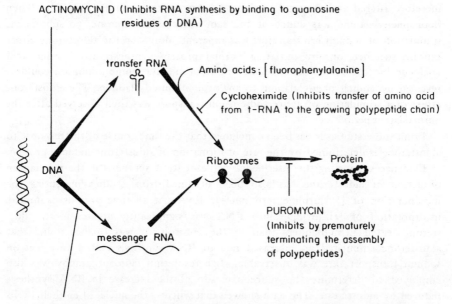

Figure 15.3   Protein and RNA synthesis and the effects of some inhibitors.

over the last few years, the short answer would appear to be that aldosterone induces protein synthesis at the level of DNA transcription, in a fashion similar to, and entirely in keeping with, that outlined for the action of estrogens, androgens and progesterone (see Chapter 14).

Antibiotic inhibitors of RNA synthesis such as actinomycin D and cordycepin were found to inhibit the stimulation of active transport by aldosterone (Fanestil, 1973). A similar inhibition of the hormonal response was found using inhibitors of protein synthesis such as puromycin and cycloheximide. All these inhibitors have their effect at different points on the pathway for protein biosynthesis (Figure 15.3), and moreover are effective in blocking the aldosterone response at concentrations of the inhibitor which have little or no effect on the basal sodium ion transport rate in aldosterone-depleted bladders. The importance of this lack of effect on the baseline sodium ion transport rate is that it indicates that these inhibitors are blocking the response to aldosterone in a specific fashion (such as inhibiting synthesis of a particular protein) rather than by some general toxic effect on the epithelial cells.

Further support for this concept of aldosterone inducing the synthesis of protein was lent by an elegant series of experiments by Edelman and coworkers involving the use of amino acid analogues, such as fluorophenylalanine and β-thienylserine. When these amino acid analogues are added normal protein synthesis continues uninterrupted, but the proteins synthesized contain for example fluorophenylalanine in place of phenylalanine (Figure 15.3). Their tertiary structure is therefore altered and they are not able to perform their normal functions. When fluorophenylalanine was added at the same time as aldosterone, no subsequent stimulation of sodium ion transport was apparent. Moreover, the aldosterone effect can be switched on, by initiating normal protein synthesis after amino acid analogue incorporation into protein. The fluorophenylalanine inhibition could be reversed by adding phenylalanine to analogue-inhibited bladders. The aldosterone effect of a stimulation of active sodium ion transport was then observed after the normal latent period.

From these studies it has been concluded that the time course of the response to aldosterone is determined by the rate of formation of aldosterone-induced protein.

Evidence supporting the intermediary role of RNA synthesis in the mechanism of action of aldosterone has also been obtained from studies measuring the incorporation of [H^3]uridine into nuclear RNA. At all time periods examined, incorporation of [H^3]uridine into RNA was significantly greater in the aldo-sterone-treated hemi-bladders than in the controls. It was further found that aldosterone stimulated an increased rate of RNA synthesis before an effect on sodium transport rate was observable. High resolution radioautography was also employed to determine the subcellular site of the increase in RNA synthesis induced by aldosterone. The data showed that whereas the nuclei of epithelial cells from control bladders were sporadically labelled with [H^3]uridine, those obtained from aldosterone-treated bladders were heavily labelled with [H^3]uridine. The evidence thus far supports the concept that aldosterone interacts with some nuclear receptor site to stimulate the rate of nuclear synthesis of some species of RNA (Fanestil, 1973). However, it is not yet clear whether this new RNA is messenger, transfer, ribosomal or some other undefined species of RNA.

Attempts to demonstrate the actual stimulation of the synthesis of a protein by aldosterone have not so far met with success. Numerous attempts to show an aldosterone-dependent increase in radioactive amino acid incorporation into protein have proved unsuccessful or at best are inconsistent and remain unreported. Clearly a new approach is needed in order to elucidate and characterize the imputed 'aldosterone-induced-protein'. Nevertheless, the data obtained by a variety of different laboratories all lend credence to the idea that aldosterone acts via induction of *de novo* protein synthesis, probably following direct involvement of nuclear RNA. The next question is how does the aldosterone-induced-protein(s) actually stimulate sodium ion transport?

VI. STIMULATION OF SODIUM ION TRANSPORT BY 'ALDOSTERONE-INDUCED-PROTEIN'

Currently three separate theories are proposed for the mechanism by which aldosterone-induced-protein stimulates active sodium transport (Figure 15.4). These theories implicate an effect of this protein either (*a*) on the ATP supply which provides the energy for the transport ATPase: '*the energy theory*', or (*b*) on the sodium ion pump itself which contains an ouabain-sensitive ATPase: '*the pump*

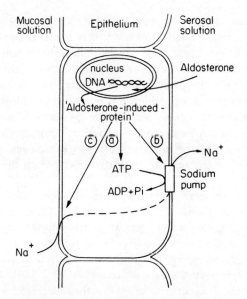

Figure 15.4 Alternative models of the aldosterone-stimulated sodium transport system in the epithelial cell; (*a*) the energy theory, (*b*) the sodium pump theory and (*c*) the permease theory.

theory' or (*c*) on a sodium permease which enhances entry of sodium ions into the epithelial cell from the mucosal side: '*the permease theory*'.

For both the 'energy theory' and the 'pump theory' the model (Figure 15.4) envisages the passive entry of sodium ions into the epithelial cell from the mucosal side (or urinary solution) coupled with active transport of the sodium ions from the intracellular to the serosal space. The energy source for the active transport step is believed to be ATP, and a Na^+-K^+-Mg^{2+} activated ATPase is considered to be the essential component of this sodium pump (Skou, 1965). It has been shown that aldosterone does not increase the activity or amount of this ATPase, and the evidence provided by Edelman and coworkers suggests that the most likely effect of the aldosterone-induced-protein is to increase the supply of ATP to the sodium ion pump (the energy theory).

Edelman and his colleagues have shown that the response to aldosterone is substrate dependent. Toad bladders pre-incubated for 15 hr are depleted of substrate and then show no response to aldosterone. However, when glucose or pyruvate was added to the medium bathing these substrate-depleted toad bladders 3 hr after the addition of aldosterone, an immediate increase in Na^+ transport was observed with no latent period. This immediate response to glucose or pyruvate implies that the aldosterone-induced-protein is synthesized during the period of substrate deficiency, but is only able to induce sodium ion transport in the presence of an appropriate substrate. After a survey of the various substrates capable of supporting aldosterone induced Na^+ transport, the conclusion has been that only precursors of oxaloacetate (e.g. glucose, pyruvate and lactate) and precursors of acetyl CoA (e.g. acetoacetate and β-hydroxybutyrate) are able to act synergistically with aldosterone – other Citric Acid Cycle intermediates were ineffective. An outline of the Citric Acid Cycle is shown in Figure 15.5 to clarify the involvement of the various substrates. Propionate, which is a precursor of succinyl CoA, does not support the stimulation of sodium ion transport by aldosterone and it was therefore suggested that the steps leading from succenate to malate are probably not involved in the aldosterone mechanism. Another important finding was that the aldosterone effect on sodium ion transport was completely dependent on an adequate O_2 supply, suggesting that oxidative metabolism mediates the steroid response.

From these data Edelman and coworkers have concluded that aldosterone stimulates a step in the Citric Acid Cycle somewhere between citrate condensing enzyme and α-oxoglutarate dehydrogenase. These studies together with those using inhibitors of the electron transport system, point to an action of aldosterone that either increases the rate of NADH production linked to conversion of citrate to α-oxoglutarate, or increases the rate of oxidation of NADH. In either case the results would be increased availability of ATP at the sodium ion pump site.

The 'pump theory' (Figure 15.4) received considerable support following the discovery that ouabain (noted for its inhibitory effect on the ATPase of the sodium ion pump) inhibited sodium ion transport in aldosterone-stimulated toad bladders considerably more than that in control bladders (Goodman et al., 1969). However it has been shown that, whereas ouabain did not inhibit the sodium ion transport of substrate-depleted bladders either in the presence or absence of aldosterone, ouabain on the other hand did inhibit (by about 20%) the sodium ion transport manifested by the aldosterone-treated bladders after they had been replenished with glucose (Fanestil, 1973). It therefore appears that the ouabain sensitivity of aldosterone-treated bladders is more likely to be associated with aldosterone involvement in the provision of energy by the cell rather than to an effect of the steroid at the level of the ouabain-sensitive ATPase of the sodium ion pump.

The 'energy and pump theories' are disputed by the proponents of the 'permease theory' (Sharp and Leaf, 1966). This group and that of Crabbé favour the concept that aldosterone-induced-protein functions to stimulate sodium ion transport by increasing sodium ion permeability at the mucosal side of the epithelial cell (see Figure 15.4). In this scheme aldosterone is believed to increase the amount of sodium ions with access to the pumping mechanism for which the sodium ion availability is envisaged as the controlling factor. The rate-limiting step for sodium ion transport is here seen as a barrier to the entry of sodium ions into the cell. In support of this view these workers have shown that the entry of sodium ions at the mucosal surface is the major determinant in the transport of sodium ions across the bladder. Removal of sodium ions from the mucosal medium was found to suppress all of the effects of aldosterone on epithelial cell metabolism, and suggested that the latter were secondary to entry of sodium ions into the cell via the mucosal surface. Amphotericin B is a polyene antibiotic that enhances entry of sodium ions into the cell through the limiting permeability barrier at the mucosal surface, and this

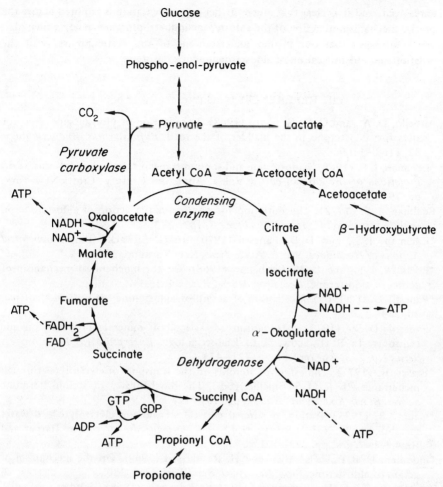

Figure 15.5 Summary of the Citric Acid Cycle and glycolytic pathway. The process of oxidative phosphorylation for the generation of ATP from reduced NAD^+ or FAD via the electron transport chain is indicated merely by the dotted lines.

antibiotic was found to stimulate sodium ion transport by the toad bladder in the absence of aldosterone. Moreover, just those same substrates (e.g. pyruvate and acetoacetate) that were found specifically to be effective in supporting the aldosterone response, were also effective in stimulating sodium ion transport after the addition of amphotericin B to the mucosal medium. As with aldosterone, the oxidation of these substrates was increased and these studies imply that these specific substrate effects are secondary to the entry of sodium ions into the tissue. Moreover, it has been suggested (Sharp and Leaf, 1966) that the substrate effects in enhancing sodium ion transport in the presence of aldosterone are secondary to an aldosterone-facilitated entry of sodium ions into the epithelial cell.

The controversy between the different schools of thought on this problem is still unresolved, and it is clear that much further experimentation is required before the precise mechanism of action of the aldosterone-induced-protein can be elucidated. It seems probable that our further understanding of this system must await the isolation and indentification of aldosterone-induced-protein.

VII. REFERENCES (*indicates review or book)

Ausiello, D. A., and G. W. G. Sharp (1968). Localization of physiological receptor sites for aldosterone in the bladder of the toad, *Bufo Marinus. Endocrinology*, 82, 1163—1169.

*Edelman, I. S. (1968). Aldosterone and sodium transport. In K. W. McKerns, (Ed.) *Functions of the adrenal cortex* Vol. 1. Appleton—Century—Crofts New York. pp. 79—133.

Edelman, I. S. (1972). The initiation mechanism in the action of aldosterone on sodium transport. *J. Steroid Biochem.*, 3, 167—172.

*Edelman, I. S., and D. D. Fanestil (1970). In G. Litwack, (Ed.) *Biochemical Actions of Hormones*, Vol. 1. Acad. Press, New York. pp. 324—331.

*Edelman, I. S., and G. M. Fimognari (1968). On the biochemical mechanism of action of aldosterone. *Rec. Prog. Horm. Res.*, 24, 1—44.

*Fanestil D. D. (1969). Mechanism of action of aldosterone. *Ann. Rev. Medicina*, 20, 223—232.

*Fanestil D. D. (1973). Mechanism of action of mineralocorticoids on ion transport. In R. O. Scow, (Ed.) Endocrinology. *Excerpta Med. Int. Congress Series No. 273*, Amsterdam. pp. 421—425.

*Fraser, R. (1971). The effect of steroids on the transport of electrolytes through membranes. In R. M. S. Smellie, (Ed.), The biochemistry of steroid hormone action. *Bioch. Soc. Symp. No. 32.* pp. 101—127.

*Gaunt, R. (1971). Action of adrenal cortical steroids on electrolyte and water metabolism. In N. P. Christy, (Ed.). *The human adrenal cortex*, Harper and Row, New York. pp. 273—301.

Goodman, D. B. P., J. E. Allen and H. Rasmussen (1969). On the mechanism of action of aldosterone. *Proc. Nat. Acad. Sci. (Wash.)*, 64, 330.

Herman, T. S., G. M. Fimognari and I. S. Edelman (1968). Studies on renal aldosterone-binding proteins. *J. Biol. Chem.*, 243, 3849—3856.

*King, R. J. B., and W. I. P. Mainwaring (1974). Mineralocorticoids. In *Steroid-Cell Interactions*. Butterworths, London. pp. 162—189.

Rousseau, G., and J. Crabbe (1972). Effects of aldosterone on RNA and protein synthesis in the toad bladder. *Eur. J. Biochem.*, 25, 550—559.

*Sharp, G. W. G., and A. Leaf (1966). Mechanism of action of aldosterone. *Physiological Reviews*, 46, 593—633.

Skou, J. D. (1965). Enzymic basis for active transport of Na^+ and K^+ across cell membrane. *Physical. Rev.*, 45, 596—617.

Ussing, H. H., and K. Zerahn (1951). Active transport of sodium as the source of electric current in the short-circuited isolated frog-skin. *Acta Physiol. Scand.*, 23, 110—127.

CHAPTER 16

Mode of action of glucocorticoids

I. METABOLIC EFFECTS OF GLUCOCORTICOIDS

The corticosteroid hormones elaborated by the adrenal cortex are essential for the maintenance of life. On the basis of survival tests with adrenalectomized animals, the mineralocorticoids (e.g. aldosterone) have the highest life maintenance potencies. Nevertheless, given an adequate salt diet and glucocorticoid therapy the adrenalectomized human can survive without mineralocorticoids.

The common, naturally occurring adrenal glucocorticoids are corticosterone, 11-deoxycorticosterone, cortisone and cortisol (also known as hydrocortisone), see Figure 6.4. In addition, several synthetic steroids have been produced with potent glucocorticoid activity and compounds such as dexamethasone, prednisolone and triamcinolone are widely used therapeutic agents (Figure 16.1). The relative biological activities of adrenocorticoids are given in Table 6.2.

Whereas the effects of mineralocorticoids are relatively straightforward being limited to effects on electrolyte balance (see Chapter 15), the actions of the glucocorticoids are much more diverse. A list of some of these metabolic effects are given in Table 16.1. From this it may be seen that the glucocorticoids affect a wide variety of metabolic events, including the regulation of carbohydrate, protein, nucleic acid and lipid metabolism. The first problem is to distinguish between those effects which occur as a direct result of the hormone action — i.e. *primary effects*,

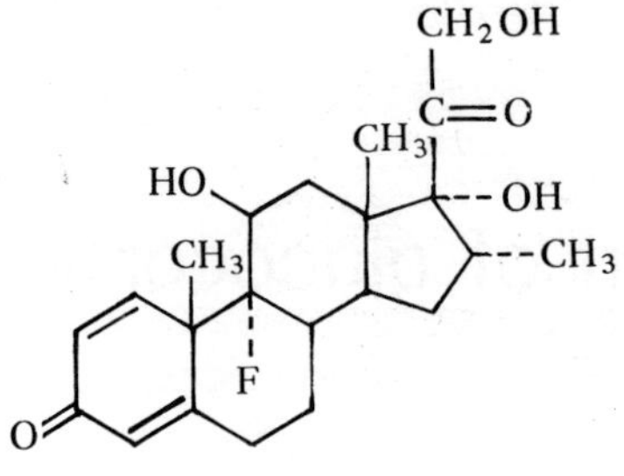

Dexamethasone
9α-Fluoro-16α-methylprednisolone

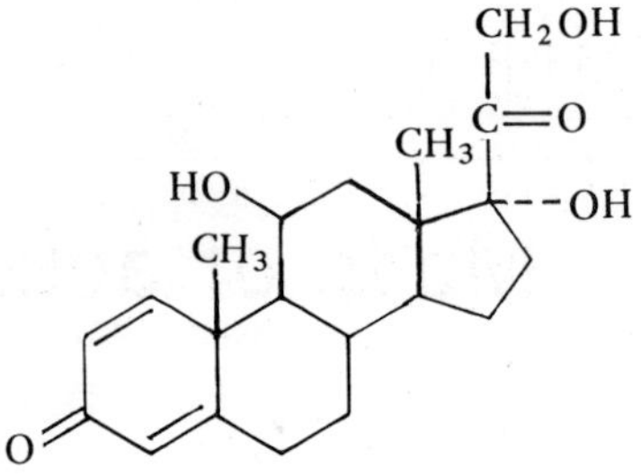

Prednisolone
1,2-Dehydrocortisol

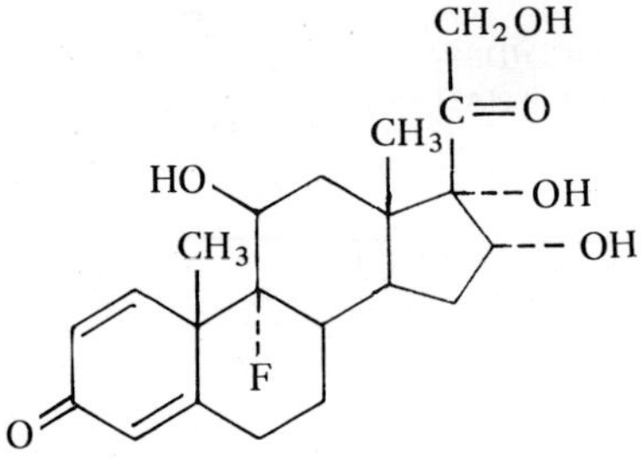

Triamcinolone
9α-Fluoro-16α-hydroxyprednisolone

Figure 16.1 Structures of synthetic steroids with potent gluco-corticoid activity. The structures of the common naturally occurring corticosteroids are shown in Figure 6.4.

and those effects which occur as a consequence of, and subsequent to, the primary effects and are in reality just *secondary effects.*

In the liver the primary effects (those which can be demonstrated in less than 2—4 hours) of the hormones may involve:

increased glycogen deposition
increased glucose production
increased uptake of aminoacids
increased synthesis of RNA and protein.

On the other hand, the increases in urea and ketone body production only became apparent at much later times after glucocorticoid administration, and almost certainly represent secondary changes that are not influenced directly by the hormones themselves. For example, increased urea production probably stems from an initial increase in the mobilization of amino acids to the liver, where the α-amino groups are then metabolized to urea. Similarly, the chronic increase in ketone bodies probably occurs as a secondary response following the increased mobilization of fat to the liver.

Table 16.1(a).
Metabolic Effects of Glucocorticoids

Effect	Time (hr)	
Liver		
Increased glycogen deposition	4—6	*in vivo*
Increased glucose production	2—6	*in vitro*
	2—6	*in vivo*
Increased amino acid uptake	2—4	*in vivo*
	1.5—2	*in vitro*
Increased RNA synthesis	2—4	*in vivo*
Increased protein synthesis	8—20	*in vivo*
Increased urea production	4—8	*in vivo*
Increased ketone body production	3—24	*in vivo*
Adipose Tissue		
Increased free fatty acid release	1—2	*in vitro*
Decreased glucose utilization	2—4	*in vitro*
Muscle		
Decreased glucose utilization	12—24	*in vivo*
Decreased protein synthesis and/or increased protein breakdown	2—4	*in vivo*
Lymphatic Tissue		
Decreased glucose utilization	2—4	*in vitro*
Decreased nucleic acid synthesis	2—4	*in vivo*
Decreased protein synthesis and/or increased protein breakdown	2—4	*in vivo*

Table 16.1(b)
Hepatic Enzyme Activities Increased by Glucocorticoids

Enzyme	Activity (% of control)	Time of Induction
Glycolytic enzymes		
Glycogen synthetase	130	4 days
Glucose-6-phosphatase	270	3—4 days
Fructose-1,6-diphosphatase	270	3—6 days
Phosphohexoisomerase	200	4—6 days
Aldolase	240	4—6 days
Phosphoglyceraldehyde dehydrogenase	180	4—8 hr
Phosphoenolpyruvate carboxykinase	300	3—5 days
Pyruvate carboxylase	250	6 hr
Amino acid metabolizing enzymes		
Alanine aminotransferase	1000	4—7 days
Tyrosine aminotransferase	800	5—12 hr
Tryptophan pyrrolase	600	3—5 hr
Threonine dehydrase	130	2 days
Urea cycle		
Arginine synthetase system	170	3—4 days
Argino succinase	150	3—4 days
Arginase	170	2—3 days

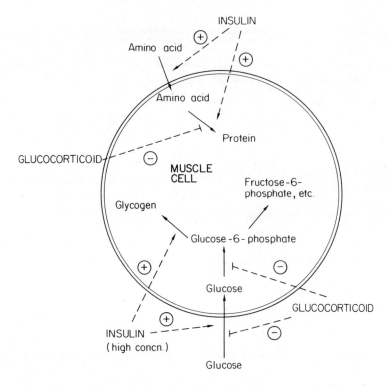

Figure 16.2 Effects of glucocorticoids and insulin on muscle cell metabolism. Stimulatory effects $-\underset{\oplus}{=}-\rightarrow$; Inhibitory effects $-\underset{\ominus}{=}-|$.

In extrahepatic tissues such as muscle and lymphatic tissue, it appears that following glucocorticoid injection *in vivo* there is a decreased incorporation of amino acid into protein. Whether this decrease in protein synthesis may be attributed to an increased breakdown of protein is debatable; however, there is little doubt that glucocorticoids do influence the metabolism of peripheral proteins at some point. The net effect is believed to be the redistribution of amino acids from muscle and other peripheral tissues to the liver. The metabolic effects of glucocorticoids (and their antagonism of the effects of insulin) on muscle are depicted in Figure 16.2.

In adipose tissue, muscle, skin and lymphatic and connective tissue, the glucocorticoids inhibit glucose utilization. However, these effects are not observed in the presence of insulin, and in the intact animal with normal insulin reserves, these effects of glucocorticoids on glucose utilization are difficult to demonstrate. In general, many of the metabolic effects of glucocorticoids are opposed by insulin (Table 16.2). Glucocorticoids can produce diabetes, while insulin prevents it; similarly the diabetes induced by the lack of insulin is counteracted by adrenalectomy or the absence of glucocorticoids. However, in higher organisms (particularly in man) the regulatory effects of glucocorticoids on the metabolism of carbohydrates are considered to be relatively less important than those of insulin.

Table 16.2.
Antagonistic effects of glucocorticoids and insulin

Glucocorticoids	Insulin
Inhibit glucose utilization	Increases glucose utilization
Promote lipid mobilization	Prevents lipid mobilization
Stimulate synthesis of specific liver enzymes	Inhibits synthesis of these liver enzymes.
Decrease protein synthesis in tissues other than liver	Stimulates protein synthesis in extrahepatic tissues.
Increase protein synthesis in liver	Decreases hepatic protein synthesis.

Although the presence of glucocorticoids is required for the normal mobilization of fuel reserves, the role of the glucocorticoids in this respect is now seen as a 'permissive' one and variations in their circulatory levels exert only marginal effects on carbohydrate homeostasis, with insulin playing the dominant role. In species lower down the evolutionary ladder however — especially in fish — the glucocorticoids are much more important in regulating metabolic processes. Cahill (1971) has provided a comprehensive review of the effects of adrenal corticosteroids on carbohydrate metabolism and the way in which insulin modulates these effects.

Homeostasis in the whole animal is maintained by counter-balancing these two hormones, and removal of either results in an increased sensitivity to the other. The present evidence suggests that insulin exerts its effect on steroid-induced gluconeogenesis, at least in part, by suppressing the biosynthesis of several key gluconeogenic liver enzymes. This concept of the antagonism between glucocorticoid induction and insulin suppression of the hepatic gluconeogenic system is outlined in Figure 16.3.

The mobilization of lipid is another important metabolic effect of the glucocorticoids, and this topic has been reviewed by Rudman and Girolamo (1971). In the adrenalectomized animal there is an obvious decrease in fat utilization and an increase in body lipid. However, several different hormones may be involved in this effect. For example, adrenalin (also known as epinephrine, Figure 16.6) is secreted by the adrenal medulla and is also a lipolytic hormone (Exton et al., 1972). It appears, therefore, that an intact adrenal is important for more than one reason in the mobilization of lipid from adipose tissue.

The hormonal regulation of adipose tissue metabolism is outlined in Figure 16.4. In the fat cell, glucocorticoids oppose the glucose uptake which is enhanced by physiologically high concentrations of insulin. This glucose is used primarily for lipid synthesis. Lipolytic agents such as adrenalin and noradrenalin stimulate membrane-bound adenylate cyclase and generate intracellular cyclic AMP, which is then believed to stimulate lipolysis. Insulin lowers the intracellular level of cyclic AMP, possibly by enhancing its breakdown by phosphodiesterase. The glucocorticoid appears to function in a permissive fashion in that it is required for the activation by cyclic AMP of the triglyceride lipase.

The complex interplay between hormones in the regulation of metabolic systems may be exemplified by the various control mechanisms involved in gluconeogenesis

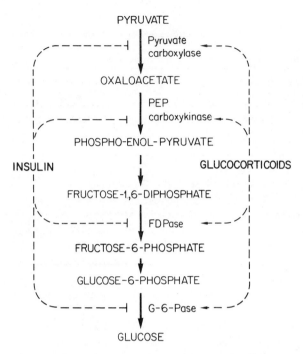

PYRUVATE

Figure 16.3 Antagonistic effects of glucocorticoids and insulin on hepatic gluconeogenic enzymes (for further details see Weber, 1968). biosynthetic pathway ⟶ ; inhibitory effect − − −⊢; stimulatory effect ⟵ − − −.

(see Exton *et al.*, 1970). In an attempt to summarize these, the scheme depicted in Figure 16.5 has been proposed to portray the processes regulating gluconeogenesis. The maintenance of a constant blood sugar concentration is here conceived as the central coordinating mechanism of hormonal control in response to a fall in blood sugar concentration, the pancreatic α-cells release glucagon and the adrenal medulla releases adrenalin. Glucagon, and to a lesser extent adrenalin, stimulate the breakdown of liver glycogen by activating liver phosphorylase, and thus tend to correct the fall in blood sugar concentration. Another effect of these two hormones is to activate lipases, thereby liberating free fatty acids and glycerol. These free fatty acids can function as inhibitors of a variety of enzymes essential to the process of glucose catabolism in the liver, while those enzymes involved in glucose synthesis from pyruvate or oxaloacetate remain unaffected. The glycerol may be utilized as a precursor of the glucose skeleton. Again, the result of this effect on lipase is to enhance glucose production. A further action of adrenalin is to bring about indirectly the release of ACTH from the pituitary, with the consequent stimulation of glucocorticoid synthesis by the adrenal (Chapter 11).

These glucocorticoid effects can be summarized as follows:

(*a*) Glucocorticoids act on peripheral tissues such as muscle and lymphoid tissue to release free amino acids, possibly by inhibiting protein synthesis in

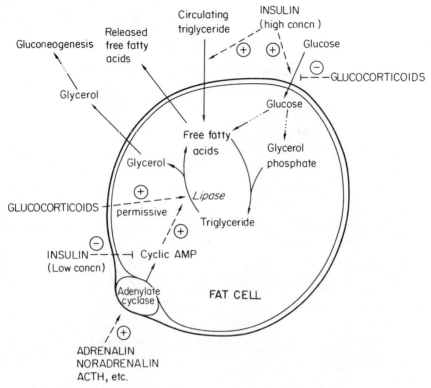

Figure 16.4 Effects of glucocorticoids and insulin on fat cell metabolism. Stimulatory effects — ⊕ — a; Inhibitory effects — ⊖ —|; Metabolic pathways — ··· →.

these tissues. The amino acids are transported in the plasma to the liver where aminotransferases and other enzymes convert them to keto acids such as pyruvate, oxaloacetate or α-oxoglutarate. These keto acids may be converted to oxaloacetate and thence to glucose via phosphoenolpyruvate. This process utilizes the capacity of existent enzymic systems for gluconeogenesis.

(*b*) Glucocorticoids have a lipolytic effect on adipose tissue releasing both glycerol, a precursor of glucose carbon, and free fatty acids which inhibit key enzymes involved in hepatic glucose catabolism (Weber *et al.*, 1966). Thus, gluconeogenesis is encouraged at the expense of glucose breakdown and utilization.

(*c*) The activities of a variety of liver enzymes involved in gluconeogenesis and aminotransfer are increased in response to glucocorticoids (see Table 16.1) thereby enlarging the hepatic capacity for gluconeogenesis.

II. ACTIONS OF GLUCOCORTICOIDS OTHER THAN THOSE ON METABOLISM

The effects of glucocorticoids on the metabolism of carbohydrate, fat and protein are of obvious fundamental importance in any discussion of the mechanism of

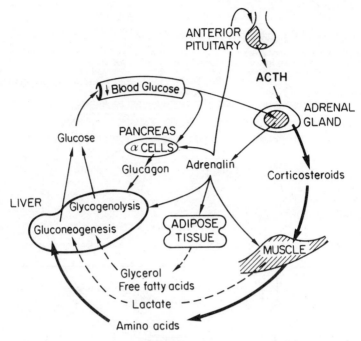

Figure 16.5 A simplified scheme for the processes of gluconeogenesis which shows the physiological processes involved in the maintenance of blood sugar homeostasis. For further details see Weber (1968).

action of the steroid hormones. Nevertheless, these are by no means their only actions.

Other actions of glucocorticoids that are of importance include the following (for a comprehensive review of these effects see David *et al.*, 1970):

A. Anti-inflammatory effect

Glucocorticoids exert a suppressive effect on inflammatory reactions. The inflammatory reaction is a local response to any tissue injury such as infection, allergy or trauma. The tissue swells with fluid and becomes red, hot and painful and this response involves the dilation of blood vessels and the migration of leucocytes from the blood stream to the site of tissue injury. The leucocytes (normally about 5 million cells/ml of blood) comprise a mixture of cells, the majority of which are neutrophils — so-called because their cytoplasmic granules remain unstained by basic or acidic dyes. These cells make up most of the cellular material in the inflammatory exudate that enters the tissue spaces through the capillary walls. Other important components of this exudate or pus are plasma proteins, inorganic salts and water. The neutrophils act as scavengers by enveloping invading bacteria or damaged tissue cells and digest them with the aid of lysosomal enzymes.

Inflammation develops from all types of injury and this includes not only local reactions as in a wound, but also more general allergic responses such as in hay-fever

Adrenalin
(epinephrine)

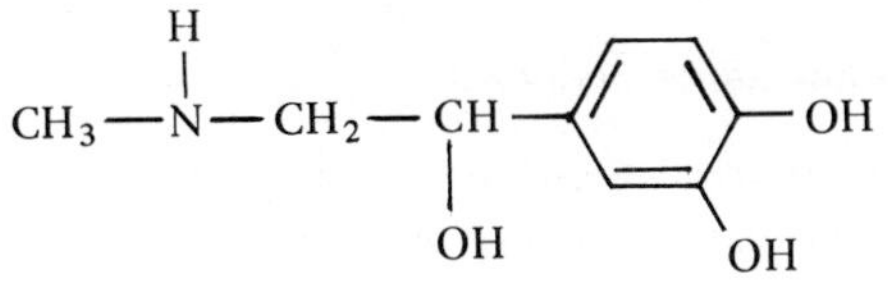

$$CH_3-\overset{\overset{\textstyle H}{|}}{N}-CH_2-\underset{\underset{\textstyle OH}{|}}{CH}-\text{(benzene ring)}-OH \quad OH$$

Histamine $\quad NH_2-CH_2-CH_2-\text{(imidazole ring)} \quad H-N \quad N$

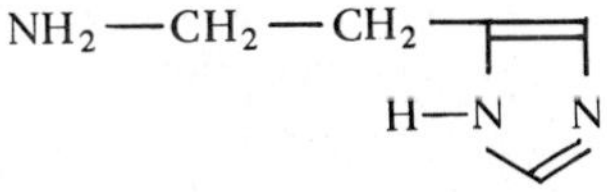

5-Hydroxytryptamine
(serotonin) $\quad NH_2-CH_2-CH_2-\text{(indole ring)}-OH$

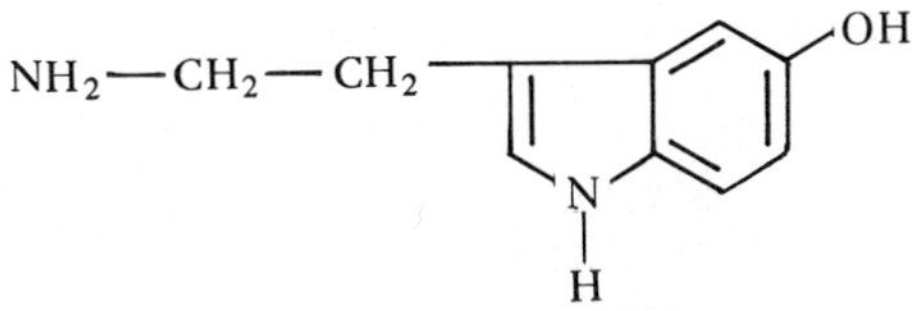

Figure 16.6 Amino acid derivatives of biological importance in relation to the action of glucocorticoids.

and asthma and auto-immune processes like rheumatoid arthritis. Allergic reactions, e.g. anaphalaxis or hypersensitivity (see Gell and Coombs, 1968), are believed to be due to the formation of a special kind of antibody. Unlike normal antibodies, these particular antibodies do not remain in the blood stream to be bound by the antigen that originally gave rise to them. Instead, they bind to mast cells which occur amongst fat cells, around blood vessels and in other loose connective tissues. Mast (or 'food-supplying') cells were designated thus by Ehrlich and their origin remains obscure; they are reportedly the prime source of histamine in the body. When mast cells which already have antibody bound to them (i.e. sensitized cells) are subjected to another dose of antigen, they respond with release of histamine. Serotonin is similarly released by the mast cells of some species. It is this histamine and other related compounds (Figure 16.6) that in asthma patients causes the contraction of smooth muscle surrounding the bronchial tubes and the consequent breathing difficulties. Histamine also increases the permeability and dilation of the capillary system. Both histamine and serotonin are known to be directly involved in the inflammatory response and to increase the permeability of small blood vessels to plasma proteins and fluid.

The precise action of glucocorticoids in suppressing these inflammatory and allergic responses is unknown, but they have been implicated at a variety of different sites. The glucocorticoids increase capillary resistance and oppose the vasodilatory action of histamine. Moreover, the liberation of histamine from the mast cells, in response to the original antigen, is inhibited – the mast cells themselves undergoing marked changes in their shape and internal structure following glucocorticoid treatment. Allergic responses such as those in asthma, hay fever and some food allergies may be greatly alleviated by the use of corticosteroids, nevertheless the mechanism is poorly understood.

B. Decreased resistance to infection

This effect may be observed following glucocorticoid therapy and is clearly linked to the anti-inflammatory effect. Diminished permeability of blood vessels with consequent limitations on leucocyte migration to the site of tissue injury has obvious consequences on the body's ability to deal with invading bacteria. In addition to this, however, there is some evidence that there may be steroid-induced changes in the intracellular ability of the neutrophils to destroy ingested micro-organisms.

C. Suppression of lymphoid function

Lymphocytes arise in the bone marrow and are found in lymphatic tissues such as the blood, spleen, lymph glands, thymus and in loose connective tissue. In lymphatic tissue, lymphocytes give rise to effector cells which either produce antibodies in response to antigens or reject transplants. The glucocorticoids rapidly inhibit protein synthesis in lymphatic tissue (Table 16.1) with the consequent liberation of protein in the form of free amino acids. The overall effect is decreased antibody formation and prolonged transplant survival with a suppression of lymphoid function. Evidence has been presented using lymphocyte cells *in vitro* (Markman *et al.*, 1967) that glucocorticoids may inhibit the transport of glucose and of precursors of protein and RNA into these cells. They may also act within the nucleus at the transcriptional level of protein synthesis, as discussed below.

III. INTRACELLULAR GLUCOCORTICOID-RECEPTOR PROTEINS

The diversity of action of glucocorticoids on different cell types, in for example stimulating the synthesis of proteins and nucleic acids in some cells while enhancing their breakdown in others, has necessitated the development of many different experimental systems for studying their mechanism of action. The properties of each system have demanded the use of techniques peculiar to that system, and have restricted the development of any unified approach in these studies. The systems which have yielded the most information include: liver, hepatoma tissue culture cells (HTC cells), fibroblasts, HeLa cells, lymphocytes and lymphoid tumours. A comprehensive survey of the use of these different cell types in studies on the intracellular binding of glucocorticoids has been published (King and Mainwaring, 1974), to which the reader is recommended for further details.

Overall, it is particularly striking that, for the binding of glucocorticoids, the observations and conclusions derived from the wide variety of different systems used are remarkably similar. The steroid enters the cell, and in each and every cell that exhibits a response to glucocorticoids, these steroids are bound specifically and with a high affinity — initially to a cytoplasmic receptor. Subsequent transfer of the steroid-receptor complex to the nucleus is a temperature-sensitive process and the complex undergoes a change in shape before combination with the nuclear chromatin. Baxter *et al.*, (1972) have provided convincing evidence that the steroid-receptor complex binds to the nuclear DNA rather than to proteins associated with the DNA. However, recent work with the estrogen receptor suggests that it binds to both DNA and non-histone protein. As to the nature of the different glucocorticoid receptors, their purification is currently being pursued in several laboratories and they appear to be rather acidic, cysteine-containing proteins.

A. Liver

The rapid effects of glucocorticoids on the liver in stimulating gluconeogenesis, and in increasing the activity of several enzymes involved in this process, such as tyrosine aminotransferase and tryptophan pyrrolase (Table 16.1), made this tissue an early candidate for studies in this field. However, the search for glucocorticoid receptors in the liver has been severely hampered by two problems peculiar to the liver system. Both the prolific metabolism of steroids by the liver (as described in Chapter 10) and the presence in liver of serum binding proteins such as albumin and transcortin (CBG), either as proteins synthesised endogenously or as contaminants from the large amounts of blood in this tissue, have made progress in the study of specific glucocorticoid receptors in the liver difficult.

Several workers have however reported the isolation of corticosteroid binding proteins from the cytoplasm of the liver cell, although the characteristics of these proteins differ widely in these different reports. After administration of $[^3H]$-cortisol *in vivo*, maximum radioactivity was found in liver about 20 minutes later, with over half of the radioactivity in the cytoplasmic fraction and less than 0.5% in the nuclei. Litwack and coworkers (1973) have isolated several glucocorticoid binding-proteins from rat liver cytoplasm, but only one of these proteins behaved in a manner consistent with it being a specific receptor. The other proteins isolated by these workers bind a large number of different molecules, including metabolites of the glucocorticoids, and therefore lack the specificity required of a receptor molecule. Similar studies (Feldman *et al.*, 1972) have demonstrated the presence of a protein in rat kidney which binds corticosterone specifically and with high affinity.

At the present time, no clear-cut evidence exists for the existence of nuclear glucocorticoid receptors in the liver.

B. Hepatoma tissue culture (HTC) cells

A stable line of hepatoma cells has been cultured that respond specifically to glucocorticoids by the induction of tyrosine aminotransferase. Tomkins and his colleagues have utilized these cells and $[^3H]$dexamethasone as an exemplary glucocorticoid in an important series of studies that have greatly enhanced our understanding of the mechanism of glucocorticoid action.

The advantages of this system as a model for steroid hormone action are that this response to glucocorticoids is relatively specific, affecting only a few cellular processes, and for dexamethasone and cortisol does not involve prior metabolism of the inducing steroid.

In early studies it was shown that there was a definite lag-period in the induction of tyrosine aminotransferase and that this induction was reversible by removal of the glucocorticoid from the culture medium. Moreover, it was found that other steroids inhibited the inductive effect of glucocorticoids, but were themselves inactive in inducing the enzyme. These studies implicated competition between these other steroids and the active glucocorticoids for specific binding sites within the cells. When cells cultured in the absence of glucocorticoid were fractionated, the receptors were localized only in the cytoplasmic fraction, but when whole cells were incubated with glucocorticoids it was found that the nucleus contained most of the specifically bound steroid. Moreover isolated nuclei were found specifically to bind glucocorticoids after addition of complexes of glucocorticoid—cytoplasmic receptor proteins. In further studies, Rousseau et al., (1973) have demonstrated that, following the binding of glucocorticoids, there is depletion of cytoplasmic receptors and associated with the concomitant nuclear binding of an equivalent number of steroid molecules. Furthermore, removal of the inducing steroid from the incubation medium brought about the dissociation of glucocorticoid from the nucleus and the return to normal levels of cytoplasmic receptor. Since these effects occurred even when protein and RNA synthesis were inhibited they are not attributable to destruction and synthesis of receptors. These findings strongly suggest that the nuclear binding of glucocorticoids is a result of the association of the steroid-cytoplasmic receptor complex itself with the nucleus, and that the receptor is unlikely to function merely as a carrier for the intracellular translocation of steroid.

A temperature-dependent two-step mechanism for estrogen action in the uterus has been proposed (see Chapter 14) whereby the cytoplasmic binding of estradiol is followed by a temperature-dependent change in the cytoplasmic receptor and the subsequent association of the receptor-complex with the nucleus. The experimental findings using the hepatoma cell support a similar sequence of events for the binding of glucocorticoids (Higgins et al., 1973). These workers have proposed a

Table 16.3.

Binding of corticosteroids to the cytoplasmic receptor of HTC cells. The characteristics of binding for each [^{3}H] steroid were calculated following a Scatchard plot (see Chapter 14) of the data. The steroids are given in order of their inductive abilities for tyrosine aminotransferase: the more active the inducer then the higher the binding affinity (i.e. the lower the K_D), whereas the number of potential binding sites remained constant (for further details see Rousseau et al., 1972, J. Mol. Biol., 67, 99).

Corticoid	Dissociation Constant (K_D; moles/litre)	Receptor site concentration (picomole/mg protein)
Dexamethasone	0.31×10^{-8}	0.66
Corticosterone	0.43×10^{-8}	0.65
Cortisol	1.10×10^{-8}	0.63
Aldosterone	2.50×10^{-8}	0.67

model in which the receptor is envisaged as an allosteric regulatory protein under the control of glucocorticoids and directly involved in the action of the hormone. The following early events are suggested: (a) glucocorticoid enters the cell and binds specifically, with a dissociation constant of about 10^{-8} M (Table 16.3), to a cytoplasmic receptor protein (size 6—8S, reduced to 4S in 0.5 M KCl); (b) the steroid-receptor complex is activated (by a process which at $0°C$ is rate-limiting); and (c) the activated steroid-receptor complex binds to a DNA-containing component of the nucleus in an interaction that eventually results in enzyme induction.

C. Fibroblasts

Glucocorticoids in low concentration inhibit the growth rate of mouse fibroblasts (e.g. L929 cells) and in such cells the most rapid observable effect of these steroids is the impairment of glucose uptake. Radioactive triamcinolone (Figure 16.1) — a particularly active glucocorticoid — has been used for studies on this system since it is not actively transported out of these cells, as are other glucocorticoids.

Studies by Aronow and Pratt and their colleagues have shown that in these cells two types of glucocorticoid binding sites are observable — one of high affinity that is saturated by about 1×10^{-8} M triamcinolone, and the other of low affinity but high capactiy that remains unsaturated even at 2×10^{-6} M. Only the high affinity receptor had the characteristics of a glucocorticoid receptor; thus the ability of different concentrations of active glucocorticoids to displace bond [3H]triamcinolone exactly paralleled their growth inhibitory capabilities in L929 cells.

The cytoplasmic receptor of L929 cells has been purified (Hackney and Pratt, 1971) and found to be a weakly acidic protein with a sedimentation coefficient of 5.5S. Despite the fact that studies in this system have focussed on the cytoplasmic receptor, it is clear that future developments in this area utilizing glucocorticoid-resistant L929 cells as well as cell-free preparations and isolated nuclei will yield valuable information on the mechanism of glucocorticoid action.

D. HeLa cells

Some sublines of HeLa cells have proved particularly useful in studies on glucocorticoid action. In these sublines the activity of enzymes such as alkaline phosphatase, ATPases and 5'-nucleotidase can be stimulated by certain glucocorticoids. Thus cortisol and prednisolone (Figure 16.1) induce alkaline phosphatase activity in HeLa 65 cells, and both Cox (1971) and Melnykovych and Bishop (1971) have employed this system for glucocorticoid binding studies.

Although at a somewhat less advanced stage, studies utilizing this experimental system have demonstrated that the glucocortical binding characteristics are similar to those obtained in other systems. The specific binding of glucocorticoids has been demonstrated in both the cytoplasmic and nuclear fractions of HeLa 65 cells. Binding was found to occur predominantly in the cytoplasmic fraction after incubating cells with cortisol at 4°C. However at 37°C the major binding site was localized in the nuclear fraction. Only inducers of alkaline phosphatase (or antagonists of this induction) have been found to exhibit competition with cortisol for these binding sites, thereby indicating the specificity of this glucocorticoid binding. Further details as to the size and nature of these receptors remain to be determined.

E. Lymphocytes and lymphoid tumours

In earlier sections of this chapter, the anti-inflammatory action of glucocorticoids and the selective destruction of lymphoid tissue by these steroids have been outlined. In several glucocorticoid-sensitive tissues (such as fat cells, skin and thymus gland), it has been shown that these steroids inhibit glucose uptake. The thymus gland in particular has been extensively used as a source of gluco-corticoid-sensitive lymphocytes, (Turnell *et al.*, 1974) which offer the advantage of very limited metabolism of glucocorticoids. It has been demonstrated that the effects on glucose uptake in these cells are steroid-specific and occur prior to major observable effects on RNA or DNA synthesis.

Besides their destructive action on normal lymphocytes, glucocorticoids also have a cytolytic effect on several malignant tumour cells derived from lymphoid tissues, and these have also provided useful systems for investigations into glucocorticoid action. In particular, the contrasting effects of these steroids on different sublines of these lymphoid tumours (e.g. glucocorticoid-insensitive sublines) have provided valuable comparative data. Inhibition of glucose uptake slows the growth of the cells and ultimately kills them. This feature is utilized in the selection of steroid resistant sublines.

A series of steroid sensitive and resistant sublines from mouse lymphoma has been developed in a number of laboratories. The cell clones were selected for their growth characteristics, maintained in continuous culture, and glucocorticoid sensitive and insensitive sublines established. The former are unable to survive in the presence of 10^{-8}M cortisol, whereas even in the presence of up to about one thousand-fold higher concentrations of cortisol, the growth of the latter sublines is unimpeded.

The glucocorticoid resistance of particular lymphoma tumour cells has been convincingly explained in terms of the absence or ineffectiveness of receptor proteins (Rosenau *et al.*, 1972). This explanation cannot hold generally. Some cells are able to grow in the presence of glucocorticoid even though they contain glucocorticoid receptors. Certain mouse myeloma cells (for which dexamethasone is cytolytic) have been fused with mouse lymphoma cells (not sensitive to dexamethasone) using the technique of cell hybridization developed by Harris and coworkers, and from the product of the fusion two different hybrid clones were grown up. These were tested for sensitivity and both were killed by glucocorticoids (Gehring *et al.*, 1972). The interesting facet of this work is that both parent cells contain specific glucocorticoid receptors as determined by [^{3}H]dexamethasone binding, and this implies that it is not only through the absence of specific glucocorticoid-receptors that these tumour cells can exhibit glucocorticoid insensitivity. It is clear that, for the hybrid myeloma—lymphoma cells, the glucocorticoid-resistance of the parent cell is due to a 'missing link' somewhere along the hormonal response system, other than at the level of the receptor concentration. In these hybrid cells, this 'missing link' is in some way overcome and the glucocorticoid-sensitivity is again apparent. From these observations it is evident that the hormonal insensitivity of tumour cells may have a variety of underlying causes, of which the presence or absence of functional receptor proteins may be but one aspect.

The studies on lymphocytes have been reviewed recently by King and Mainwaring (1974) who have detailed the important binding studies of Munck and his colleagues and the thermodynamic approach pioneered by Schaumberg and coworkers. Definitive evidence has been provided by these investigators for the specific high-affinity binding of glucocorticoids in lymphocytes. In keeping with the mechanism pertaining in other systems, the binding of glucocorticoids is held to occur via a two-stage process. A glucocorticoid complex is formed initially with a cytoplasmic receptor which undergoes a temperature-dependent change followed by translocation of the entire complex to the nucleus. Moreover the specific mechanism observed for glucocorticoid binding in lymphocytes of thymus gland origin has been shown to be similar to that in lymphocytes derived from other sources. The presence of high affinity receptors in different populations of lymphocytes is shown in Table 16.4.

F. Other systems

The mammary gland, brain tissue, cultures of chick embryo retina and foetal lung have also been developed as useful systems for studying the glucocorticoid mechanism. For further details consult King and Mainwaring (1974).

Table 16.4.
Distribution of high affinity glucocorticoid receptors in blood cells originating from different tissues (for further details see Schaumburg and Crone, 1971).

Cell Type	Tissue of origin	Dissociation constant for corticosterone (M)	Number of receptor sites (p moles per mg protein)
Lymphocytes	Thymus gland (rat)	1.7×10^{-8}	148
	Thymus gland (chicken)	1.4×10^{-8}	47
	Bursa of Fabricius (chicken)	1.6×10^{-8}	52
	Peripheral blood (chicken)	1.5×10^{-8}	58
	Peripheral blood after removal of thrombocytes (chicken)	1.2×10^{-8}	107
Erythrocytes	Peripheral blood (chicken)	1.8×10^{-8}	2
	Peripheral blood (sheep)	not measurable	< 1

IV. MOLECULAR PROCESSES FOLLOWING STEROID-RECEPTOR INTERACTION IN THE NUCLEUS

Data from a wide variety of different systems have now accumulated to support the concept that glucocorticoids act via a stimulation of nuclear RNA synthesis and an increase in the rate of production of particular cellular proteins. Although the subtleties and intimate details of this process are far from clear, nevertheless the general mechanism proposed is similar to that envisaged for the estrogens, androgens and progesterone (see Chapter 14).

The result of glucocorticoid action is to induce the synthesis of enzymes or other proteins. It is by means of some of these newly-synthesized proteins that the destructive effect of the glucocorticoids occurs in cells where these steroids act in a catabolic manner. However, regardless of whether a particular cell-type responds in an anabolic or a catabolic fashion, a consistent uniformity in the processes for the initial interaction at the cell nucleus (via steroid-receptor: chromatin complexes) has been observed in different cell systems. The nuclear binding of the glucocorticoids is one of the first observable phenomena in each system, and there is always a subsequent delay in the hormonal response, during which period inhibitors of protein and RNA synthesis are invariably effective in suppressing the response.

In the liver, the stimulation by glucocorticoids of tyrosine aminotransferase and tryptophan pyrrolase activity is preceded by a marked increase in the appearance of various RNA species and, in particular, by the transfer of some RNA sequences derived from heterogeneous nuclear RNA (also termed messenger-like RNA and DNA-like RNA) to the cytoplasm. Moreover, an early effect on the activation of nuclear RNA polymerase has been found (Yu and Feigelsen, 1971), and studies on solubilized preparations of liver RNA polymerase (Sajdel and Jacobs, 1971) have demonstrated in particular a stimulation of the nucleolar form of the enzyme — RNA polymerase A (also termed RNA polymerase I). Since the nucleolus is the site of ribosome synthesis, an early effect of glucocorticoids on the synthesis of precursors of ribosomal RNA is evident. However, the mechanism for this activation of liver RNA polymerase remains unknown and the liver system in particular is bewilderingly complex. A wide variety of agents can stimulate tyrosine aminotransferase activity: NH_4^+ ions, various L- and D-amino acids, insulin, glucagon, cyclic AMP and adrenalin can all stimulate the synthesis of this enzyme in liver and clearly it is not under the unique control of the glucocorticoids. For a further understanding of the mechanism, it is essential to resort to simpler models.

As indicated previously, tissue culture systems such as HTC and HeLa cells provide exceptionally informative systems, in which glucocorticoids effect the sythesis of only a few, well-characterized proteins. From their studies using HTC cells, Tomkins and his colleagues have proposed a model that envisages a post-transcriptional control system for tyrosine aminotransferase induction by glucocorticoids. (For a review of post-transcriptional control processes see Hogan, 1974).

In the HTC system (see above, Subsection IIIB), it has been found that about 30 minutes after adding the steroid, RNA required for synthesis of tyrosine aminotransferase (presumably mRNA) accumulates, and after about 60 minutes an increase in the rate of synthesis of the enzyme is detectable. The initial increase in synthesis of the enzyme is inhibited by low doses of actinomycin D (0.1 μg/ml) that inhibit mRNA synthesis. However, if the glucocorticoid is removed and high doses of actinomycin D (5 μg/ml) are added either simultaneously or some time after removal of the steroid, then the tyrosine aminotransferase level increases ('superinduction') or remains constant for some hours: this despite the fact that following straightforward removal of the steroid hormone after full enzymic induction, the amount of tyrosine aminotransferase declines steadily to the basal levels within a few hours. This paradoxical or 'superinductive' effect of inhibitors of macromolecular synthesis has been noted in a wide variety of bacterial, plant and animal systems. Tomkins *et al.*, (1972) have listed some eighty such observations thereby pointing to a fairly common control system for gene expression operating by post-transcriptional mechanisms. One interpretation of the superinductive effect of actinomycin D is that RNA synthesis is required not only to induce enzyme synthesis, but also to shut it off as well (deinduction). Tomkins has incorporated this into a model (Figure 16.7) which has received much attention and envisages the involvement of two genes for tyrosine aminotransferase synthesis: one for the mRNA of this inducible enzyme, and another for a labile repressor molecule which combines reversibly with the mRNA for the enzyme. The repressor may both block

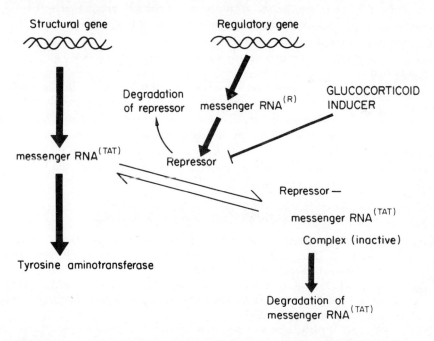

Figure 16.7 A model for the post-transcriptional control of tyrosine aminotransferase and messenger RNA regulation in hepatoma cells. For further details see text and Tomkins *et al.* (1969), *Science*, **166**, 1974.

translation of this mRNA and enhance its degradation. In this scheme, gluco-corticoids could stimulate tyrosine aminotransferase synthesis entirely at the transcriptional level by promoting the synthesis of the mRNA for tyrosine aminotransferase and also blocking synthesis of repressor molecules. Alternatively, Tomkins has proposed that the steroid hormones could act entirely post-transcriptionally by inactivating the repressor, thereby allowing the accumulation of mRNA for the enzyme. Low doses of actinomycin D would preferentially inhibit the synthesis of mRNA for the enzyme, while high doses will also inhibit synthesis of the labile repressor. Under these circumstances degradation of mRNA (via repressor complexes) is limited and the rate of tyrosine aminotransferase synthesis is increased. Since the mRNA for the enzyme is now stable, synthesis of the enzyme may then proceed for an extended period in the absence of inducing glucocorticoid and while RNA synthesis is blocked.

There is little direct or conclusive evidence supporting these ideas about glucocorticoid action at either the transcriptional or post-transcriptional level. However, the observation that steroid–receptor complexes bind to DNA provided very strong suggestive evidence that at least some (if not all) regulation occurs at the transcriptional level. Moreover, Kenney *et al.*, (1973) have provided further evidence against the concept of post-transcriptional control in this system. These workers have measured the rate of tyrosine aminotransferase synthesis under superinduction conditions and at no time have they observed stimulation or maintenance of aminotransferase synthesis in actinomycin-treated cells. It is now evident that the manner in which the data for the rate of enzyme synthesis are expressed is crucial to these observations, and the careful work of Kenney and coworkers appears to place in jeopardy the intriguing model proposed by Tomkins (Figure 16.7).

On balance it now seems that the action of glucocorticoids in the various systems that have been studied is directly comparable with that presently believed to occur for other steroid hormones in their target tissues. The steroid hormones are believed to pass firstly through the cell membrane and bind to specific cytoplasmic receptor proteins. These steroid–receptor complexes then rapidly migrate into the nucleus where they interact with binding sites on the DNA and affect the transcriptional processes of the cell.

V. REFERENCES (*indicates review or book)

Baxter, J. D., G. G. Rousseau, C. Benson, R. L. Garcea, J. Ito and G. M. Tomkins (1972). Role of DNA and specific cytoplasmic receptors in glucocorticoid action. *Proc. Nat. Acad. Sci. U.S.*, 69, 1892–1896.

*Cahill, G. F. (1971). Action of adrenal cortical steroids on carbohydrate metabolism. In N. P. Christy, (Ed.) *The Human Adrenal Cortex* Harper & Row, New York. Chap. 6, pp. 205–239.

*Cox, R. P. (1971). Early events in hormonal induction of alkaline phosphatase in human cell culture: hormone cell interaction and its dependence on DNA replication. *Ann. N.Y. Acad. Sci.*, 179, 596–610.

*David, D. S., M. H. Grieco and P. Cushman (1970). Adrenal glucocorticoids after 20 years. A review of their clinically relevant consequences. *J. Chron. Dis.*, **22**, 637–711.

*Exton, J. H., L. E. Mallette, L. S. Jefferson, E. H. A. Wong, N. Friedman, T. B. Miller and C. R. Park (1970). The hormonal control of hepatic gluconeogenesis. *Recent Prog. Horm. Res.*, **26**, 411–461.

Exton, J. H., N. Friedmann, E. H. Wong, J. P. Brineaux, J. D. Corbin and C. R. Park (1972). Interaction of glucocorticoids with glucagon and epinephrine in the control of gluconeogenesis and glycogenolysis in liver and of lipolysis in adipose tissue. *J. Biol. Chem.*, **247**, 3579–3588.

*Feldman, D., J. W. Funder and I. S. Edelman (1972). Subcellular mechanisms in the action of adrenal steroids. *Am. J. Med.*, **53**, 545–560.

Gehring, U., B. Mohit and G. M. Tomkins (1972). Glucocorticoid action on hybrid clones derived from cultured myeloma and lymphoma cell lines. *Proc. Nat. Acad. Sci. U.S.*, **69**, 3124.

*Gell, P. G. H., and R. R. A. Coombs (Eds) (1968). *Clinical Aspects of Immunology*. 2nd ed. Blackwell, Oxford.

Hackney, J. F., and W. B. Pratt (1971). Characterization and partial purification of the specific glucocorticoid-binding component from mouse fibroblasts. *Biochemistry*, **10**, 3002–3008.

Higgins, S. J., G. G. Rousseau, J. D. Baxter and G. M. Tomkins (1973). Early events in glucocorticoid action. Activation of the steroid receptor and its subsequent specific nuclear binding studied in a cell-free system. *J. Biol. Chem.*, **248**, 5866–5872.

Hogan, B. (1974). Post-transcriptional control of protein synthesis. In R. Weber, (Ed.), *The Biochemistry of Animal Development* Vol. 3. Academic Press, New York. Chap. 5.

Kenney, F. T., K.-L. Lee, C. D. Stiles and J. E. Fritz (1973). Further evidence against post-transcriptional control of inducible tyrosine aminotransferase synthesis in cultured hepatoma cells. *Nature New Biology*, **246**, 208–210.

*King, R. J. B., and W. I. P. Mainwaring (1974). Glucocorticoids. In *Steroid-Cell Interactions*. Butterworths, London. Chap. 5, p. 102–161.

Litwack, G., R. Filler, S. A. Rosenfield, N. Lichtash, C. A. Wishman and S. Singer (1973). Liver cytosol corticosteroid binder II, a hormone receptor. *J. Biol. Chem.*, **248**, 7481–7486.

*Markman, M. H., S. Nakagawa and A. White (1967). Studies on the mode of action of adrenal steroids on lymphocytes. *Recent Prog. Horm. Res.*, **23**, 195.

Melnykovych, G., and C. E. Bishop (1971). Specific binding of cortisol in subcellular fractions of HeLa cells: temperature dependence and effects of inhibitors. *Endocrinology*, **88**, 450–455.

*Munck, A. (1968). Effects of hormones at the cellular level. In V. H. T. James, (Ed.), *Recent Advances in Endocrinology*, 8th ed. Churchill. Chapter 5, p. 139.

Rosenau, W., J. D. Baxter, G. G. Rousseau and G. M. Tomkins (1972). Mechanism of resistance to steroids: glucocorticoid receptor defect in lymphoma cells. *Nature New Biol.*, **237**, 20–24.

Rousseau, G. G., J. D. Baxter, S. J. Higgins and G. M. Tomkins (1973). Steroid-induced nuclear binding of glucocorticoid receptors in intact hepatoma cells. *J. Mol. Biol.*, **79**, 539–554.

*Rudman, D., and M. D. Girolamo (1971). Effect of adrenal cortical steroids on lipid metabolism. In N. P. Christy, (Ed.) *The human adrenal cortex* Harper & Row, New York. Chap. 7, p. 241—255.

Sajdel, E. M., and S. T. Jacobs (1971). Mechanism of early effect of hydrocortisone on the transcriptional process: stimulation of the activities of purified rat liver nucleolar RNA polymerases. *Biochem. Biophys. Res. Comm.,* 45, 707.

Schaumburg, B. P., and M. Crone (1971). Binding of corticosterone by thymus cells, bursa cells and blood lymphocytes from the chicken. *Biochim. Biophys. Acta,* 237, 494—501.

Tomkins, G. M., B. B. Levinson, J. D. Baxter and L. Dethlefsen (1972). Further evidence for post-transcriptional control of inducible tyrosine aminotransferase synthesis in cultured hepatoma cells. *Nature New Biol.,* 239, 9—14.

Turnell, R. W., N. Kaiser, R. J. Milholland and F. Rosen (1974). Glucocorticoid receptors in rat thymocytes. Interactions with the antiglucocorticoid cortexolone and mechanism of its action. *J. Biol. Chem.,* 249, 1133—1138.

*Weber, G. (1968). Action of glucocorticoid hormone at the molecular level. In K. W. McKerns, (Ed.), *Functions of the Adrenal Cortex*, Vol. II. Appleton—Century—Crofts, New York. Chap. 27, pp. 1059—1135.

Weber, G., H. J. Hird-Convery, M. A. Lea and N. B. Stamm (1966). Feedback inhibition of key glycolytic enzymes: action of free-fatty acids. *Science,* 154, 1357.

Yu, F. L., and P. Feigelson (1971). Cortisone stimulations of nucleolar RNA polymerase activity. *Proc. Nat. Acad. Sci. U.S.,* 68, 2177—2180.

Appendix

A-I. REACTIONS OF SYNTHETIC UTILITY

The reactions discussed in this section have found wide application in laboratory syntheses in which one steroid is converted into another. The area of total synthesis of steroids, where the molecule is built up from simple materials, is not dealt with in this book since it is primarily of interest to the organic chemist and is better left to texts in that field.

Alcohol and ketone groups are the two most common functional groups in steroids and their interconversions are therefore of considerable interest to the steroid chemist. The net overall effect in such a reaction is always the transfer of hydrogen. The manner in which hydrogen is removed or added depends on the reagent which promotes the reaction. In most cases hydrogen does not appear as the element but as a proton (H^+) or a hydride ion (H^-).

The complex hydrides of certain metals such as aluminium and boron are able to reduce ketones to alcohols very efficiently. This is accomplished by the transfer of a hydride onto the carbonyl carbon of the free ketone; the proton is derived from water which is added to the reaction (or may already be present in some cases). Lithium aluminium hydride ($LiAlH_4$) is one of the best known reagents of this type. One molecule of reagent is capable of reducing four molecules of ketone, since all four of the hydrogens on the aluminium can react as H^-.

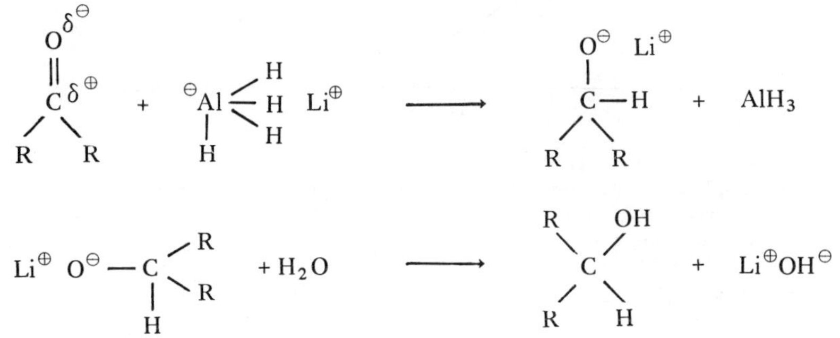

Most steroidal ketones are completely reduced by metal hydrides; however, there is the question of the stereochemistry of the resulting alcohol. Since a new asymmetric carbon atom is generated, two epimeric alcohols are possible. In general, it has been found that the equatorial alcohol is produced in greatest amount. For example, if we look at the reduction of a ketone at C-3 in the 5α series, we find that 91% of the product is the equatorial 3β and only 4% is the 3α (the remaining 5% are unidentified materials). The reduction of a C-3 ketone in the 5β series gives similar results; however, here the 3α is the equatorial isomer and is the major product.

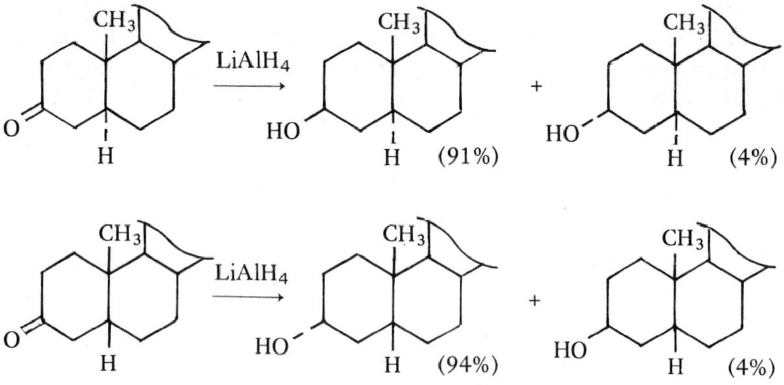

This selectivity is due to steric factors. In general a reagent will approach a steroid from the most open side and this is where the hydride will come from in this case. If one were to examine models of the above two examples, it could be readily seen that in the 5α series the α side is least hindered and that the hydride will come from that side. In the 5β series the reverse is true. At certain positions the choice for the reagents' approach is not as clear and the result is a more even mixture.

The aluminium ion also plays a part in the reduction of ketones. There is a polarization of charge on the carbonyl group such that the oxygen is negative and the carbon is positive. The Al^{3+} is attracted to the oxygen and the hydride is thereby brought into close proximity to the carbon, facilitating the whole reaction. Aluminium bound to three alkoxyl groups can also be used to reduce ketones; however, a source of hydride must be supplied. This is accomplished by adding an excess of a simple alcohol which is oxidized to the corresponding ketone in the process; the aluminium functions as a catalyst in this instance.

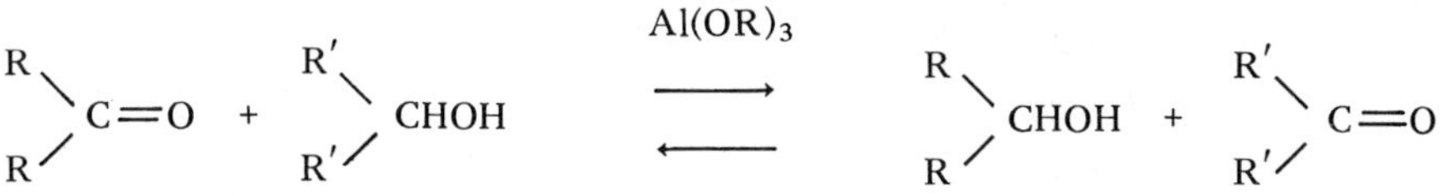

$$\begin{array}{c} R \\ \diagdown \\ \diagup \\ R \end{array} C{=}O \ + \ \begin{array}{c} R' \\ \diagdown \\ \diagup \\ R' \end{array} CHOH \quad \xrightarrow[\longleftarrow]{\ Al(OR)_3\ } \quad \begin{array}{c} R \\ \diagdown \\ \diagup \\ R \end{array} CHOH \ + \ \begin{array}{c} R' \\ \diagdown \\ \diagup \\ R' \end{array} C{=}O$$

The reaction is an equilibrium process and its direction can be reversed by providing an excess of $R_2'CO$.

The function of the aluminium ion seems to be to bring the reactants together in such a manner that hydride can be transferred with a minimum of energy. The reactive complex, or transition state can be depicted as follows with the aluminium, the two oxygens, the two carbons and the carbinol forming a six-membered ring:

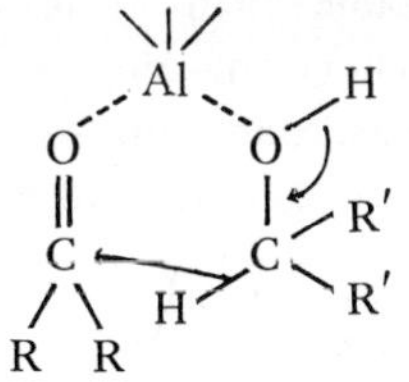

A simultaneous shift of bonds (electrons) leads to a transfer of hydride, hence the reduction–oxidation process. In general the stereochemical course of this type of reduction is the same as in the metal hydrides and for the same reasons.

Other metal ions can bring about oxidation of alcohols. However, they are not catalysts like Al^{3+} since they are reduced in the reaction. One of the best such reagents for steroidal alcohols is Cr^{6+} which is reduced to Cr^{3+} in the process. In contrast to the reduction reactions above, an asymmetric centre is destroyed so that

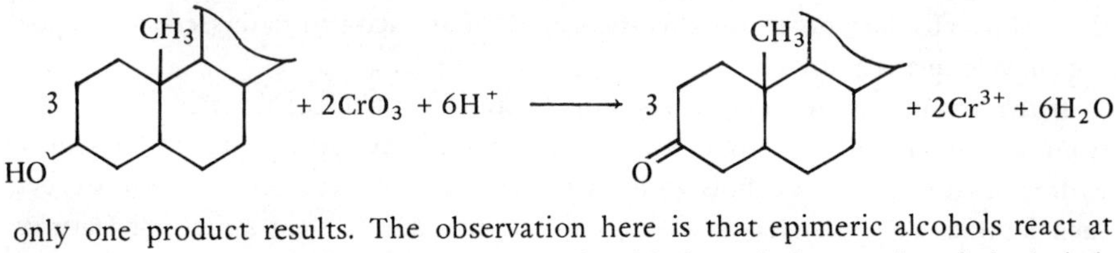

$$3 \cdots + 2CrO_3 + 6H^+ \longrightarrow 3 \cdots + 2Cr^{3+} + 6H_2O$$

only one product results. The observation here is that epimeric alcohols react at quite different rates. The relative rates of oxidation of three pairs of alcohols is given in Table A.1.

The first question of interest is why the axial alcohols react faster than their epimeric equatorial counterparts? Secondly, one would like an explanation for the

Table A.1.
Oxidation Rates*

Position of the Hydroxyl			Conformation
$3\beta = 1.0$	$6\alpha = 20$	$11\alpha = 7.0$	equatorial
$3\alpha = 3.0$	$6\beta = 36$	$11\beta = 60$	axial

*Rates are relative to the 3β hydroxyl.

differences in rates at different positions. A possible answer lies in an examination of the transition state which has been proposed for this reaction. There is evidence that the alcohol forms an ester with H_2CrO_4 (a hydrated form of CrO_3) which then breaks down in such a manner that the ketone and reduced chromium result.

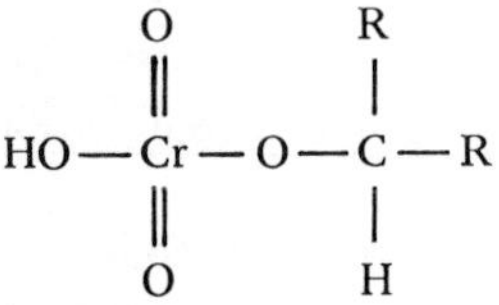

Chromate Ester

Equatorial esters are more stable than axial, since there are no 1,3 diaxial interactions which means they will not decompose as quickly to form the products. This theory could also answer the second point since the 1,3 interactions increase in intensity in going from 3α to 6β to 11β, therefore giving a general increase in rates.

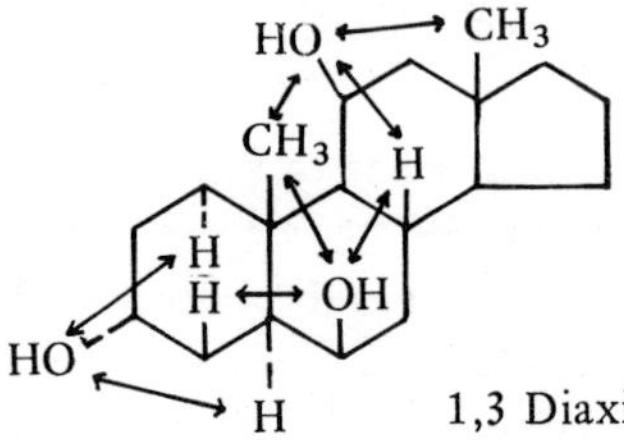

1,3 Diaxial Interactions

3α encounters two mild OH–H interactions, 6β has two OH–H and one OH–CH_3 interactions, while 11β has two OH–CH_3 and one OH–H interactions. Although there is no absolute proof for this theory, all of the data to date seem to support the above explanations.

If the conditions are suitable, it is possible to effect a direct transfer of hydrogen from an alcohol to a ketone. Certain ketones of the quinone type can remove hydrogen from allylic alcohols without the aid of a catalyst. As one might expect, such ketones are polarized as all ketones are, but due to their structural features, the positive charge on the carboxyl carbon is quite high. The other factors contributing to the success of this reaction is the greater reactivity of allylic alcohols.

DDQ Oxidation

Dichlorodicyanoquinone (DDQ) is a good example of this type of oxidizing agent. Both the chloro and cyano groups have the ability to withdraw electrons from the ring creating a positive charge which will be centred at the carbonyl carbons. This apparently serves the same purpose as the Al^{3+} in the previous case. The quinone is reduced to the corresponding hydroquinone in the process.

The role of the double bond adjacent to the hydroxyl is not well established; however, it is believed that it stabilizes the transition state. If an unstable charged species can distribute its charge over several atoms, it can be produced with less energy. There are other examples of reactions at allylic positions which proceed much more easily than their saturated counterparts. The above mechanism could also apply if a negative charge were generated by initial removal of H^+. It is sometimes very difficult to determine which process is operating.

Charge Distribution During Oxidation

The reactivities of carbon–carbon double bonds are due in a large measure to their π electron systems. Any reagent which is seeking electrons (electrophilic) to produce a more stable situation will react with a double bond in some fashion. Very often, but not always, such reagents contain a positively charged centre.

The addition of HCl or HBr to double bonds best exemplifies this type of reaction. The proton first attacks the π electron to form a new carbon–hydrogen bond. This leaves the other carbon with a deficiency of electrons (carbonium ion). The chloride ion then forms a covalent bond with this second carbon to complete the reaction.

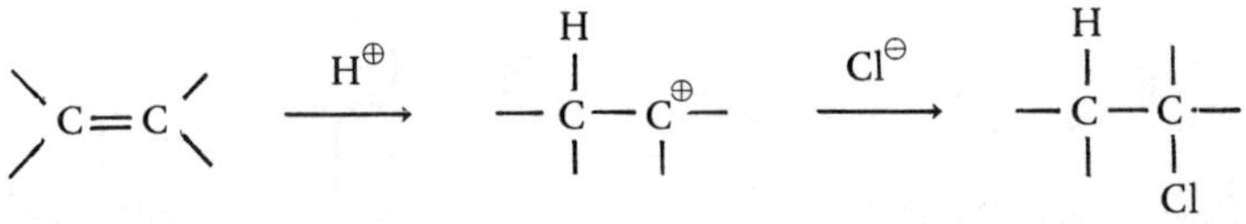

Addition to a Double Bond

In an analogous manner, hydrogen can be added to a double bond. Here, however, a catalyst is required probably to polarize the hydrogen and/or the double bond so that they will react.

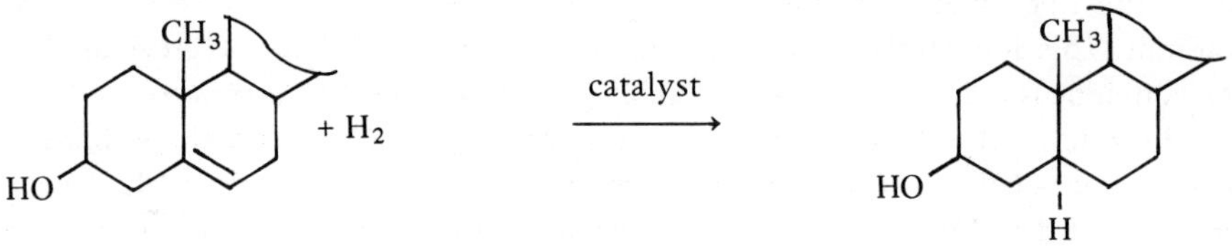

Reduction of a Double Bond

The usual catalysts are platinum or palladium which are recovered unchanged at the end of the reaction. These reductions are often stereoselective: that is, the hydrogen will be added from the least hindered side of the steroid. In the case of the 5,6 double bond shown above, addition proceeds from the α-side, giving a compound of the 5α series.

Reagents such as hydrogen peroxide can produce OH^+ in solution and this is a powerful electrophilic agent. It will react vigorously with double bonds to give two alternative products depending upon the pH of the solution. In a basic medium a three-membered ring containing oxygen (an epoxide) is obtained. In the presence of acid, a 1,2-glycol is the product. For unconjugated double bonds, derivatives of hydrogen peroxide such as peracetic (CH_3-COOH) or perbenzoic ($\phi-COOH$) are used.

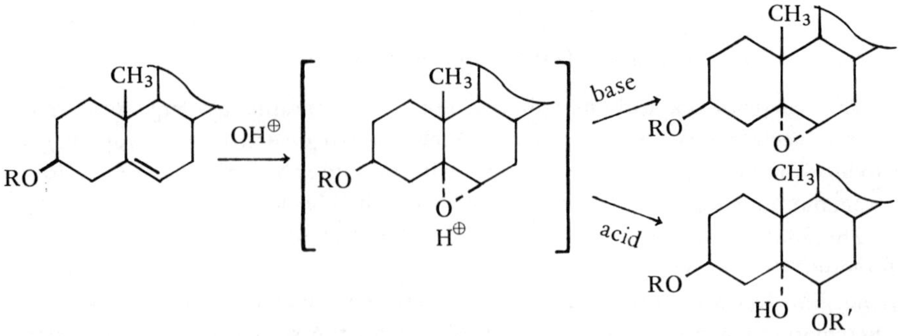

Peracid Oxidation

An important consideration for anyone undertaking to perform a reaction on a steroid is selectivity. Almost every biologically active steroid has at least two functional groups and care has to be taken that a reagent intended for one group does not react with any of the others. Very often the other groups may be of the same type and there are only subtle differences in reactivity due to steric factors which can be utilized. A knowledge of the relative rates of reaction, such as is described in Table A.1 on the chromic acid oxidation of hydroxyls, can be useful in choosing conditions which will allow only the desired reaction to occur.

A more general approach to this problem is the use of protecting groups. In this method, the groups which are not to be reacted, are converted to some derivative which is stable under the conditions the molecule will be subjected to. Afterwards, they are removed and the net effect is the desired change only.

An example of such a procedure is the reaction of the 5,6 double bond with OH⁻ in the presence of a 3β-hydroxyl. Peracids will also oxidize alcohols although this is not a satisfactory method for other reasons. However, this means that the hydroxyl must be protected during the reaction. Esters are stable under the conditions of the procedure and can be easily cleaved afterward, hence they make a useful protecting group.

Simple esters of steroidal alcohols such as the acetate or benzoate can be prepared most conveniently by means of the anhydride or acyl halide.

Ester Formation

A mild base such as a pyridine is needed to speed up the reaction and maintain the appropriate pH.

Primary alcohols react very rapidly, whereas tertiary alcohols do not esterify except at high temperatures or other extreme conditions. Among the secondary alcohols there are more subtle differences in the rates of esterification, equatorial alcohols generally being more reactive. This is a consequence of their sterically less crowded situation. All of these factors can be utilized in performing selective esterifications of polyhydric steroids.

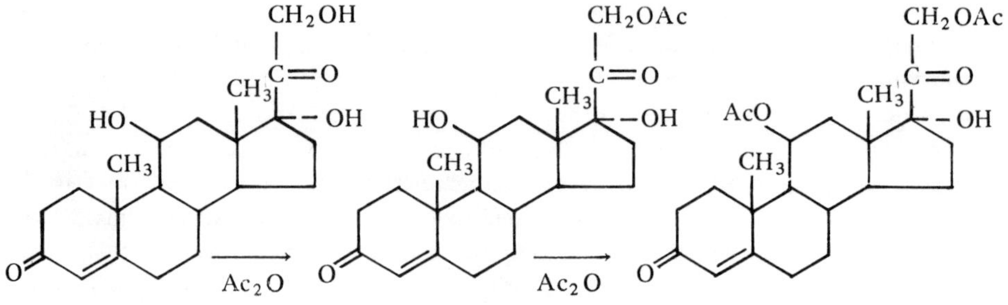

| Cortisol | 21-Monoacetate | 11,21-Diacetate |

Cortisol contains a primary, a hindered secondary and a tertiary hydroxyl group. The first will acylate with extreme ease and the reaction can be stopped at the monoacetate stage. Continued reaction with the secondary hydroxyl produces a diacetate which will not esterify further under the usual conditions. Often one can reverse esterification in a stepwise fashion by carefully controlled saponification. If applied to the above case, for example, the 11β monoacetate would be obtained.

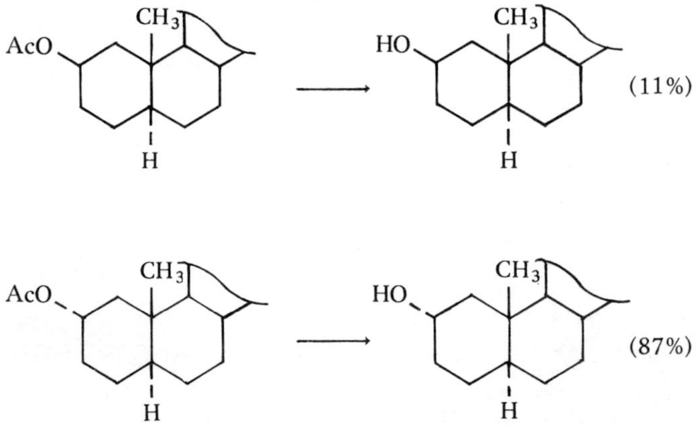

(11%)

Steric Effects in
Saponification

(87%)

Stereochemical differences between esters can sometimes be utilized for selective purposes. Equatorial esters can be hydrolized at a more rapid rate than their axial counterparts. When subjected to identical reaction conditions, the epimeric acetates at position 2 exhibit an eight-fold difference in the extent of cleavage. Apparently the rate-determining step in the hydrolysis does not reflect relief of 1,3 diaxial interaction as in the case of chromic acid oxidation of alcohols. Instead the greater accessibility of equatorial groups to attacking reagents is the dominant factor.

Hydroxyl groups can be protected by an alternative method, using dihydropyrane (DHP). This molecule can be considered to be the cyclic enol ether of 5-hydroxyvaleraldehyde which is formed by loss of water from the unstable intermediate hemiacetal.

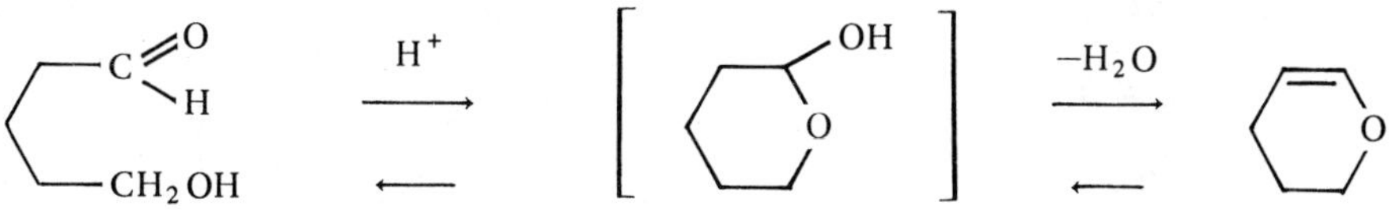

Hemiacetal   'DHP'

The reaction with an alcohol group proceeds as though it was an addition to the double bond, giving an acetal as the product. This reaction is similar to the equilibrium which exists between the cyclic and chain forms of the hexoses in carbohydrate chemistry.

The utility of tetrahydropyranyl (THP) ether derivatives lies in the fact that they are stable to hydride, Grignard reagents and other basic substances. They are readily removed by treatment with mild acid and as such cannot be used as protecting groups under acidic conditions. This reaction seems contradictory to the fact that

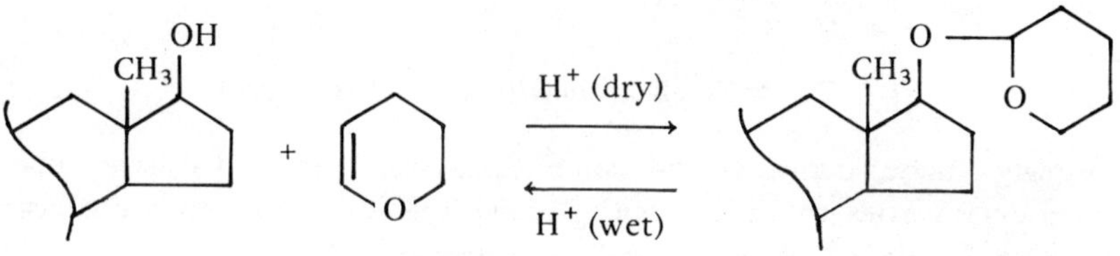

'DHP'   'THP' Ether

acid is required as catalyst for their formation; however, the difference in conditions is the presence of water. Under anhydrous conditions the equilibrium is shifted toward ether formation while water is required for cleavage.

An analogous reaction occurs between ketones and alcohols. Under anhydrous acidic conditions two molecules of an alcohol condense with a ketone to form a ketal.

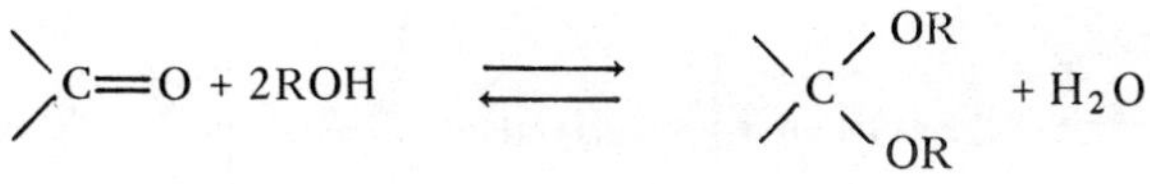

Ketal Formation

A more stable derivative is obtained if both hydroxyl groups reside on the same molecule in a 1,2 relationship; for this purpose ethylene glycol is most convenient and leads to cyclic ethylene ketal derivatives. Like the DHP derivative above, these compounds are stable to basic conditions while they are cleaved in acidic media if water is present.

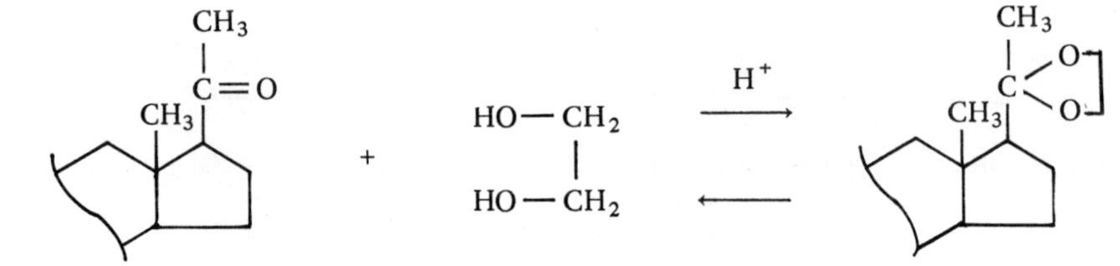

Cyclic Ketalization with a Steroidal Ketone

Occasionally, a steroid may contain a 1,2 glycol system in which case it can form a ketal derivative with acetone.

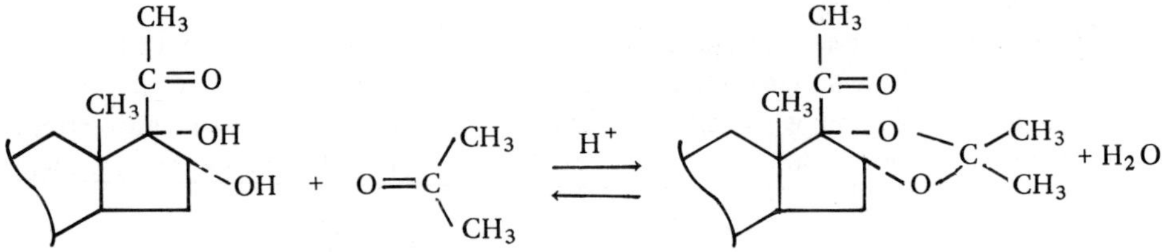

Cyclic Ketalization with a Steroidal Glycol

Interestingly, these derivatives in some cases were found to have superior therapeutic properties to their parent glycols. Acetonide derivatives can also be formed with 1,3 glycols of which there are a number of examples in the corticoid field where the 17,21-dihydroxy-20-one system is often present.

A-II. REACTIONS USED IN ASSAYING STEROIDS

The condensation reactions between ketones and various derivatives of hydrazine are well known throughout the field of organic chemistry, and there are several different types of steroid assays based on these condensations. The fundamental reaction involves attack by the electron rich amino group upon the positively charged carbonyl carbon.

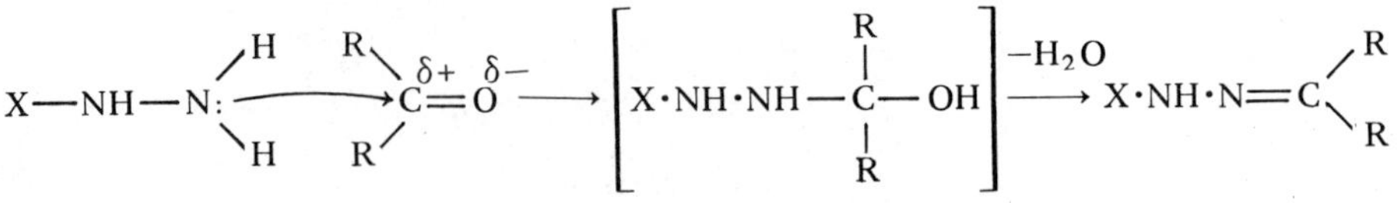

Hydrazone Formation

Hydrazine itself (X=H) will undergo this reaction; however, the resultant hydrazones have no analytically useful properties. These reactions are summarized in Table A.2.

The phenylhydrazones and their nitro analogues are deeply coloured so that small amounts can be measured spectrophotometrically. Since all ketonic materials

Table A.2.
Derivatives of Steroidal Ketones and NH_2NH-X

Derivative	X	Formula	Assay
Hydrazone	H−	$R_2C{=}NHNH_2$	None
Phenylhydrazone	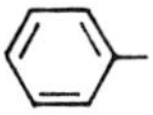	$R_2C{=}NHNH-$ 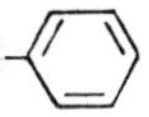	Porter-Silber*
2,4 Dinitrophenyl-hydrazone	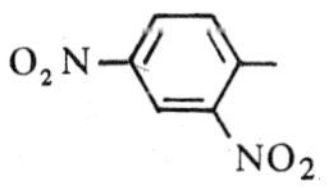 $O_2N-$$-NO_2$	$R_2C{=}NHNH-$$-NO_2$ ... NO_2	Brays Reagent
Thiosemicarbazide	$\overset{S^{35}}{\overset{\|}{-C}}-NH_2$	$R_2C{=}NHNH-\underset{\underset{S^{35}}{\|}}{C}-NH_2$	Double isotope method*

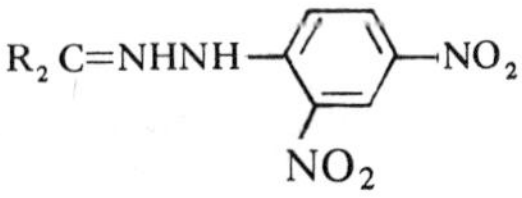

*See Chapter 2.IV for applications.

will react, interfering substances must be removed from biological extracts before meaningful assays can be made.

The assay based upon the reaction with phenylhydrazine is known as the *Porter–Silber Assay* (see Table 2.1). By adjusting the conditions of the reaction, some selectivity amongst various steroidal keto groups can be achieved. The most successful application of this reaction has been in the measurement of steroids containing $17\alpha,21$-dihydroxy-20-one side chain. Here the reaction with phenyl hydrazine is very rapid and an intense chromophore with a typical spectrum is produced. The course of this reaction is not a simple condensation with the 20-ketone. Instead, it is preceded by a rearrangement resulting in a net loss of water from the side-chain and giving a 21-aldehyde group. Interestingly, only the aldehyde reacts with the phenylhydrazine even when there is an excess of reagent.

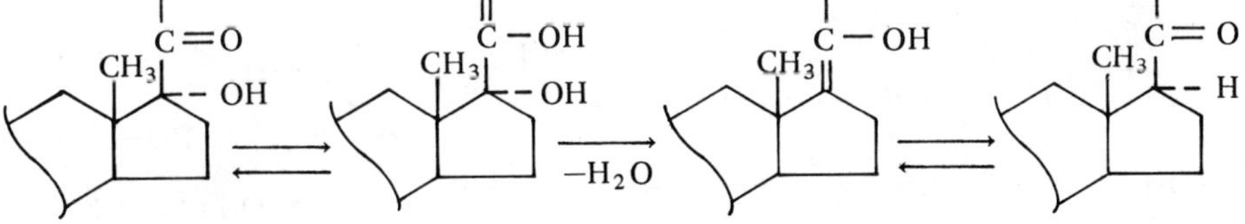

Rearrangement During the Porter–Silber Assay

Steroidal ketones will condense with *m*-dinitrobenzene to give a complex which is oxidized to give an intensely coloured chromophoric system. All of the compounds shown in the reaction below have been isolated and evidence given for their structures. The first step involves removal of a proton from the methylene group α to the ketone *via* the enol. This participation of the enol was demonstrated by isolation of the product when a 3-ketone was used. The reaction was mainly at position 2 which is the direction of enolization. The intermediate complex is then oxidized by a second molecule of *m*-dinitrobenzene as evidenced by the isolation of the reduction product, *m*-nitroaniline. This reaction is used in the *Zimmermann Assay* and has found its best application in the measurement of 17-oxosteroids (see Chapter 2.IV).

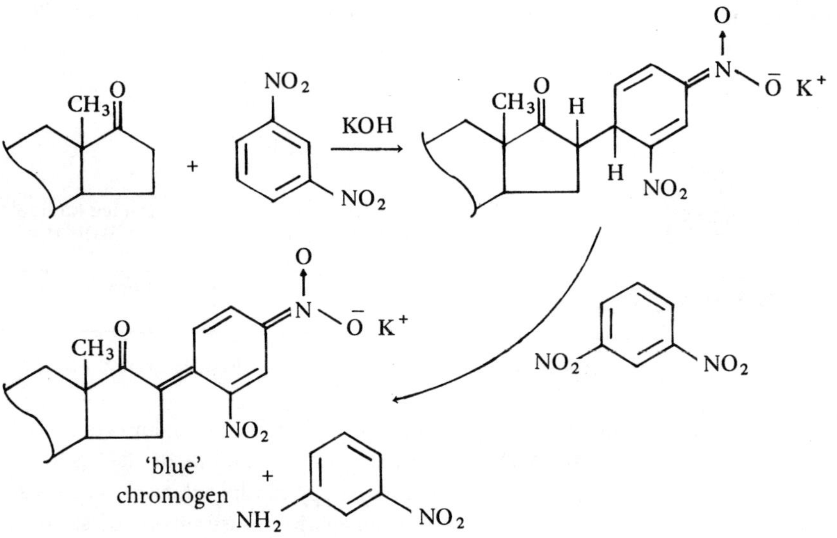

The Zimmermann Assay

The use of the Zimmermann reaction has been extended to the corticoid field by the use of reagents which can readily cleave off the side-chain to give products with a 17-keto group. Periodic acid has been extensively used in the carbohydrate field for the cleavage of 1,2-glycols. It apparently forms a cyclic complex which then breaks down to give two carbonyl functions and reduced iodine.

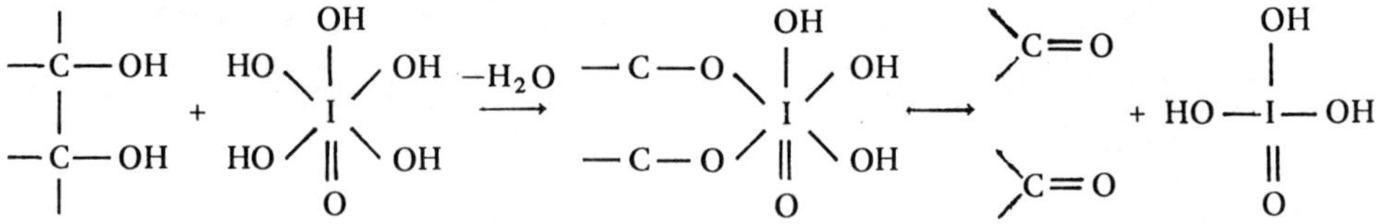

Periodate Cleavage

17-Hydroxy-20-oxo steroids can thus be converted to 17-oxo steroids, if the prior reduction of the 20-ketone is performed to generate a glycol. The product can then be assayed by the Zimmermann reaction. The same type of reaction sequence can be carried out using sodium bismuthate as the cleaving agent. Certain advantages have been claimed for this reagent and many laboratories prefer it to periodate.

Conversion to a Zimmermann Sensitive Derivative

Esters formed from steroidal alcohols and benzene-sulphonic acid derivatives have been used in double isotope derivative assays (see Chapter 2.IV). 'Pipsyl chloride' (*p*-iodobenzenesulphonyl chloride), for example, has been applied in the assay of estrone.

Pipsyl Derivative Formation

The reaction is analogous to esterification with an acyl halide. Both isotopic iodine and sulphur have been used in this method.

The reducing power of the 21-hydroxy-20-keto steroid grouping can be employed for assay purposes in the same fashion as α-ketols found in the carbohydrates. Some of the same reagents can be used for both steroids and sugars. A particularly useful one for quantitative studies is the reduction of a tetrazolium salt to a coloured product known as formazan.

Colourless (tetrazolium)   Coloured (formazan)

The nature of the colour depends upon the R groups; the most popular one for steroids is the derivative which gives a blue colour. The procedure is often referred to as the *Blue Tetrazolium Assay*.

A-III REACTIONS OF BIOSYNTHETIC SIGNIFICANCE

In this sub-section several reactions from synthetic organic chemistry and their mechanisms are discussed because of their relevance to an understanding of the biological reactions of steroids. Much of the emphasis is on the reactions leading to the formation of the steroid ring system.

Condensation reactions between derivatives of carboxylic acids and molecules with active methylene groups are well known in organic chemistry. Malonic ester contains such an active methylene and will react with acetate to give a reactive intermediate which can be decarboxylated to give acetoacetic ester.

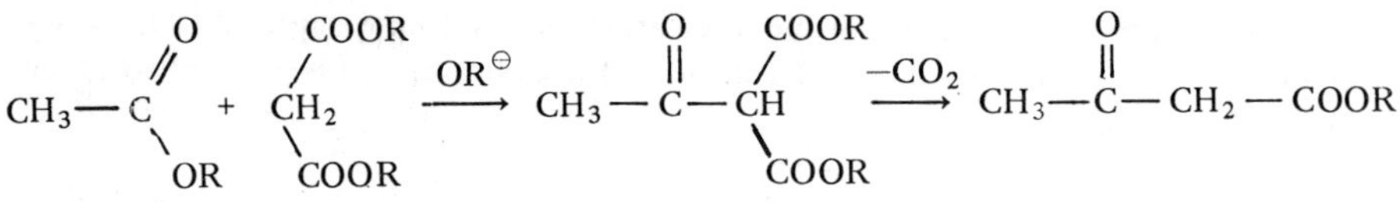

$$CH_3-C \overset{O}{\underset{OR}{\diagup\diagdown}} + \overset{COOR}{\underset{COOR}{CH_2}} \xrightarrow{OR^{\ominus}} CH_3-C-\overset{COOR}{\underset{COOR}{CH}} \xrightarrow{-CO_2} CH_3-C-CH_2-COOR$$

Ester Condensation

The reaction is usually carried out in the presence of a basic catalyst and requires heat. A proton is removed from the active methylene and the resulting anion attacks the acetate carbonyl.

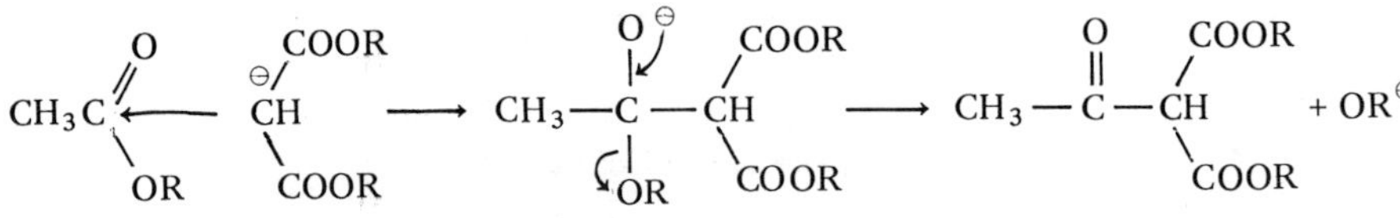

$$CH_3C \overset{O}{\underset{OR}{\diagup\diagdown}} \overset{COOR}{\underset{COOR}{\underset{\ominus}{CH}}} \longrightarrow CH_3-C-\overset{COOR}{\underset{COOR}{CH}} \longrightarrow CH_3-C-\overset{COOR}{\underset{COOR}{CH}} + OR^{\ominus}$$

One of the ester groups is then saponified and the resulting carboxylate group lost as carbon dioxide. The resulting enolate then acquires a proton from the alcoholic medium and ketonizes to give the product.

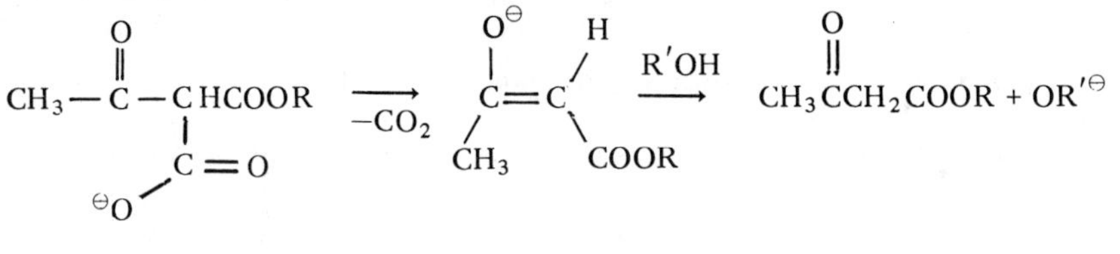

$$CH_3-C-CHCOOR \xrightarrow{-CO_2} \overset{O^{\ominus}}{\underset{CH_3}{C}}=\overset{H}{\underset{COOR}{C}} \xrightarrow{R'OH} CH_3CCH_2COOR + OR'^{\ominus}$$

The biological counterpart of this reaction, and how it is used in building some of the intermediates in steroid biosynthesis, is described in Chapter 4.

The polymerization of olefins is a process which has been exploited by the chemical industry to produce plastics. This type of reaction plays an important role in nature also. If an olefin is attacked by an electrophilic species, the π electrons will form a bond with it and a carbonium ion will be generated. If there is no more olefin present, the carbonium ion reacts in a similar fashion being electrophilic itself.

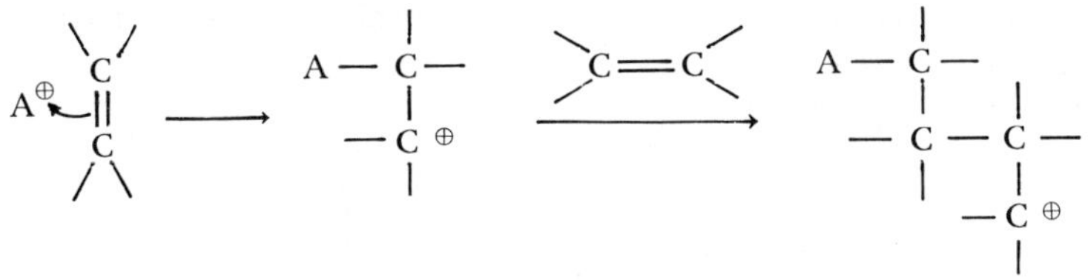

Olefin Polymerization

The chain will thus be propagated until some other species reacts with the carbonium terminating the reaction.

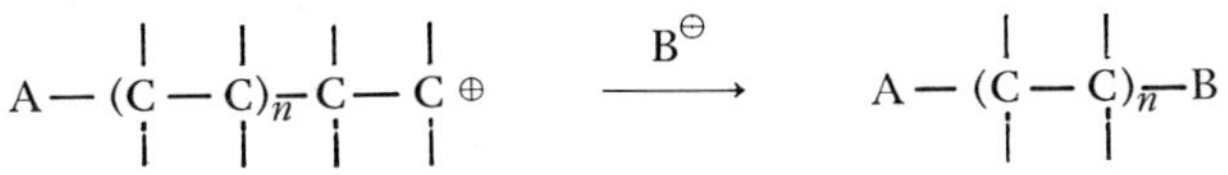

Chain Termination

The length of the resultant chain will depend (among other things) on factors such as concentration. In the biological polymerizations discussed in Chapter 4, enzymic factors probably determine chain length and there are other major differences from the above model reaction.

Polyunsaturated olefin chains will cyclize to form a ring if the double bonds are properly located, and if an electrophilic species is present.

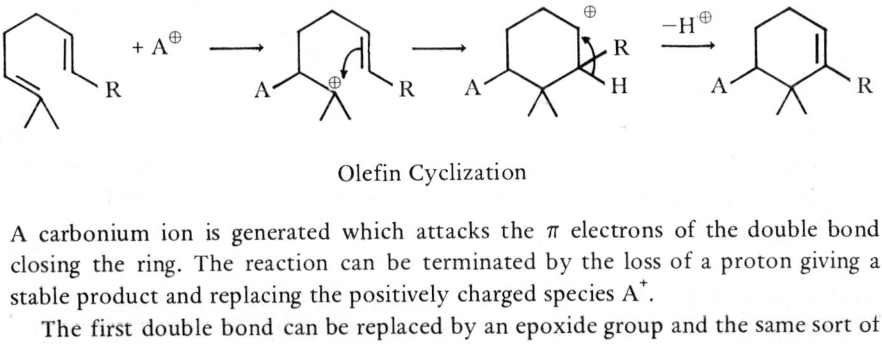

Olefin Cyclization

A carbonium ion is generated which attacks the π electrons of the double bond closing the ring. The reaction can be terminated by the loss of a proton giving a stable product and replacing the positively charged species A^+.

The first double bond can be replaced by an epoxide group and the same sort of cyclization will occur. The oxide can be opened to give a carbonium ion in a manner similar to the double bond.

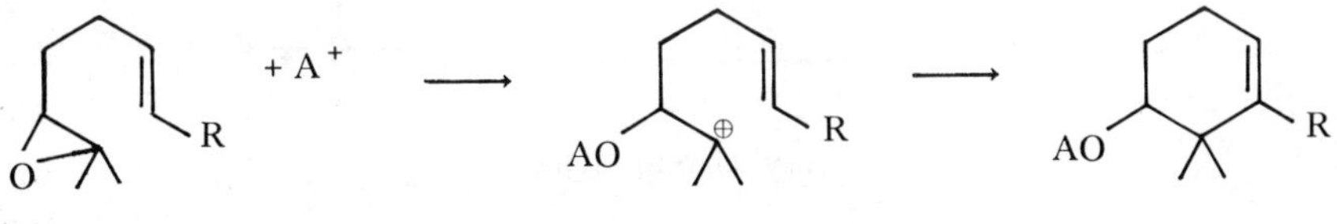

Oxide Cyclization

Recent evidence indicates that in nature the oxide precursor is by far the most prevalent.

A somewhat analogous reaction in a mechanistic sense is the migration of a double bond within the steroid ring system. A steroid with a double bond at the 7 position readily isomerizes to the 8,14 position when treated with acid.

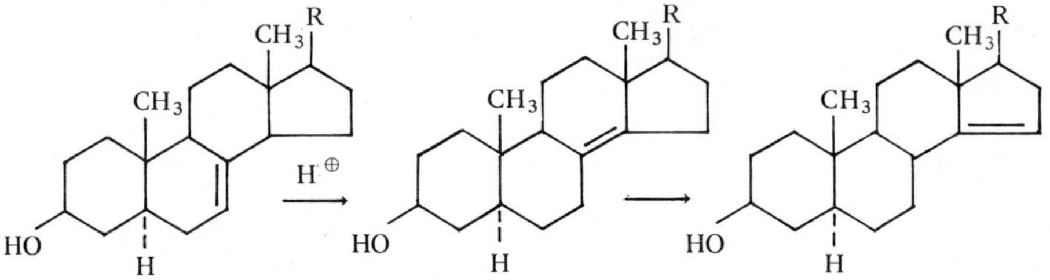

Double Bond Isomerization

In some cases (depending upon the nature of the R group) the unsaturated system may migrate as far as the 14,15 position. The course of migration depends upon subtle differences in the stability of the product.

The mechanism of double bond migration proceeds *via* carbonium ion intermediates. A proton adds to the system and a proton from another position is lost.

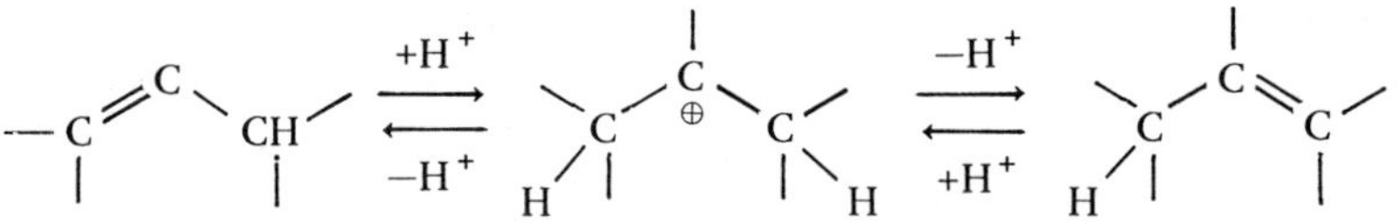

Mechanism of Isomerization

All of the reactions are reversible; therefore the distribution of products represents the relative stabilities of each. This of course applies where the catalyst is not selective, such as protons. If the reaction is enzymically catalized this may not be the case.

The positive charge of a carbonium ion can be neutralized by migration of an adjacent group with its pair of electrons as well as by the loss of a proton as illustrated above.

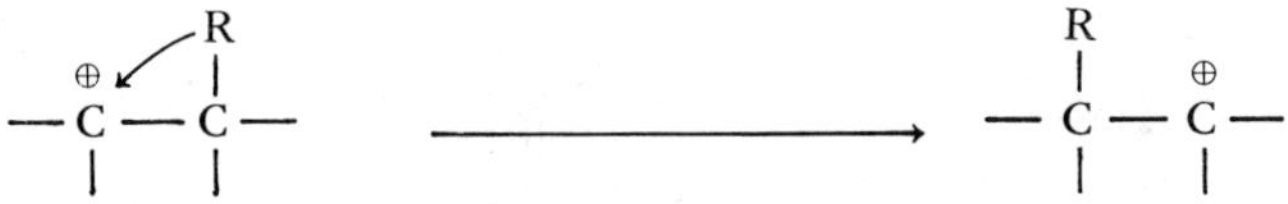

Alkyl Group Migration

This of course generates a new carbonium ion which must somehow be neutralized. Many groups are capable of such migrations; however, there is a definite order of reactivity. Hydrogen is the most labile and methyl is also easily moved; other alkyl groups migrate with greater difficulty. Stereochemical factors are also important since migrations occur more readily if the group is properly oriented. An example of methyl migration which is the basis of the *Kägi–Miescher Reaction* is given at the end of Chapter 2.III.

Ketones will react with peracids in such a manner that they are cleaved between the carboxyl and one of the α-groups. Thus, the 17β-acyl group in the steroids can be cleaved to give a 17-hydroxy acetate.

The conversion is always stereospecific since the 17α-acyl side-chain leads to a 17α-hydroxy acetate. This reaction closely parallels one of the biosynthetic pathways leading from the pregnane to the androstane series (Chapter 4).

REFERENCES

See Chapter 1, page 15.

Index